KV-387-743

MEDICAL LIBRARY
ODSTOCK HOSPITAL
SALISBURY SP2 8BJ

Salisbury District Hospital Library

T03443

Library
Education Centre
Salisbury District Hospital
Wilts
SP2 8BJ

LIBRARY & INFORMATION SERVICE
ODSTOCK HOSPITAL
SALISBURY SP2 8BJ

To be renewed or returned on or before the date marked below:

29. MAY 1992	08. SEP 97	04. NOV 04
	17. FEB 98	12. OCT 06
	10. AUG 98	6 H 06.
10. MAR 1993	17. SEP 98	06. MAR 09
6|5|93	10. FEB 99	-8 FEB 2010
24. JUL 95	12. APR 00	12. JAN 12.
15. NOV 95	30. MAY 01	03. APR 12.
27. MAR 96	22. MAY 02	13 JL 12
09. SEP 96	08. MAY 03	07. AUG 12.
26. FEB 97	-1 NOV 2017	04 12. 12.

PLEASE ENTER ON LOAN SLIP: 10 DEC 14.

AUTHOR: BURGHARDT, E.

TITLE: COLPOSCOPY: CERVICAL PATHOLOGY:
TEXTBOOK AND ATLAS

ACCESSION NO:	CLASS MARK:
1182	WP 400

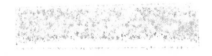

Colposcopy
Cervical Pathology

Textbook and Atlas

2nd, revised and enlarged
edition

Erich Burghardt

*Translated by and
with the collaboration of
Andrew G. Östör*

*Foreword by
Richard F. Mattingly*

415 mostly colored illustrations
28 tables

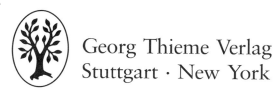

Georg Thieme Verlag
Stuttgart · New York

Thieme Medical Publishers, Inc.
New York

1991

Erich Burghardt, M.D.
Professor and Chairman
Dept. of Gynecology and Obstetrics
University of Graz
Auenbruggerplatz 14
8036 Graz
Austria

Andrew G. Östör, M.D.
Dept. of Pathology
Royal Women's Hospital
132 Grattan Street
Carlton
Victoria 3053
Australia

Library of Congress Cataloging-in-Publication Data

Burghardt, E. (Erich)
    [Kolposkopie, spezielle Zervixpathologie. English]
    Colposcopy, cervical pathology : textbook and atlas /
    Erich Burghardt ; translated by and with the collaboration
    of Andrew G. Östör. –– 2nd rev. and enl. ed.
       p.   cm.
    Translation of: Kolposkopie, spezielle Zervixpathologie.
    Includes bibliographical references and index.
    ISBN 3-13-659902-0. –– ISBN 0-86577-348-3
    1. Colposcopy. 2. Cervix uteri-Diseases. 3. Colposcopy-
    Atlases. 4. Cervix uteri––Diseases––Atlases.
    I. Östör, Andrew G.
    II. Title.
    [DNLM: 1. Cervix Uteri––pathology. 2. Colposcopy.
    WP 470 B958ka]
    RG107.5.C6A8613 1991
    618.1'45––dc20
    DLC
    for Library of Congress   91-528
                                                                  CIP

Cover design: Renate Stockinger, Stuttgart

Some of the product names, patents and registered designs referred to in this book are in fact registered trademarks or proprietary names even though specific reference to this fact is not always made in the text. Therefore, the appearance of a name without designation as proprietary is not to be construed as a representation by the publishers that it is in the public domain.

This book, including all parts thereof, is legally protected by copyright. Any use, exploitation or commercialization outside the narrow limits set by copyright legislation, without the publisher's consent, is illegal and liable to prosecution. This applies in particular to photostat reproduction, copying, mimeographing or duplication of any kind, translating, preparation of microfilms, and electronic data processing and storage.

© 1991 Georg Thieme Verlag, Rüdigerstrasse 14,
D-7000 Stuttgart 30, Germany
Thieme Medical Publishers, Inc., 381 Park Avenue South,
New York, N.Y. 10016

Typesetting by R. Hurler, D-7311 Notzingen
Printed in Germany by K. Grammlich, D-7401 Pliezhausen

ISBN 3-13-659902-0   (GTV, Stuttgart)
ISBN 0-86577-348-3   (TMP, New York)
                                    1 2 3 4 5 6

This book is a revised and enlarged edition of an translation from the 1st German edition, published and copyrighted 1984 by Georg Thieme Verlag, Stuttgart, Germany. Title of the German edition: Kolposkopie, spezielle Zervixpathology.

Important note: Medicine is an ever-changing science undergoing continual development. Research and clinical experience are continually expanding our knowledge, in particular our knowledge of proper treatment and drug therapy. Insofar as this book mentions any dosage or application, readers may rest assured that the authors, editors and publishers have made every effort to ensure that such references are in accordance with the state of knowledge at the time of production of the book.
Nevertheless this does not involve, imply, or express any guarantee or responsibility on the part of the publishers in respect of any dosage instructions and forms of application stated in the book. Every user is requested to examine carefully the manufacturers' leaflets accompanying each drug and to check, if necessary in consultation with a physician or specialist, whether the dosage schedules mentioned therein or the contraindications stated by the manufacturers differ from the statements made in the present book. Such examination is particularly important with drugs that are either rarely used or have been newly released on the market. Every dosage schedule or every form of application used is entirely at the user's own risk and responsibility. The authors and publishers request every user to report to the publishers any discrepancies or inaccuracies noticed.

Foreword to the First Edition

The time is long overdue for the publication of an authoritative textbook on the cervix that combines a detailed description of cervical pathology with the morphologic expression of disease, as seen by the colposcope. This detailed and beautifully illustrated text is the product of a wealth of material from an author, a pathology laboratory, and a clinic that are internationally recognized for their contribution to the field of cervical neoplasia. Few gynecologists in the present era have a thorough understanding of the subtle pathologic changes in the cervix that may mask, precede, or accompany the development of clinical cancer. This detailed textbook transposes the epithelial and vascular changes in the cervix into a visual transparency that can be easily understood and visualized through the magnifying lenses of the colposcope. Within the pages of this monograph, the student of this subject will find three textbooks blended into one that includes: the field of cervical pathology, an atlas of colposcopy that mirrors each pathologic lesion, and a clinical interpretation of the significance of these lesions by an author who is a clinician, a pathologist, and an authority in both fields.

The text fills a void that is clearly evident in a period of medicine that has become "gadget oriented." Medical societies have been organized around various instruments that have been idolized by an ever-increasing national and international membership. Yet, few clinicians have an in-depth understanding of the underlying disease processes. This opus, which represents the lifetime work of the author and his predecessors, has no equal. It has its roots in the classic writings of Robert Mayer and other distinguished pathologists which set the stage for the field of gynecologic pathology, and stems from the setting where the colposcope itself was first developed by Hinselmann in 1925. Within the confines of this text, one can appreciate the fine-tuning of the historic and current thinking of the microscopic changes of the cervix as demonstrated by the colposcope. These interpretations are based on a precise definition of the pathologic lesions in the cervix.

The interested reader may ask why it has required more than a half-century for this compendium to evolve since the original description of the colposcope by Hinselmann in 1925. More important, one might ask why the English-speaking countries were late in adopting the technique of colposcopy for the study of cervical neoplasia. This text, which is not the first atlas to be published on this subject, emphasizes that the original classifications of Hinselmann and his followers were encumbered by a complex and over-detailed morphologic terminology that was impractical for the clinician's use. It was not until the nomenclature was simplified and illustrated by Coppleson and co-workers (1971), and Kolstad and Stafl (1972), that the diagnostic value of colposcopy became recognized and widely utilized in North America. Only recently has this diagnostic modality been adopted in the United Kingdom. So it is with the wheels of progress; new innovations require the test of time and clinical use before they are accepted and implemented.

While the reader may be persuaded to accept the author's lucid description, illustration, and interpretation of the histologic and colposcopic lesions, there are still some legitimate differences of opinion between continents regarding their treatment. For example, this text clearly defines and illustrates the division of microinvasive carcinoma into "early stromal invasion" and "microcarcinoma." Although there can be no misinterpretation regarding these two entities, as discussed in this text, these are residual terms from the German literature that remain regional, rather than international in use. In North America, a malignancy that extends beneath the basement membrane is defined less precisely as either microinvasion (≤ 3 mm) or invasive. One might anticipate that the international classification of microinvasive cervical cancer will be clarified promptly by the Cancer Committee of the International Federation of Gynecology and Obstetrics (FIGO). Until that time, it is unlikely that the recommendation for treatment of microcarcinoma that encourages the use of therapeutic conization will be adopted on an international basis, despite the favorable results of the Graz clinic.

One of the major strengths of this work is the perfection in photomicrography and histologic details of the illustrations in each chapter. The quality of the text is exemplified in the histologic magnification of each cellular abnormality and the comparison with the colpophotograph of the colposcopic lesion. This comparison provides clarity of the underlying cervical lesion to the most uninformed novice. These features are the hallmark of the author's current and previous publications.

This text is a welcome addition to an international library on this subject. It will be of particular interest to the resident-in-training, the practicing clinician, the clinical researcher and for those gynecologists who are specifically interested in colposcopy. It provides an important link between the diagnosis of the earliest manifestation of cervical neoplasia and a rational approach toward treatment.

Milwaukee,
Wisconsin (USA),
Late
March 1984

Richard F. Mattingly, M.D.
Professor and Chairman
Department of Gynecology and Obstetrics
Medical College of Wisconsin
Milwaukee, Wisconsin, USA

Preface by the Translator to the First Edition

I entered the field of gynecologic pathology in 1973 when the English version of Burghardt's classic monograph "Early Histological Diagnosis of Cervical Cancer" (Thieme, Stuttgart, and Saunders, Philadelphia 1973) was published. I first met Erich Burghardt in 1977 in Graz during a study tour and I spent several months in his department in 1979–1980. Our collaboration produced a recent article (Burghardt, E., A. G. Östör: Site and origin of squamous cervical cancer: a histomorphologic study. Obstet. Gynec. 62 [1983] 117).

The idea of translating this book arose in October 1982 when Professor Burghardt was a guest lecturer in Sydney. It may be asked why, not being a professional translator, I undertook this arduous task. I believe this book makes a fundamental contribution to the practice of colposcopy and to its histopathologic basis. Colposcopy, introduced by Hinselmann some 50 years ago, has been largely ignored by English-speaking medical communities until recently. However, their new concepts have resulted in some unwarranted and unwelcome trends in the practice of colposcopy. This book will restore the balance.

It will be shown that the role of colposcopy is not to predict the histologic diagnosis, but to delineate the extent of the lesion on the cervix and to select the best area for biopsy. The colposcope cannot replace the microscope for two major reasons. First, invasion, or at least microinvasion, cannot always be excluded by cytology and colposcopy. And second, the same colposcopic picture may be produced by different histologic changes, each of which may have different biologic significance. This fact, however, will be appreciated only if one performs colposcopy in the Burghardt way *routinely* on *all* patients. Through such a routine, it soon becomes clear that the well-known patterns of punctation, mosaic, and keratosis are frequently expressions of a completely benign but specific epithelial change, characterized microscopically by hyperkeratosis, parakeratosis, acanthosis, and elongated stromal papillae, alone or in combination which in German is designated "abnormes Epithel." Because the strictly translated term "abnormal epithelium" does not distinguish between the benign and the premalignant, no equivalent term has found its way into the English colposcopic and pathologic literature, which dismiss it merely as "metaplastic." Furthermore, English-speaking colposcopists do not recognize the significance of this type of epithelium because selection of patients ensures that there is no opportunity to study colposcopically the cervices of women with normal smears, in whom such epithelium is frequent.

Neither the term "abnormally differentiating epithelium" suggested in the aforementioned monograph (Burghardt 1973) nor the appelation "abnormally maturing epithelium" used in our article (Burghardt and Östör 1983) overcome the problem associated with the word "abnormal." The designation "acanthotic epithelium" employed in this book was proposed by Professor Richard Kempson of Stanford University, California, during an animated conversation between him, the author, and the translator. This term is again not ideal, as acanthotic epithelium, while always acanthotic, frequently also shows parakeratosis or keratinization. However, it avoids premalignant connotation and is established in dermatology.

Acanthotic epithelium provides the key to the understanding of the discrepancy between colposcopic and histologic diagnosis, and obviates the hypothesis of premalignant colposcopic changes predating those of histology (Stafl, A., R. F. Mattingly: Angiogenesis of cervical neoplasia. Obstet. Gynec. 41 [1973] 168).

The importance of conization is also stressed. This procedure has attracted notoriety during the last two decades because of indiscriminate use and alleged complications. In English-speaking countries it has been largely superseded by so-called conservative, superficial ablative methods. It will be seen, however, that if carried out for the correct indications and by competent physicians, the complication rate is acceptable. Furthermore, only a cone biopsy (properly processed and examined) provides full assessment of all the histopathologic changes in the cervix. All other therapeutic measures destroy the tissues. The drawback of target biopsies as opposed to cone biopsy is that "'tis but a part we see, and not a whole" (Alexander Pope).

This book is the culmination of a lifetime devoted to the study of preinvasive and early invasive carcinoma of the cervix. Professor Burghardt has succeeded in bridging the ever-increasing gap between the laboratory and the bedside, having had rigorous training in all the disciplines required for this purpose: cytology, surgical pathology, colposcopy, and gynecology. It is little appreciated that it was he who first attributed diagnostic importance to aceto-white epithelium (Burghardt, E.: Über die atypische Umwandlungszone. Geburtsh. u. Frauenheilk. 19 [1959] 676).

I am indebted to Dr. Ruth Davoren, cytopathologist at the Royal Women's Hospital, Melbourne, and Dr. Vernon Hollyock, the doyen of colposcopists in this city, both of whom have read the translation and made numerous valuable suggestions. My mother, Mrs. Magdalena Östör, has helped with the German language, and to her I am grateful. The final responsibility of course is mine, and I hope I have avoided the pitfalls epitomized by the French savant who compared translations with women: "Lorsqu'elles sont belles, elles ne sont pas fideles." My thanks also to Mrs. Kathleen Cassidy, whose expertise on the word processor made my task so much easier. Finally, I would like to express my gratitude to my wife Elizabeth and children Andrew, Jr., and Charlotte, who have kept their patience while I have often lost mine during the work's long gestation.

Melbourne, Australia, January 1984   *Andrew G. Östör*

Preface by the Author to the First Edition

Routine colposcopy was instituted at the Graz Frauenklinik by my teacher Ernst Navratil in 1947. This date coincided with the introduction of cytologic diagnosis. In 1950 we acquired a modern surgical pathology laboratory devoted primarily to the study of early cervical cancer. Emphasis was placed on the examination of serial sections of ring biopsies and later of conization specimens. From the beginning of 1954 I had the opportunity to be at the forefront of these developments. Following a year of combined clinical and laboratory duties, I was appointed to the colposcopy outpatient clinic. Within two years I performed approximately 20,000 examinations. This experience was particularly valuable, as I also had the opportunity to interpret all the cytology smears and biopsies that I took. I also examined the serial sections from ring biopsies and conization specimens, not only for the first two years, but also for the following decades.

While accumulating knowledge and experience I participated in the historic evolution of colposcopy, witnessing its hesitant beginning and later, especially during the last 10 years, its stormy international course. The breakthrough was due no doubt to better international communication and exchange of ideas. Although textbooks as recently as 1960 have rejected colposcopy as "cumbersome and troublesome," its value is now undisputed. Controversies are centered merely on the indications for the colposcopic examination. While in Europe and South America, colposcopy is accepted as an essential part of every gynecologic examination, in English-speaking countries its use is selective. This is due to the propagation of colposcopy not as a basic diagnostic modality, but as one which enables the taking of a directed target biopsy and consequently the avoidance of conization, a measure which is primarily cost-saving. During the last few years, colposcopy has found further application in the evaluation of vaginal adenosis and that of the seemingly more frequent condylomatous lesions. Colposcopy has thus become regarded as a special diagnostic tool; this was never intended. Typically, history repeated itself: as discussed later, some current concepts of morphogenesis of cervical carcinoma are mainly based on colposcopy, as envisaged by Hinselmann.

With colposcopy well established, every effort should be made to reinstate the method's original role and to reconcile it with the other means of diagnosis, in particular that of histology. This is the aim of this book. With the careful correlation of the colposcopic and histologic findings, it will be shown how easy it is to resolve seemingly difficult problems. The enormous scope for colposcopic research will also be demonstrated. The fact that cervical lesions arise not only in histologically but also in colposcopically recognizable and assessable fields with constant distributions leads us to discuss topics that are ignored or poorly discussed in the present colposcopic literature. It is hoped that in addition to its instructive value, this book will provide the stimulus for further study.

The future prospects for colposcopy have become clear during the last few years. Originally it was intended to devote a chapter to "functional colposcopy" to be written by Otto Baader. This undertaking was interrupted by the untimely death of this eminent colposcopist. He left, however, many photographs that he partly took with his unique equipment during a study leave at our clinic. Thanks to the friendly cooperation of Mrs. Elsa Baader, who placed at our disposal her husband's material, previous publications, and notes, it was possible to complete this chapter (Chapter 12).

For Figure 13.1 (vaginal adenosis), I would like to thank Dr. Stefan Seidl, Hamburg; we had no experience of this lesion.

This book could not have been written without the assistance of my colleagues, all of whom I thank warmly. First of these is Dr. Hubert Schreithofer. He undertook the task of documenting colpophotographically every lesion on the cervix prior to conization, as well as a number of benign lesions. Most of the colpophotographs reproduced here have come from this collection. The fascinating job of correlating colposcopic and histologic findings in conization specimens was given to Dr. Wolf Dieter Schneeweiss. His schematic representation of the complex colposcopic and histologic findings is entirely original (Chapter 15). In the selection of the microphotographs, I had the valuable assistance of University Dozent Dr. Jürgen Hellmuth Pickel. And not the least, I would like to extend my special gratitude to the translator, Dr. Andrew Östör, who undertook this task with great expertise. He was confronted not only by the challenge of translating the German text into the best possible English, but also with the production of a text with scientific appeal to the English-speaking reader. It is thus more proper to refer to him as a collaborator, rather than merely a translator. Dr. Östör was also the first critical reader of the text. His observations and advice have also been incorporated into the German version. This collaboration between author and translator can only be regarded as unique.

Last but not least, my thanks go to all the staff of Georg Thieme Verlag, who are responsible for the realization of this book. They have troubled themselves to produce the best possible result.

Graz, Austria, January 1984   *Erich Burghardt*

Preface to the Second Edition

The success of the first edition of this book has made a new edition necessary. Almost all the chapters have been expanded in light of new knowledge. Additions include the most recent data on human papillomavirus (HPV) infection of the cervical epithelium, the current terminologies employed by FIGO (Féderation Internationale de Gynécologie et d'Obstétrique) and the International Federation for Cervical Pathology and Colposcopy, and a new chapter on "Colposcopy in Pregnancy." Also, the references have been brought up to date.

It has not proved necessary to change the essential postulates laid down in the first edition. This applies to the cautious evaluation of superficial destructive therapy as well as to the adoption of colposcopy as a routine screening tool. The recent success enjoyed by laser conization and diathermy loop excision in fact militates against superficial ablative therapy, while the current advocates of cervicography admit what colposcopists have known for decades, namely, that the optimal way to detect early cervical cancer is to combine direct visual methods and cytology in routine practice.

Particularly gratifying was the acceptance of the long-opposed concept that cervical lesions need not be confined to the transformation zone, but may also occur outside it. The contrary view, as mentioned in the critical discussion of the "atypical transformation zone" in the first edition, is obsolete. The concept of the atypical transformation zone, formerly considered to be of overriding importance, no longer appears in the new colposcopic terminology of 1990.

The encouraging feedback from the readership reinforced the principle on which the book was based, namely that true expertise in colposcopic diagnosis rests on an appreciation of the underlying histology.

The pictorial content has also been improved. A number of illustrations have been replaced and new ones have been added. Of the 78 new figures, nine are microphotographs and the remainder are color colpophotographs, 30 of which are in the new chapter "Colposcopy in Pregnancy." The new colpophotographs were taken by my colleague Dr. F. Girardi, an expert in his own right, who also advised me on human papilloma virology based on his research done in collaboration with Prof. H. Pfister from the Virology Institute of the University of Erlangen. As in the first edition, Dr. A. Östör has provided an excellent translation. I am also grateful to Prof. H. Pickel for help with the cervical pathology and to Dr. K. Tamussino for editorial assistance.

Graz, January 1991   *Erich Burghardt*

Table of Contents

1

Introduction

The primary aim of this book is to instruct. Every gynecologist should be familiar with colposcopy, and this monograph is intended to act as both a textbook and a manual, incorporating basic principles and detailed descriptions of the various appearances, to be consulted as the latter are encountered. The colposcopic image is a magnified view of the living tissue, the substructure of which is revealed only by the microscope. The histologic picture, however, should not be regarded merely as a static finding, but also as a certain stage of development of the dynamic process that leads from normal colposcopic appearances to the early stages of cervical cancer. Only with this knowledge of the morphogenesis of carcinoma can an isolated colposcopic finding be placed in its proper context. Two chapters are devoted to basic histopathologic principles, written so that, with the help of illustrations, previous understanding of the subject is not required. The first of these, Chapter 3, describes the growth and development of various abnormalities of cervical epithelia, based on meticulous morphometric investigations, and culminates in a hypothesis of cervical carcinogenesis. Chapter 4 lays the histologic foundation of colposcopic manifestations and addresses the question of how tissue changes at the microscopic level determine colposcopic configuration. A certain degree of overlap between these chapters is inevitable.

The histologic studies are based on the methodical examination of numerous serial step sections obtained from more than 5000 conizations. This unique material provides a complete evaluation of all existing lesions in the cervix, both in single sections (Figs. 3.15, 4.40, 4.46, 4.47, 19.1, 19.2, 20.4 and 20.7) and in serial sections (Fig. 20.7) in continuity. Furthermore, this is the only method that allows study of frequently coexisting lesions, their mutual relationship, their extent, and their growth patterns. For those so trained it soon becomes clear how conclusions drawn from a variety of sophisticated techniques may be misleading when applied to theories of morphogenesis. It is well to remember the admonition of the great pathologist Ribbert: "Only he who has completely familiarized himself with the growth processes of carcinomas can apply himself successfully to the study of their genesis."

A firm grasp of histology paves the way for the meaningful interpretation of the colposcopic appearance. The relevant sections of Chapter 11 should not be read without prior or simultaneous consultation of Chapters 3 and 4. Chapter 13 addresses colposcopic changes in pregnancy and the role of colposcopy in pregnancy. Of special importance is Chapter 15, which deals with colposcopic-histologic correlation and details the complexity of the colposcopic findings and how these are based on a corresponding variety of histopathologic changes. This subject is curiously neglected in the literature.

Consideration is next given to the consequences of the colposcopic and histologic findings, i.e., the histopathologic evaluation of the colposcopically abnormal cervix, the results of which determine therapeutic decisions. The controversy currently raging about the proper treatment of these lesions, engendered by the undue attention given to the so-called conservative methods, should not be an insurmountable barrier. Although the various treatment modalities may achieve the same rate of therapeutic success, and the particular method used often depends on local preferences and the type and availability of health care services, it is nevertheless important to know the exact success rate of each. To avoid serious mistakes, one must not employ treatment methods that result in destruction of tissue without a firm grasp of colposcopic and histopathologic principles. It is hoped this book will help to avoid such errors.

The subsequent chapters describe the use of the colposcope, the positioning of the patient, the choice of instruments, the colposcopic examination and the documentation and terminology of the findings.

The reader is urged to begin with Chapter 2, a historical survey that outlines the discovery of the colposcopic method, its current status, and its future prospects. By detecting the earliest lesions, colposcopy should enable the physician to gain the upper hand in the constant battle against the ravages of cervical cancer.

2

Historical Survey

Colposcopy has a checkered history. In addition to the initial technical teething problems, the new concepts encountered considerable opposition, making the course of its acceptance stormy. Accordingly, during the last 50 years, the colposcopic method has enjoyed a doubtful reputation, and its value and application have been continually questioned. During its long gestation, the body of knowledge engendered by colposcopy was forgotten until its recent "rediscovery." At least some of the difficulties were due to the fact that most of the colposcopic literature was in German and thus inaccessible to the medical world at large.

In 1924 Hinselmann was asked to write the chapter, "Etiology, Symptoms and Diagnosis of Uterine Cancer" in the third edition of the *Handbook of Gynecology*, edited by Veit and Stöckel (20). Hinselmann faced this challenge most admirably. He was struck by the limitations of palpation and naked-eye examination in the early diagnosis of cervical cancer, which he believed could be improved only by optical aids. He felt it imperative to "provide an intense light source for the magnified image without sacrificing binocular vision" (20). By 1925 he reported the construction of the first colposcope (16):

> For this purpose I have attached a light source to the Leitz binocular dissecting microscope. Using a longer working distance and intense illumination, the vagina and portio can be enlarged more than 3.5 times. According to the length of the vagina and the accessibility of the portio, these structures can be enlarged from 10.5 to 30 times. I have enjoyed using this equipment more and more in the last few months. It enables the study of all diseases of the vulva, vestibule, vagina and portio in a way which was not hitherto possible. I have attached the optical system to a stand which allows movement in every direction, and have also supplied a small screw for fine adjustment.

Until this time a cervical tumor the size of a pigeon's egg was regarded as early. After the invention of the colposcope, Hinselmann was able to state that "with regard to the so-called early cancers, we can say that colposcopy enables detection of considerably earlier cases. Even a tiny dot-like tumor should not escape detection. In principle, we can detect lesions as small as one would care to think of" (20). Later the accusation was made that in his search for the elusive "dot-like" tumor Hinselmann misinterpreted the hitherto unknown and only colposcopically visible surface epithelial lesions on the cervix. This was not entirely fair. Hinselmann was of course familiar with the work of Schauenstein (41), Schottlander and Kermauner (42), and his teacher von Franqué (11–13) described surface carcinoma (intraepithelial carcinoma or what we now call carcinoma in situ) as well as the surface epithelial changes found at the periphery of invasive carcinoma. Hinselmann had also identified the latter changes as the preinvasive portions at the periphery (*Randbelag*) of invasive cancers and had urged their colposcopic study (20, 22).

All remaining epithelial lesions were designated by Hinselmann as *leukoplakia*. The problem of leukoplakia was of special interest at that time, even single cases having been reported. Von Franqué (12) described six cases of leukoplakia of the portio in 1907, four of which "progressed" to invasive carcinoma in the absence of any treatment. Hinselmann (18) also encountered two cases of leukoplakia that on histologic examination proved to be small invasive carcinomas. These and similar observations prompted Hinselmann (20) to conclude that "to date there are no cases of leukoplakia of the portio which have not been cancerous." Hinselmann realized of course that many cases of leukoplakia had to be followed over a number of years to determine if they all progressed to carcinoma. Although he posed the question whether leukoplakia was the only manifestation of precancer, he immediately provided the answer that it was. His reasoning culminated in the conclusion that "exceptionally with the naked eye but certainly with the colposcope, it is possible to detect epithelial changes which appear as leukoplakia and which in time may progress to carcinoma" (20).

Accordingly, lesions that could be detected only by colposcopy were also termed "leukoplakia". Given that these lesions were clearly demarcated from, and whiter than normal squamous epithelium, important colposcopic criteria for the recognition of preinvasive and early invasive carcinoma of the cervix were laid down. By 1927 Hinselmann had already stated a view still current—that it is of special significance that leukoplakia apparently always appears in the transformation zone. Thorough appreciation of the transformation zone is therefore a prerequisite for the understanding of "leukoplakia" (17, 20). However, by 1928 Hinselmann (19) realized that "leukoplakia may involve the original squamous mucosa of the portio", that is, an epithelial abnormality may occur outside the transformation zone, an object of controversy at the present time.

Hinselmann (22) evaluated his colposcopic findings by rigorous histologic study. A large number of amputated cervices were processed by serial sectioning. This was undoubtedly a great achievement and proof of his dedication. He subsequently attempted to correlate colposcopic and histologic findings, which, however, resulted in considerable confusion and was largely responsible for the slow dissemination and acceptance of his method. The peculiar histologic terminology he devised was misleading, being heavily biased by the colposcopic viewpoint, which stated that only colposcopy could provide the key to the understanding of cervical carcinogenesis (21, 24).

Hinselmann opened up a completely new field and based his ideas on appearances never seen before. His train of thought is easy to follow. By studying leukoplakia, Hinselmann (25) discovered fine new patterns under the keratin: *punctation*, which he designated as *ground* of leukoplakia, as well as *Felderung*, now known as *mosaic*. Histologic studies of these changes revealed that they were due to certain disturbances of the epithelial architecture. As distinct from normal cervical squamous epithelium, epithelium from areas of punctation or mosaic was characterized by tall stromal papillae interdigitating with bulky epithelial pegs and frequently parakeratosis or keratinization.

These characteristic features were shared by two different kinds of epithelia. In the first type, the normal glycogen-containing layers were replaced by a wide band of prickle cells showing no atypia. In the second type, the whole thickness of the epithelium consisted of more or less atypical and undifferentiated cells. The latter type corresponded to what we now call cervical intraepithelial neoplasia (CIN) and was regarded by several authors even then as a precursor of cervical carcinoma (38, 40–42). We must remember that Hinselmann's starting point was the colposcopic finding. Biopsies from colposcopic areas of leukoplakia, mosaic, or punctation returned not only atypical epithelium, but also epithelium that could be distinguished from normal cervicovaginal squamous epithelium only by its disturbed maturation. Even today it is understandable that Hinselmann (23) regarded these colposcopically similar changes merely as different stages of the same disease process. He designated minimally altered epithelium as *simple atypical* (see "acanthotic epithelium" below) and that showing carcinomatous atypia as *markedly atypical*. Hinselmann regarded the colposcopic appearances of leukoplakia, punctation, and mosaic as indicators of malignant transformation and referred to these collectively as the *matrix area* (22, 24) of carcinoma.

Hinselmann realized that both simple and markedly atypical epithelium could lack tall stromal papillae and epithelial bud formation and could display only hyperkeratosis. Thus Hinselmann (21, 24, 25) incorporated all the various epithelial lesions and growth patterns into his histologic terminology. Confusing at first sight, this classification, using various headings and symbols, was designed to reduce all the colposcopic and histologic changes to a common denominator. It is surprising how such a complicated nomenclature could have been adopted by such a large number of German-speaking pathologists.

Criticism, however, was not lacking. The Swiss pathologist Askanazy (1) was quick to point out that the word *atypical* could be used only in a cancerous context in German. Instead of simple and marked atypia, he recommended the terms *abnormal* and *atypical epithelium*. This proposal was adopted by the Zurich school (14) but proved to be no better, as in English the terms abnormal and atypical are essentially synonymous*. Nevertheless, this distinction was an important milestone in both colposcopic and histologic diagnosis (see below). In his monograph, which appeared in 1950, Glatthaar (14) classified the squamous epithelial abnormalities from a cytologic point of view. He subdivided atypical epithelium (Hinselmann's marked atypia) according to the degree of atypia into *unruhiges (restless) epithelium, atypical epithelium,* and *surface carcinoma*. These correspond, of course, to the modern equivalents of mild, moderate, and severe dysplasia/carcinoma in situ. Glatthaar also addressed the problem of the *abnormal* epithelium in great detail. He correctly distinguished among reactive, dysontogenetic, and regenerative forms of abnormal epithelium. Disagreeing with other authors, especially Wespi (43), he regarded the regenerative type of abnormal epithelium in the transformation zone (which arose by metaplasia) as a precursor of squamous carcinoma and the *unruhiges* epithelium (now called mild dysplasia) as an *intermediate mutable stage* between abnormal and atypical epithelium. This gave rise to the concept of stepwise evolution of cervical squamous epithelium. Subsequent investigation showed, however, that simple atypia (acanthotic epithelium) played no part in cervical carcinogenesis. The studies of Hinselmann's pupil Dietel (8), who wrote on the subject with Focken, were particularly instructive; he followed 390 women with matrix areas (first diagnosed by Hinselmann and his coworkers) from 1 to 23 years and did not see a single case of malignant transformation of acanthotic epithelium. It was concluded that the likelihood of malignant change of acanthotic epithelium was no greater than that of normal squamous epithelium of the cervix.

This was a decisive breakthrough in colposcopy. It transpired that many *matrix areas* (characterized by leukoplakia, punctation, or mosaic) did not carry any premalignant connotation. By 1952 Novak (36) had already expressed the view that "between the first two grades of four described by Hinselmann and actual cancer there is a wide gap, almost as wide as that between normal epithelium and cancer".

---

* Abnormal epithelium is termed "acanthotic epithelium" in this book; it was called "abnormally differentiating in my previous monograph (3) and "abnormally maturing" in our review article (Burghardt E, Östör AG. Site and origin of squamous cervical cancer: a histomorphologic study. Obstet Gynecol 1983;62:117). For difficulty with translating this term, see also Translator's foreword.

This essentially correct, yet at that time controversial, opinion was formulated with no knowledge of the basic principles of colposcopy. Complete evaluation of acanthotic epithelium is of course impossible without full appreciation of the colposcopically visible lesions on the cervix. It should therefore be pointed out that acanthotic epithelium is not discussed, or is referred to merely as metaplastic epithelium, in highly specialized textbooks of physiology and pathology of the cervix (7) and even in textbooks of colposcopy.

We now know that acanthotic epithelium is essentially due to a disturbance of differentiation or maturation, and may develop both in the course of metaplasia and during the regeneration of original squamous epithelium (3). In either case, acanthotic epithelium is a basic tissue pattern that arises in a manner similar to that of atypical epithelium. Acanthotic epithelium is therefore a model that contributes to the understanding of the genesis of atypical epithelium, just as appreciation of its colposcopic appearance is essential for the understanding of colposcopy.

In the course of the so-called rediscovery of colposcopy, this historical evolution has been mostly forgotten. It appears that all the mistakes that have been made in the past must be repeated and that one must go through the whole learning process again. The old concept of the *matrix area* has been replaced by the "new concept" of the *atypical transformation zone* (7, 9), which in turn gives rise to the suggestion that atypical colposcopic appearance may biologically predate the histologic changes. This misconception does not matter as long as colposcopy is used predominantly for the evaluation of abnormal smears and not for routine diagnosis. In the first instance, it is inevitable that the colposcopist will see changes that are always, or nearly always, due to histologically atypical lesions. He or she will therefore come to the conclusion that specific colposcopic findings such as punctation or mosaic always indicate a premalignant state. For colposcopists so trained, it must be surprising and difficult to understand when these same colposcopic findings have no corresponding histologic significance. Only more recent colposcopic literature addresses the "vexatious problem of atypical colposcopic appearances associated with histology of trivial significance" (7), but without finding a satisfactory explanation. The introduction of the concept of the original transformation zone (7) complicates rather than simplifies the problem, the solution of which lies in traditional colposcopy.

Pari passu with the development of colposcopy, new theories of the morphogenesis of cervical carcinoma had to evolve. According to early histopathologic concepts, squamous cell carcinoma arose by "dedifferentiation" of single mutant cells situated in any layer of preexistent squamous epithelium (13). It was soon pointed out, however (9, 27) that only the immature, pluripotential cells of the basal (germinative) layer could participate in any epithelial transformation, including malignant transformation. Fischer-Wasels (9) attributed particular importance to the role of metaplasia in this regard. He referred to the latter process as *indirect metaplasia*, to stress that one type of epithelium did not simply change to another. In the case of columnar epithelium, it is the as yet undifferentiated subcolumnar or reserve cell that leads to the development of squamous epithelium (3). The very existence of metaplasia or indirect metaplasia has been debated for some time, its occurrence being flatly denied by Robert Meyer (30), the leading gynecologic pathologist of the time. Meyer proposed an active spread of squamous epithelium that undermined and eventually peeled off the columnar epithelium. Even today, such expressions as "the squamous epithelium shows active downgrowth into the glands" linger as relics of his teaching; this appearance can be simply explained by squamous metaplasia (10). Hinselmann also spoke of a "tactical ingrowth" of squamous epithelium into the glands, even though he was fully aware of the important role metaplasia played in the process of transformation (19). It was Wespi (43) who stressed the role of metaplasia in cervical carcinogenesis; his concepts are still valid today. Later, Glatthaar (14) reached the same conclusions.

It is remarkable how the growth of science is always punctuated by extreme views. Originally it was thought that squamous neoplasms could arise only from native squamous epithelium, whereas now there is a tendency to regard metaplastic epithelium as the sole precursor of invasive squamous carcinoma 7, 39). If this were true, however, the cervix would be an exception to all other organs (such as the vagina and vulva) that normally harbor squamous epithelium and squamous carcinoma.

As described in Chapter 3, cervical carcinoma may arise in various ways. In any case, the cells that undergo malignant transformation are undifferentiated cells capable of multiplication, be they the basal cells of squamous epithelium or the subcolumnar cells of the endocervical mucosa.

These theories, in turn, have been put into question by evidence of the role of viral infection in cervical carcinogenesis. While viruses are at least an important cofactor in carcinogenesis, the simple concept of the incorporation of viral DNA into the genome of the host cell, causing an irreversible mutation to a malignant stem cell, is in sharp conflict with the manifest phases in the morphogenesis of cervical cancer. Viruses have also refocused attention on the squamous epithelium, in which either condylomas or atypical lesions can arise, according to the type of virus. Colposcopy will be able to help clarify a number of problems in this field.

The new discipline of *cytology*, introduced by the classic monograph of Papanicolaou and Traut (37), revolutionized the early diagnosis of cervical cancer and at the same time almost brought about the collapse of colposcopy. The success of cytology was swift. It gained widespread acceptance, not only in the Anglo-Saxon world, where it was the only method for detecting early cervical cancer, but surprisingly also in Europe after the Second World War. Until this time, colposcopy had not made a similar breakthrough even in German-speaking countries. It was expected that colposcopy would be entirely replaced by cytology, which was simpler and more practical. For the fact that this did not happen we can thank those true pioneers who played down the relative merits of the various methods and realized that **all** modalities should be used in concert to perfect early diagnosis and to prevent invasive cancer. The names of Mestwerdt (29), Wespi (43), Limburg (28) Navratil (31, 32), and Held and co-workers (15) come to mind.

These men championed the cause of colposcopy as a method that allowed direct observation of the site of developing cancer, a facility denied by indirect cytologic sampling. Experience has shown that of the two methods, cytology, when practiced by experts, is more accurate. This is due to the fact that approximately 15% of carcinomas develop exclusively in the endocervical canal, out of reach of the colposcope. Because of sampling error and misinterpretation of findings, even cytology was estimated to have a false-negative rate of approximately 10%. Detailed studies (2, 4, 5, 33−35), especially those from Graz between 1954 and 1960, have shown that the best results could be achieved only by the *combination of the two methods* (see Tables 17.1 and 17.2). To this end, a unique diagnostic policy was formulated, consisting of routine colposcopic examination of every patient coupled with colposcopically directed cytologic smears, as described in Chapter 17.

Thanks to increasing international communication and new insights, colposcopy underwent at first a hesitant, but later an enthusiastic, revival outside Europe, especially in the United States. Objections were raised not only to the colposcopic theories (36) but also to the time thought to be required by the technique and its cost-effectiveness. It was not so much as a necessity but as a way of closing a diagnostic loophole that colposcopy eventually succeeded. Cytology detected an abnormality but gave no indication of its location. Histologic clarification thus depended on blind biopsy or conization. The ability of colposcopy to obtain a biopsy specimen from the right area and to reduce the number of conizations was responsible for its eventual acceptance. The indication for colposcopy, however, became highly selective; it was limited to the evaluation of abnormal smears rather than to its use as a routine diagnostic tool. The decisive role this played in the further development of colposcopic practice did not become evident till some time later. Since the colposcopic images encountered in these circumstances almost always corresponded to some atypical histologic change, the colposcopist's interpretation of the normal and pathologic appearance of the cervix became distorted and one-sided. Concepts of cervical carcinogenesis became similarly biased. Conversely, categorization of colposcopy as a specialized endoscopic tool to be used only in selected cases overrated its value. But the establishment of special colposcopy clinics where patients were examined for periods of up to 15 minutes gave rise once more to the fears which had previously been expressed that the method was costly and time-consuming. The future will decide which way the pendulum will swing: whether colposcopy will be used selectively or whether it will form an integral part of every gynecologic consultation, always augmenting the speculum examination with the naked eye. In the latter case, what every gynecologist who uses colposcopy as a routine knows will be proven time and again, that the procedure can be time-effective and that it improves diagnostic accuracy.

References

1 Askanazy N. [Cited in reference 14 below.]

2 Bajardi F, Burghardt E, Kern H, Kroemer H. Nouveaux résultats de la cytologie et de la colposcopie systématiques dans le diagnostic précoce du cancer du col de l'utérus. Gynécol Prat 1959;5:315.

3 Burghardt E. Early histological diagnosis in cervical cancer. Stuttgart: Thieme; Philadelphia: Saunders, 1973.

4 Burghardt E, Bacaj T. L'associazione sistematica della colposcopia e della colpocito-cariologia nella diagnosi precoce del cancro della portio. Minerva Ginecol 1956;8:1.

5 Burghardt E, Bajardi F. Ergebnisse der Früherfassung des Collumcarcinoms mittels Cytologie und Kolposkopie an der Univ.-Frauenklinik Graz 1954. Arch Gynäkol 1956;187:621.

6 Coppleson M. The transformation zone. In: Burghardt E, Holzer E, Jordon JA, eds. Cervical pathology and colposcopy. Stuttgart: Thieme, 1978:5.

7 Coppleson M, Pixley E, Reid B. Colposcopy. Springfield, IL: Thomas, 1978.

8 Dietel H, Focken A. Das Schicksal des atypischen Epithels an der Portio. Geburtshilfe Frauenheilkd 1955;15:593.

9 Fischer-Wasels B. Metaplasie und Gewebsmißbildung. In: Bethe N, ed. Handbuch der normalen und pathologischen Physiologie, vol. 14:2. Berlin: Springer, 1927:1211.

10 Fluhmann CF. The cervix uteri and its diseases. Philadelphia: Saunders, 1961.

11 von Franqué O. Das beginnende Portiokankroid und die Ausbreitungswege des Gebärmutterhalskrebses. Z Geburtshilfe 1901;44:173.

12 von Franqué O. Leukoplakia und Carcinoma vaginae et uteri. Z Geburtshilfe 1907;60:237.

13 von Franqué O. Anatomie, Histogenese und anatomische Diagnostik der Uteruscarcinome. In: Veit J, Stöckel W, eds. Handbuch der Gynäkologie, vol. 6:1. Munich: Bergmann, 1930:1.

14 Glatthaar E. Studien über die Morphogenese des Plattenepithelkarzinoms der Portio vaginalis uteri. Basle: Karger, 1950.

15 Held E, Schreiner WE, Oehler I. Bedeutung der Kolposkopie und Cytologie zur Erfassung des Genitalkarzinoms. Schweiz Med Wochenschr 1954;84:856.

16 Hinselmann H. Verbesserung der Inspektionsmöglichkeiten von Vulva, Vagina und Portio. Münchner Med Wochenschr 1925;72:1733.

17 Hinselmann H. Der Begriff der Umwandlungszone der Portio. Arch Gynäkol 1927;131:422.

18 Hinselmann H. Zur Kenntnis der präcancerösen Veränderungen der Portio. Zentralbl Gynäkol 1927;51:901.

19 Hinselmann H. Das klinische Bild der indirekten Metaplasie der ektopischen Zylinderzellenschleimhaut der Portio. Arch Gynäkol 1928;133:64.

20 Hinselmann H. Die Ätiologie, Symptomatologie und Diagnostik des Uteruscarcinoms. In: Veit J, Stöckel W, eds. Handbuch der Gynäkologie, vol. 6:1. Munich: Bergmann, 1930:854.

21 Hinselmann H. Beitrag zur Ordnung und Abteilung der Leukoplakien des weiblichen Genitaltraktes. Z Geburtshilfe 1932;101:142.

22 Hinselmann H. Ausgewählte Gesichtspunkte zur Beurteilung des Zusammenhanges der "Matrixbezirke" und des Karzinoms der sichtbaren Abschnitte des weiblichen Genitaltraktes. Z Geburtshilfe 1933;104:228.

23 Hinselmann H. Einführung in die Kolposkopie. Hamburg: Hartung, 1933.

24 Hinselmann H. Die klinische und mikroskopische Frühdiagnose des Portiokarzinoms. Arch Gynäkol 1934;156:239.

25 Hinselmann H. Die Kolposkopie. In: Klinische Fortbildung. Neue Deutsche Klinik 1936; suppl. 4:717.

26 Hinselmann H. Die Kolposkopie. Wuppertal: Girardet, 1954.

27 Krompecher E. Der Basalzellenkrebs des Uterus. Z Geburtshilfe Gynäkol 1919;81:299.

28 Limburg H. Die Frühdiagnose des Uteruscarcinoms. Stuttgart: Thieme, 1956.

29 Mestwerdt G. Atlas der Kolposkopie. Jena: Fischer, 1953.

30 Meyer R. Die Epithelentwicklung der Cervix und Portio vaginalis uteri und die Pseudoerosio congenita. Arch Gynäkol 1910;91:579.

31 Navratil E. Vergleich zwischen Zytologie und Kolposkopie in der Entdeckung von Frühkarzinomen. Acta Union Int Cancer 1958;14:286.

32 Navratil E. Colposcopy. In: Gray LA, ed. Dysplasia, carcinoma in situ and microinvasive carcinoma of the cervix uteri. Springfield, IL: Thomas, 1964:228.

33 Navratil E, Bajardi F, Burghardt E. Weitere Ergebnisse der Krebsfährtensuche an der Univ.-Frauenklinik Graz. Wien Klin Wochenschr 1959;71:781.

34 Navratil E, Burghardt E, Bajardi F. Ergebnisse der Erfassung präklinischer Karzinome an der Univ.-Frauenklinik Graz. Krebsarzt 1956;11:193.

35 Navratil E, Burghardt E, Bajardi F, Nash W. Simultaneous colposcopy and cytology used in screening for carcinoma of the cervix. Am J Obstet Gynecol 1958;75:1292.

36 Novak E. Gynecologic and obstetric pathology. Philadelphia: Saunders, 1952.

37 Papanicolaou GN, Traut HF. Diagnosis of uterine cancer by the vaginal smear. New York: Commonwealth Fund, 1943.

38 Pronai K. Zur Lehre von der Histogenese und dem Wachstum des Uteruscarcinoms. Arch Gynäkol 1909;89:596.

39 Reid B, Coppleson M. Natural history: recent advances. In: Jordan JA, Singer A. The cervix. London: Saunders, 1976.

40 Rubin IC. The pathological diagnosis of incipient carcinoma of the uterus. Am J Obstet Gynecol 1910;62:668.

41 Schauenstein W. Histologische Untersuchungen über atypisches Plattenepithel an der Portio und an der Innenfläche der Cervix uteri. Arch Gynäkol 1908;85:576.

42 Schottländer J. Kermauner F. Zur Kenntnis des Uteruskarzinoms. Berlin: Karger, 1912.

43 Wespi H. Early carcinoma of the uterine cervix: pathogenesis and detection. New York: Grune and Stratton, 1949.

3

Histopathology of Cervical Epithelium

Histologic Terminology

The nomenclature of atypical forms of cervical squamous epithelium is currently in a state of flux. Some prefer the terminology proposed by the First International Congress of Exfoliative Cytology held in Vienna in 1961, which distinguished between dysplasia and carcinoma in situ. Supporters of the more recent term *cervical intraepithelial neoplasia* see no need to differentiate between these, all atypical squamous epithelia being included in the one designation. Neither scheme has attempted to define other alterations of squamous or columnar epithelium. The terminology employed in this book is outlined here.

Squamous Epithelium

The cervix is normally covered by a stratified glycogen-containing squamous epithelium, referred to as

> *normal squamous epithelium,*

which may be native to the site or may have been newly formed; in the former case we speak of

> *original squamous epithelium.*

The squamous epithelium of the cervix and vagina may show *disturbed maturation* without atypia, which is designated

> *abnormal epithelium*

in German. As there is no clear distinction between the words *abnormal* and *atypical* in English, the term

> *acanthotic epithelium*

will be applied to this type of squamous epithelium (see p. 13). The squamous epithelium may display marked atypical proliferation of its basal layers, which are sharply demarcated from the normal superficial ones; this change is referred to as

> *atypical basal hyperplasia.*

When atypical cells are distributed in the middle and superficial zones of the epithelium as well (i.e., there is full-thickness involvement), the general term

> *atypical epithelium*

is applied. According to the degree of architectural disturbance and cellular and nuclear atypia, *atypical epithelium* may be further classified as

> *carcinoma in situ*

when the changes are maximal and

> *dysplasia*

when they are less pronounced.
Dysplasia may be further subdivided into

> *mild dysplasia,*
> moderate dysplasia, and
> *severe dysplasia.*

Currently there is a tendency to include all atypical epithelia under the one designation. Indeed the distinction between *dysplasia* and *carcinoma in situ* is not clear. As they represent essentially the same disease process, a two-tier division is artificial, and the all-inclusive term

> *cervical intraepithelial neoplasia* (CIN)

has been suggested (103). Even within this framework, three different grades are recognized, each of which has its exact counterpart in the old scheme:

CIN grade 3 = severe dysplasia and carcinoma in situ
CIN grade 2 = moderate dysplasia
CIN grade 1 = mild dysplasia

Invasive Lesions

The first sign of *invasion* is the appearance of tongues of epithelium extending from the base into the stroma. These are not visible with the naked eye in histologic sections, and measure only fractions of a millimeter. This lesion is called

> *early stromal invasion.*

With deeper invasion, the small tumor becomes macroscopically visible in the histologic section and is referred to as

> *microcarcinoma.*

It has been suggested that the volume of such tumors should not be greater than 500 mm³ (13, 16, 19, 21). According to the new FIGO classification, however, depth of invasion should not be more than 5 mm and the horizontal spread must not exceed 7 mm, giving a maximal area of 35 mm². The method of measurement is described on p. 19.

Finally there are

> *clinically invasive carcinomas,*

which are diagnosed by the simple methods of inspection and palpation.

Columnar Epithelium, Squamous Metaplasia, and Ascending Healing

The single-layered tall columnar mucus-secreting epithelium that covers and lines the endocervical mucosa and its glands (or crypts) is referred to as

> *normal columnar epithelium.*

The appearance of rows of cuboidal cells under the columnar epithelium heralds the process of

> *squamous metaplasia.*

While the cells remain single-layered, they are designated as

> *subcolumnar cells*
> or
> *reserve cells.*

When these multiply and become stratified, we speak of

> *metaplastic epithelium.*

The metaplastic process may be atypical from its inception, giving rise to

> *atypical metaplasia.*

Thin, poorly stratified, immature metaplastic epithelium has no distinguishing features when the columnar epithelium has been shed from its surface. The appearance may be identical to tongues of original squamous epithelium that extend from the periphery to cover a true erosion, as in wound healing. This process has been called

> *ascending healing.*

Initially this type of epithelium is also thin, having only a few layers, but it will eventually attain normal thickness. Should a biopsy be taken from such a nonspecific epithelium, it may not be possible to determine whether the process is *metaplastic* or is due to *ascending healing*, and is best referred to simply as

> *regenerating epithelium.*

Finally, the columnar epithelium itself may undergo *atypical proliferation*, to resemble well-differentiated adenocarcinoma, in which case we speak of

> *adenocarcinoma in situ.*

Cervical Squamous Epithelium and Its Pathology

Normal Squamous Epithelium

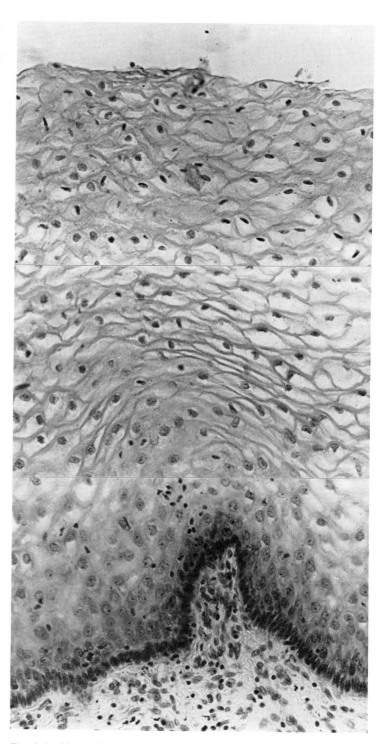

Fig. 3.**1 Normal squamous epithelium.** Almost the whole thickness of the epithelium is taken up by cells with clear cytoplasm containing glycogen. Note the prominent single-layered basal row and the short stromal papilla

Normal cervicovaginal squamous epithelium is stratified, *contains glycogen* (Fig. 3.1), and is arranged in several layers. A single row of basal cells supports a band of prickle cells with a thick layer of large polygonal cells above. The surface is covered by a slender layer of flattened cells. Normal squamous epithelium is nonkeratinized. Short stromal papillae extend into the epithelium at regular intervals. The epithelial-stromal junction is straight.

Acanthotic Epithelium

Acanthotic epithelium is characterized by *disturbed maturation* of the squamous epithelium *without atypia*. The epithelium lacks glycogen and resembles *epidermis*. Almost the full thickness of the epithelium is composed of prickle cells, and the basal layer is no longer sharply demarcated. The surface is cornified, its appearance ranging from parakeratosis to obvious keratinization. Occasionally a stratum granulosum may be present. The stratum lucidum of the skin, however, is never seen (Fig. 3.2). The stromal papillae are usually tall and slender, contain blood vessels, and their tips extend close to the surface. The papillae interdigitate with the plump epithelial rete pegs (Fig. 3.3). The appearance resembles *acanthosis* of the epidermis. The junction between acanthotic and normal squamous epithelium is always *sharp* (see Fig. 3.63 a).

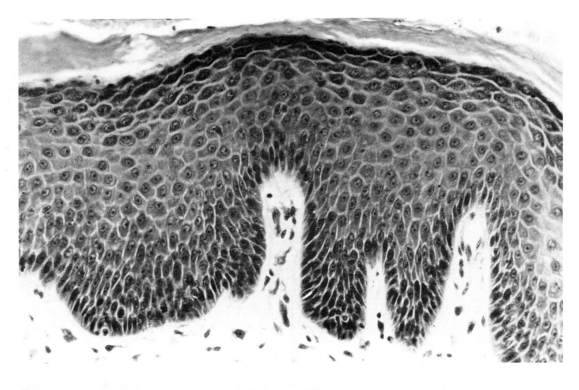

Fig. 3.**2 Acanthotic epithelium,** characterized by acanthosis (thickening of the prickle cell layer), a stratum granulosum, and keratinization. The cells do not contain glycogen. The stromal papillae are elongated

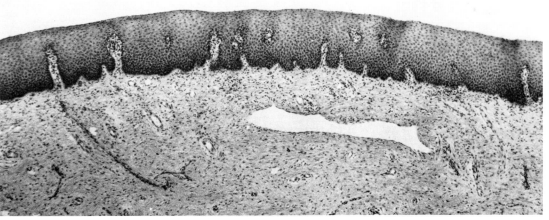

Fig. 3.**3 Acanthotic epithelium.** Tall stromal papillae interdigitate with plump epithelial pegs

Atypical Squamous Epithelium
= Dysplasia and Carcinoma in Situ
= Cervical Intraepithelial Neoplasia

The hallmark of this epithelium is the proliferation of *atypical cells*. There is variation in the size and shape of cells and their nuclei, the latter being enlarged and hyperchromatic. Mitoses are increased. The epithelial architecture is disturbed, with loss of polarity of the cells (Fig. 3.4). The surface often shows some degree of parakeratosis or keratinization. Stratification may completely disappear, the whole thickness of epithelium being composed of a uniform population of atypical cells (Fig. 3.5). As with acanthotic epithelium, the stromal papillae are often tall, and the rete pegs bulky (Fig. 3.6), but occasionally these features may be lacking (Fig. 3.7). Again, as with acanthotic epithelium, the border between atypical and normal epithelium is sharp (see Fig. 3.63b). Should several different types of atypical epithelium coexist on the same cervix, which is not uncommon, the borders between them are also clearly delineated (see Figs. 3.64 and 3.65a−c).

According to the degree of cellular atypia and disturbance of epithelial architecture, several *grades* of severity can be recognized. *Mild dysplasia*, or *CIN 1*, is characterized by only slight nuclear and cellular atypia, with preservation of stratification (Fig. 3.8). When borders between individual atypical cells and between cell layers become indistinct, the appearance is that of *severe dysplasia, carcinoma in situ*, or *CIN 3* (Figs. 3.5 and 3.6).

The histologic manifestations of the various grades of dysplasia and carcinoma in situ are protean, and correspond to the rich variety of invasive carcinoma (9). If the atypical epithelium has a uniform appearance throughout its full thickness, then it is said to be poorly differentiated (Fig. 3.5). If distinct layers can still be recognized, or there is evidence of surface keratinization, or both, the lesion is well differentiated (Fig. 3.4).

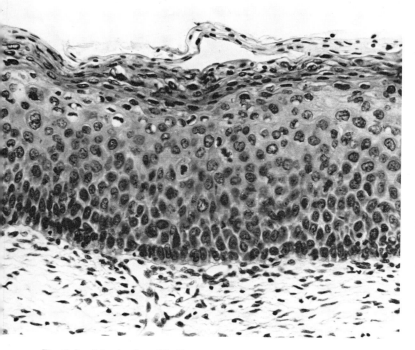

Fig. 3.4 Atypical epithelium.
The nuclei are pleomorphic and hyperchromatic. Mitoses are increased. Some degree of cellular layering, however, is preserved. There is a moderate degree of parakeratosis. The appearances are those of moderate dysplasia (CIN 2)

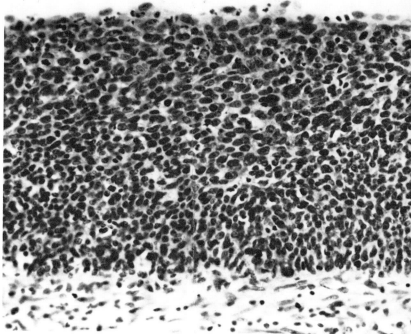

Fig. 3.5 Atypical epithelium.
The nuclei are closely packed together and are markedly atypical. There is complete loss of cellular polarity and layering. The changes are those of undifferentiated carcinoma in situ (CIN 3)

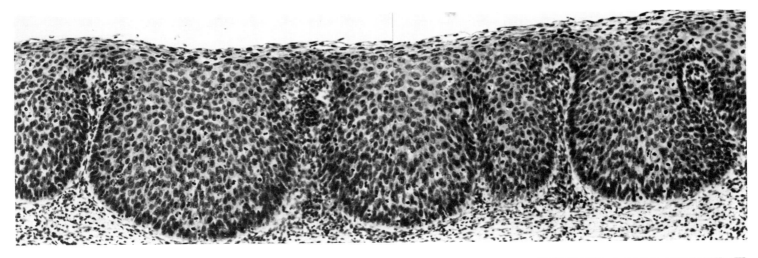

3.7

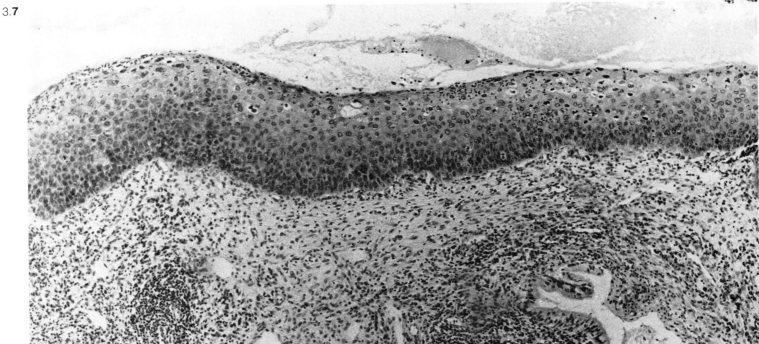

3.8

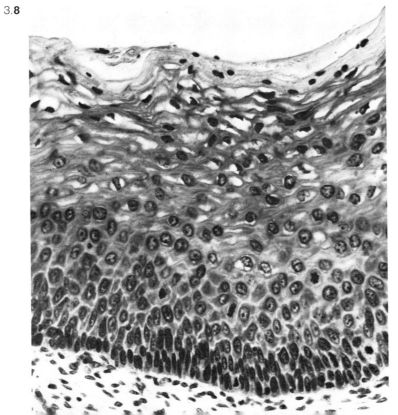

Fig. 3.**7 Moderately dysplastic epithelium** (CIN 2) of uniform thickness, undisturbed by stromal papillae

Fig. 3.**8 Atypical epithelium** with only mild increase in cellularity, atypia, and mitoses, best seen in the basal layers. There is little disturbance of polarity. The picture is that of mild dysplasia (CIN 1)

◁ Fig. 3.**6** The epithelium shows high-grade atypia. The elongated stromal papillae subdivide the epithelium to give it a "baggy pants" appearance. There is increased cellularity with increased mitoses. The basal layer is still discernible, and the surface shows parakeratosis. This is moderately differentiated carcinoma in situ (CIN 3)

Atypical Basal Hyperplasia

In atypical basal hyperplasia, the changes are confined to the lower third or half of the epithelium and are *sharply demarcated* from the normal superficial layers. The atypia is marked, and mitoses are frequent (Fig. 3.9). In *simple basal hyperplasia*, the band-like layer, due to proliferation of basal cells with only mildly hyperchromatic and enlarged nuclei, merges imperceptibly with the layers above (Fig. 3.10).

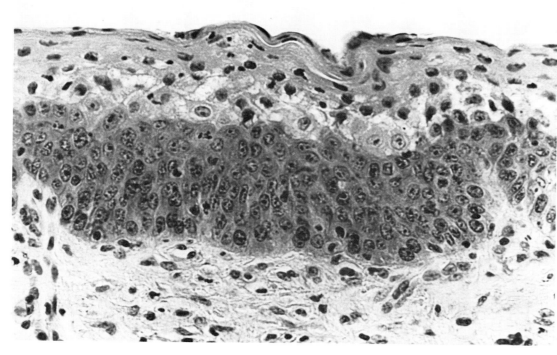

Fig. 3.**9** **Atypical basal hyperplasia.** The atypical basal half is clearly demarcated from the superficial normal half

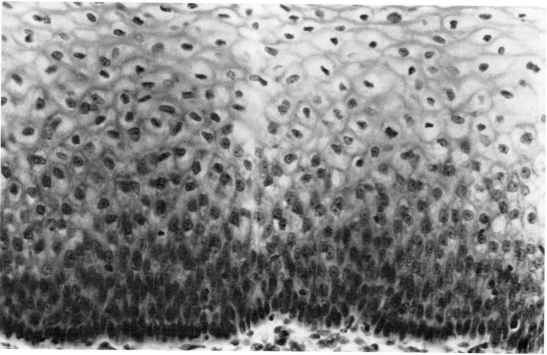

Fig. 3.**10** **Simple or reactive basal hyperplasia.** The basal layers show increased cellularity, but the cells lack atypia and mitoses. The transition to the normal superficial layers is gradual

Microinvasive Carcinoma (Stage Ia)

The most recently published FIGO terminology divides microinvasive carcinoma (Stage Ia) into Stages Ia 1, or early stromal invasion, and Ia 2, or microcarcinoma (38). The rationale for such a distinction is the fact that microcarcinoma is significantly larger than early stromal invasion, and consequently its clinical behavior may be different.

Early Stromal Invasion (Stage Ia 1)

The elongated and sometimes arborizing stromal papillae, associated with acanthotic, but above all atypical, epithelium accentuate the rete pegs, which may appear quite irregular (Fig. 3.11). Involvement of the endocervical crypts or glands by atypical squamous epithelium may give rise to a similar appearance (Fig. 3.12). Both appearances may be mistaken for genuine stromal invasion, a diagnostic pitfall with tragic consequence.

The histologic criteria of early stromal invasion have been well known for more than 30 years (3, 9, 34, 114). These take the form of round, club-shaped or finger-like projections extending from the base of the atypical epithelium into the underlying stroma (Fig. 3.13). The invasive tongues are distinctly different from the parent epithelium in that the cells are enlarged, with bigger and paler nuclei and abundant eosinophilic cytoplasm, giving the impression of higher differentiation. Alternatively, these features may be viewed as degenerative. It is then conceivable that the invasive foci are disrupted and destroyed by the body's defense mechanisms.

The stroma surrounding the invasive buds is never normal. It is edematous and is infiltrated to a greater or lesser extent by round cells, usually lymphocytes (Fig. 3.14). Epithelial buds surrounded by normal stroma must never be mistaken for signs of invasion.

It is important to realize that invasion may arise not only from carcinoma in situ but also from dysplasia, even from mild dysplasia. In such cases, characteristic histologic features have been described (3, 9).

Fig. 3.**11** **Carcinoma in situ** (CIN 3). The markedly elongated stromal papillae accentuate epithelial peg formation

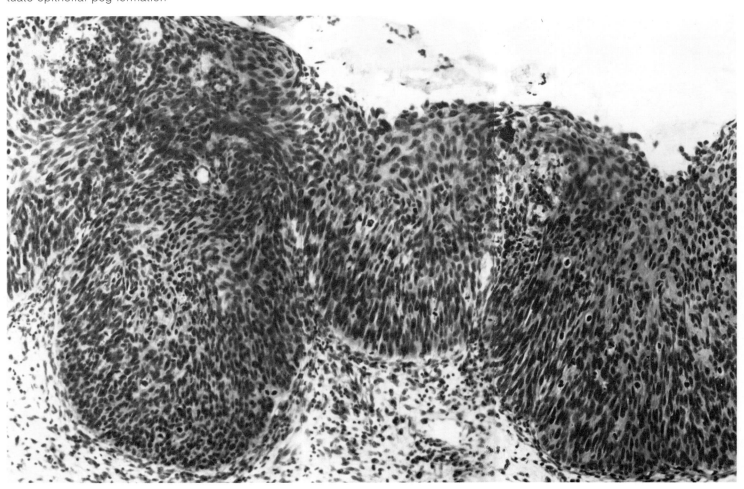

3.12

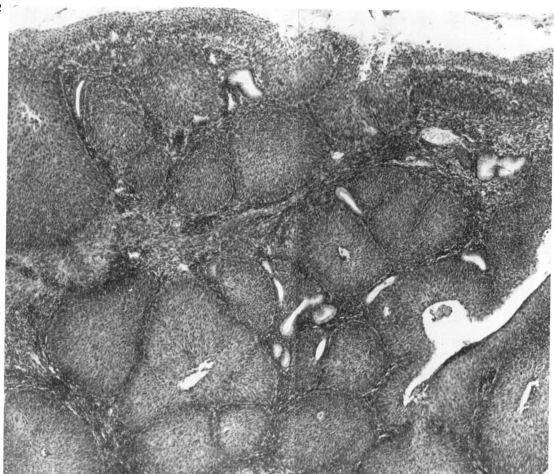

Fig. 3.12 Carcinoma in situ (CIN 3) with extensive glandular involvement. Islands of normal columnar epithelium remain. There is no evidence of invasion

Fig. 3.13 Early stromal invasion. The invasive peg is better differentiated than the parent epithelium, and shows distinct eosinophilia. The surrounding stroma is loose, edematous, and infiltrated by round cells (from Wien Klin Wochenschr 1978;90:477)

Fig. 3.14 Carcinoma in situ (CIN 3) involving the surface and crypts. The dark nuclei-rich epithelium around the gland openings appears as white cuffs colposcopically. An invasive focus arises from the base of the stout epithelial phalanx, which plugs a gland crypt

3.13

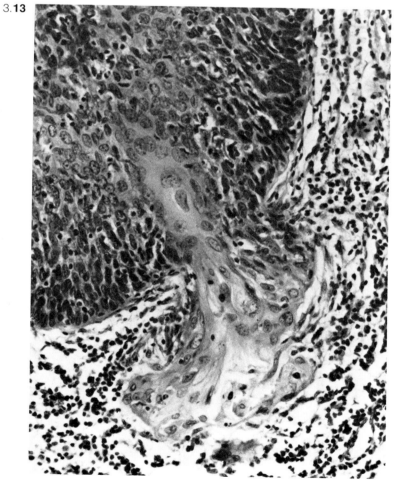

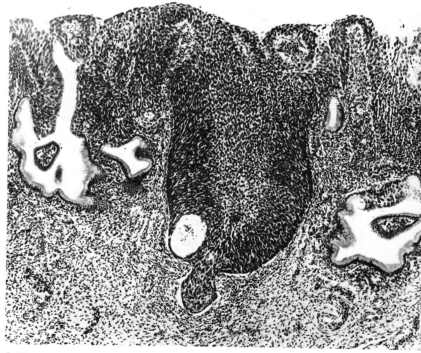

3.14

3.15

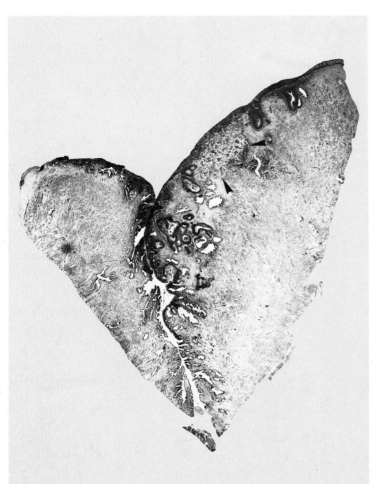

Fig. 3.**15** **Conization specimen containing a microcarcinoma** arising from the surface of the cervical lip *(right, arrows)*. The depth of invasion is 4 mm, and the surface spread is 7 mm. The glands extend for a distance of 7 mm into the stroma, and are extensively involved by carcinoma in situ

Fig. 3.**17** This microcarcinoma with a diffuse, net-like pattern is associated with a distinctive stromal reaction restricted to the invasive area. The individual invasive foci show cytoplasmic clearing, as in early stromal invasion

3.16

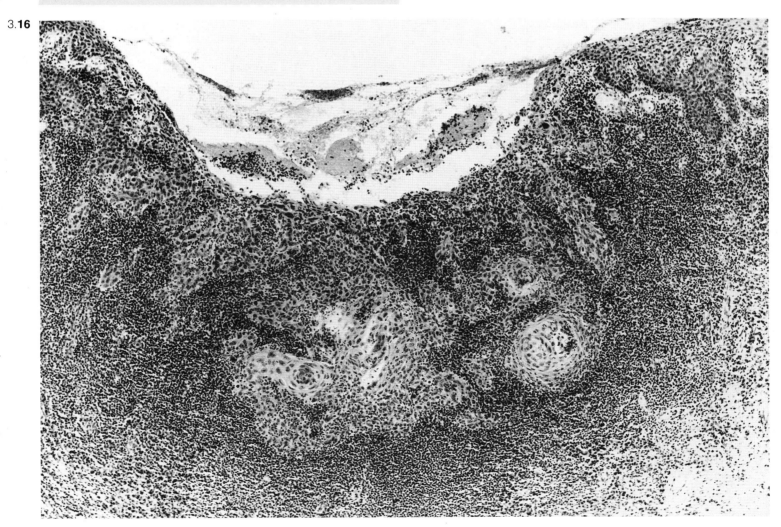

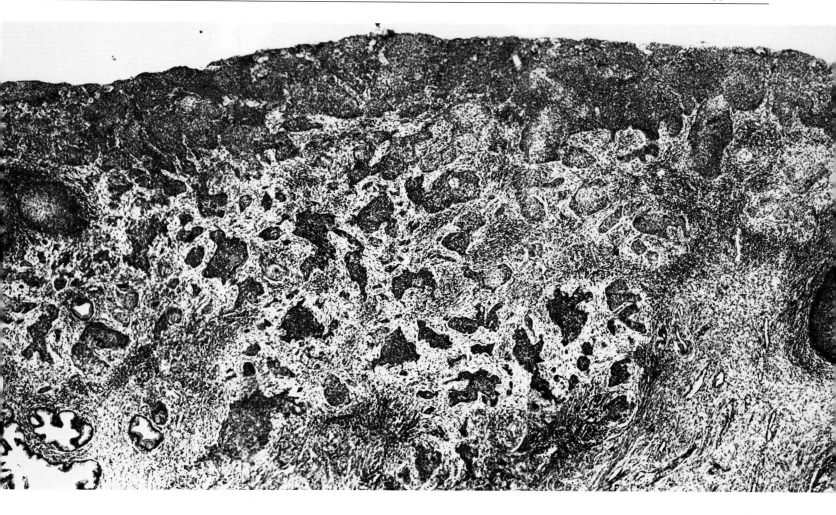

Microcarcinoma (Stage Ia 2)

Microcarcinoma is a small invasive tumor (Fig. 3.15). It has been suggested that the volume of microcarcinoma should be defined as not more than 500 mm³ (16, 21). According to the 1987 FIGO definition (38), the upper limit is given by measuring the two largest dimensions in any given section. The depth of invasion should not be more than 5 mm, and the horizontal spread must not exceed 7 mm. One can then estimate the volume by assuming that the third dimension does not exceed the greater of the two previous diameters by more than 50%. Suppose the depth of invasion is 5 mm and the surface spread 7 mm, then the breadth is calculated as 10.5 mm. The area is therefore 35 mm² and the hypothetical volume 368 mm³ (5×7×10.5). Many authors still believe that the definition should depend on the depth of invasion, which should not be greater than 5 mm. However, some microcarcinomas show wide horizontal spread without deeply invading the stroma; measuring only the depth of invasion does not indicate their real size. Furthermore, there is a close relationship between the volume of a tumor and its metastatic potential (12, 17, 23, 83, 124).

Like clinically invasive carcinomas, microcarcinomas may exhibit kaleidoscopic growth patterns and various degrees of differentiation. Well-differentiated microcarcinomas can be shown to arise from dysplastic epithelium (Fig. 3.16). The stroma investing microcarcinomas is similar to that associated with early stromal invasion, and has a rich capillary network. The focal degenerative changes resemble those seen with early stromal invasion (Fig. 3.17). The presence of capillary-like space involvement by tumor does not change the diagnosis, but should always be noted (38). There are no foolproof criteria that distinguish such involvement from artifacts due to tissue shrinkage.

Fig. 3.**16** **Well differentiated microcarcinoma with scattered epithelial pearls.** The surface epithelium from which the carcinoma originates shows moderate dysplasia (CIN 2). Note the dense, round-cell stromal reaction

Clinically Invasive Carcinoma

Large, clinically obvious carcinomas display several growth patterns. They may be

> *exophytic,*
> *endophytic,*

or a combination of the two, i.e.,

> *partly exophytic and partly endophytic.*

Of diagnostic importance are

> *tumors confined to the endocervical canal.*

Exophytic carcinoma is usually only superficially invasive (Fig. 3.18), its bulk growing into the vaginal lumen and cap-

ping the cervix like a mushroom. Such tumors are classically soft, friable, and subject to contact bleeding.

Endophytic carcinomas (Fig. 3.19) extensively infiltrate the stroma without exhibiting much surface growth. If they are not excessively large, there is little disturbance in the size or shape of the cervix. Even histologically, one sees only a flat ulcer surrounded by normal or abnormal squamous epithelium. If some of the tumor is still covered by epithelium, the eroded area gives no indication of its true size. The surface of an endophytic tumor may be rough, papillary, and granular, as in ulceration (Fig. 3.20).

The surfaces of the *partly endophytic, partly exophytic* tumors (Fig. 3.21) are usually ulcerated. In spite of their exophytic component, they may deeply infiltrate the underlying stroma. A purely *endocervical tumor* (Fig. 3.22) cannot be seen

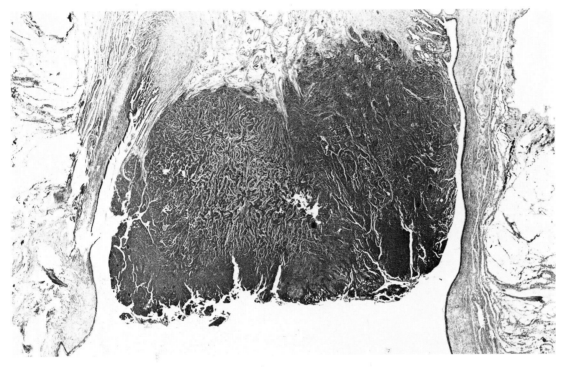

Fig. 3.18 Large surface section of the whole cervix and vaginal cuff, obtained at radical abdominal hysterectomy, containing a superficially invading exophytic squamous cell carcinoma

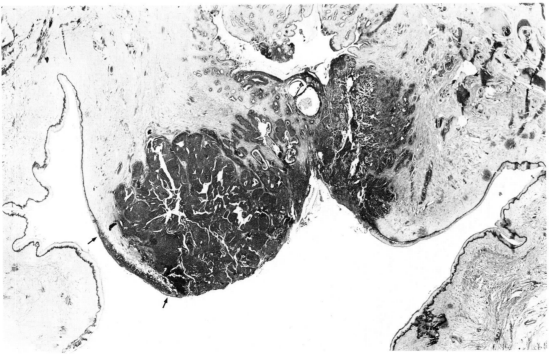

Fig. 3.19 Large surface section of the whole cervix, vaginal fornices, and cuff removed by radical abdominal hysterectomy, containing an entirely endophytic squamous cell carcinoma (left). The surface is ulcerated, and the tumor is bordered by carcinoma in situ (arrows)

Fig. 3.21 Large section of the whole cervix, vaginal fornices, and cuff, taken after radical abdominal hysterectomy, containing a partly exophytic and partly endophytic squamous cell carcinoma, arising mostly on the right side in the illustration. The vaginal portion is ulcerated

on inspection; it distorts and enlarges the cervix according to its size.

The *microscopic forms* of cervical carcinoma are many and varied and may be classified according to the grade of differentiation, nuclear size, cell type, or growth patterns.

First, one must distinguish between squamous cell carcinoma (Fig. 3.23; see also Fig. 3.26) and the less common adenocarcinoma (Fig. 3.24). The mixed adenosquamous type is less frequent than in the endometrium. Both the squamous and glandular components may be well differentiated, the epithelium showing distinct squamous differentiation and well-formed glands (Figs. 3.26 and 3.24). At the other end of the spectrum, there are solid tumors composed of cells with a monotonous appearance that diffusely invade the stroma, the histogenetic classification of which is no longer possible (Fig. 3.25).

Cellular stratification is relatively well preserved in well-differentiated squamous cell carcinomas, having a basal layer of densely packed nuclei, an intermediate zone, and a parvicellular surface layer (Fig. 3.26). The appearance may closely mimic that of moderate or mild dysplasia. Typically, keratin pearls may be seen. The resemblance between moderately differentiated squamous cell carcinoma and classical carcinoma in situ may be striking (Fig. 3.23). In spite of marked cellular and nuclear atypia, the tumor nests are unmistakably squamous. It is much more difficult to classify tumors that grow in narrow slender strands or columns (Fig. 3.27); if they show no suggestion of acinus formation, they are probably of squamous origin.

3.**20**

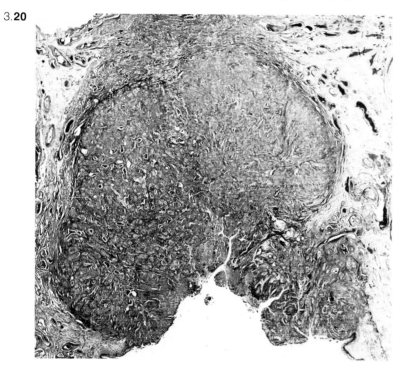

3.**22**

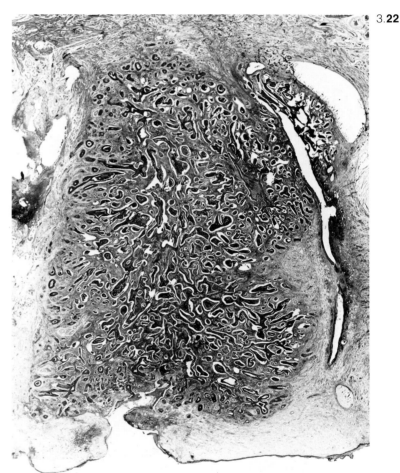

3.**21**

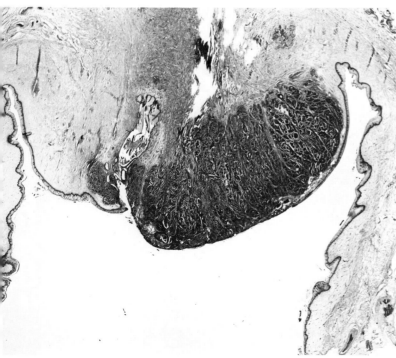

Fig. 3.**20 Large surface section of the whole cervix and vaginal cuff,** obtained by radical abdominal hysterectomy, containing a predominantly endophytic squamous cell carcinoma, the surface of which is fissured and ulcerated

Fig. 3.**22 Large surface section of the whole cervix,** from radical abdominal hysterectomy, containing a squamous cell carcinoma located entirely within the endocervical canal. Note that the squamous epithelium covering the ectocervix and lower portion of the endocervical canal is entirely normal

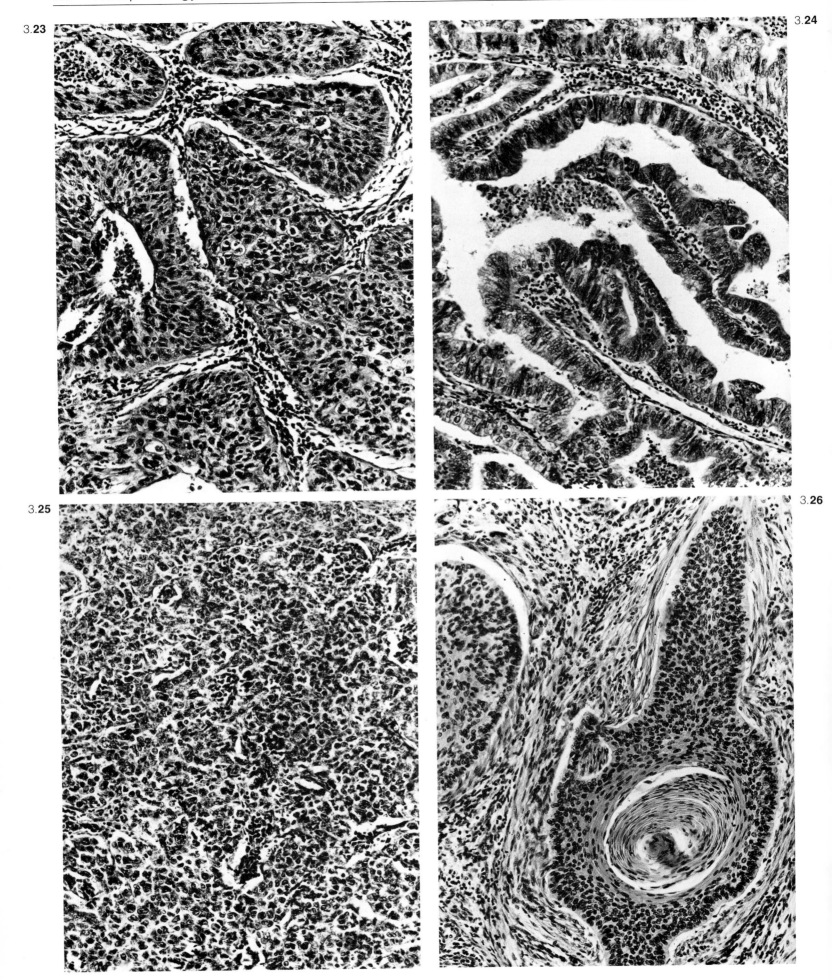

There are also other variants. It is important, yet little appreciated, that large, solid tumors not uncommonly display two or three microscopically different components, which are clearly demarcated from each other (Fig. 3.28), just as different forms of intraepithelial neoplasia frequently coexist (see Figs. 3.65 a–c).

Cervical adenocarcinoma is easily recognized as such, and can usually be distinguished from endometrial adenocarcinoma. The well-differentiated forms retain their resemblance to normal columnar epithelium in that the cells are tall and clear and contain abundant cytoplasm. The glands lie back to back, with virtually no stroma between them (Fig. 3.24). Mitoses are numerous and are situated mostly near the luminal surface.

The stromal reaction to invasive squamous tumors is variable, ranging from a well-preserved stroma containing only a light round cell infiltrate (Fig. 3.26) to a loose netlike stroma containing a dense population of mixed inflammatory cells (Fig. 3.23).

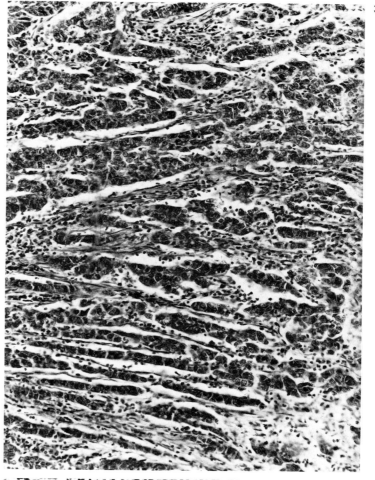

3.27

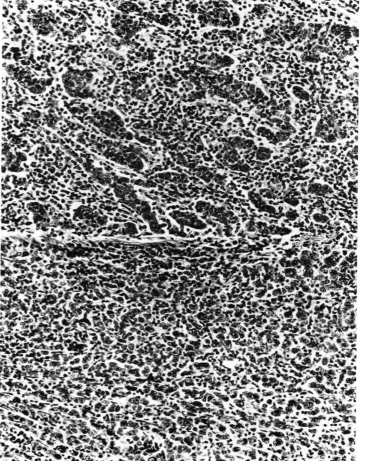

3.28

Fig. 3.23 Invasive carcinoma. A squamous differentiation is clearly recognizable

Fig. 3.24 Invasive adenocarcinoma. The neoplastic glands are reminiscent of normal mucin-producing endocervical glands

Fig. 3.25 Solid, undifferentiated carcinoma. Its histogenesis is unclear

Fig. 3.26 Well-differentiated squamous cell carcinoma. There is preservation of polarity, the surface shows parakeratosis, and there are a number of keratin pearls. The stroma is essentially unchanged and contains only a light chronic inflammatory infiltrate

Fig. 3.27 "Indian file" pattern of poorly differentiated cervical carcinoma, the histogenesis of which is uncertain; nevertheless, it is probably of squamous origin. Cell polarity and stratification are lost. The stroma is edematous, and contains a round cell infiltrate

Fig. 3.28 The undifferentiated carcinoma below is clearly delineated from the one above, which displays a different, trabecular pattern

Condylomatous Lesions

There are five different histologic types of condylomas (75–77):

    (1) papillary,
    (2) spiked,
    (3) flat,
    (4) inverted, and
    (5) atypical (78).

Like simple papilloma, *papillary condyloma* (Fig. 3.29) is essentially a fibroepithelial proliferation, but its etiology is probably different. The architecture is highly papillary, with thickened epithelium forming excrescences supported by a scaffolding of elongated and delicate stromal stalks rich in blood vessels (Fig. 3.30); the latter are best seen in tangentially cut sections. The surface often shows a variable degree of keratinization. The epithelial make-up is squamous, with a distinct basal layer, covered by a thick layer of prickle cells that in turn is surmounted by a zone of cells with clear cytoplasm, reminiscent of normal cervical squamous epithelium (Fig. 3.31). The similarity to the "empty" normal glycogen-containing cells is due to perinuclear haloes offset by the rather dense cytoplasm.

These cells are often binucleated or multinucleated, and are referred to as *koilocytes* (47, 69). They are characteristic of the viral condylomas and may show marked nuclear abnormalities. Koilocyte-like cells without nuclear enlargement or hyperchromasia are found in inflammation, especially with trichomonads (69).

In *spiked condylomas* (Fig. 3.32), the elongated and slender stromal papillae containing blood vessels push upward and indent the thickened epithelium to produce small undulations or fully developed "spikes". The epithelial architecture is similar to that of the papillary condyloma. Cells showing koilocytosis predominate in the superficial layers, but are also found in the midzone. The surface shows parakeratosis, with retention of pyknotic nuclei in the keratin.

The viral etiology of dysplasia of the cervix has been suspected since 1958 (123). More recently, the *flat condyloma* (Figs. 3.33 and 3.34) has attracted a great deal of attention. It is distinguished from other intraepithelial lesions by the presence of koilocytes and human papillomavirus (HPV) antigen (82, 122). These cells, with their perinuclear haloes, nuclear pleomorphism, and dense cytoplasm, are found in the middle and superficial zones of the epithelium, accompanied by cells showing only a mild degree of atypia. Pronounced atypia and atypical mitoses, however, are lacking, and some of the cells

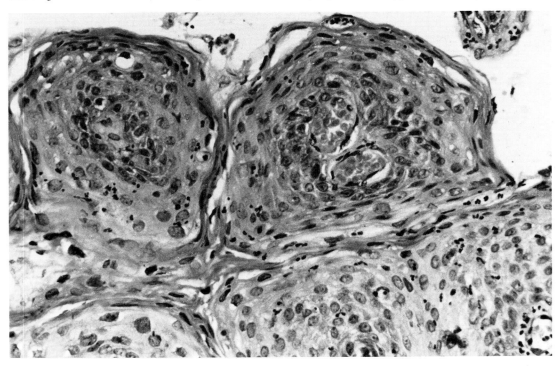

Fig. 3.29 Segment of papillary condyloma, the stromal stalks of which contain prominent blood vessels. Only an occasional koilocyte is present

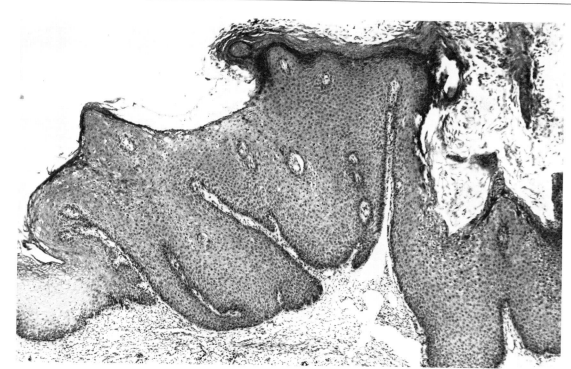

Fig. 3.**30** **Condyloma** showing papillary excrescences
and marked hyperkeratosis of
its surface

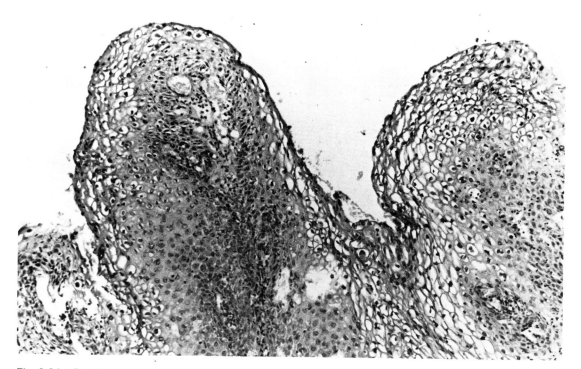

Fig. 3.**31** **Papillary condyloma.** The normal architecture
of the squamous epithelium is
disturbed. Most of the cells
with clear cytoplasm contain
glycogen

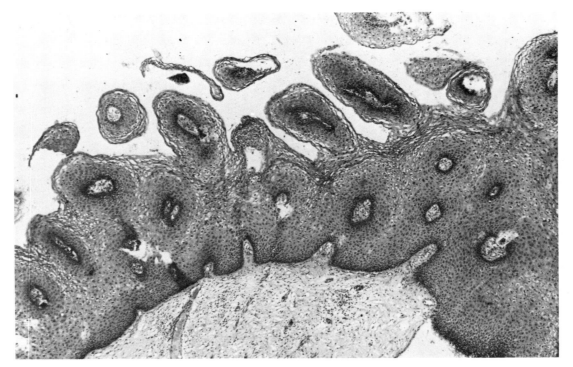

Fig. 3.**32** **Segment of a spiked condyloma** character-ized by numerous fine, finger-like epithelial projections. Some of the cells in the sur-face layers contain glycogen; others are koilocytes

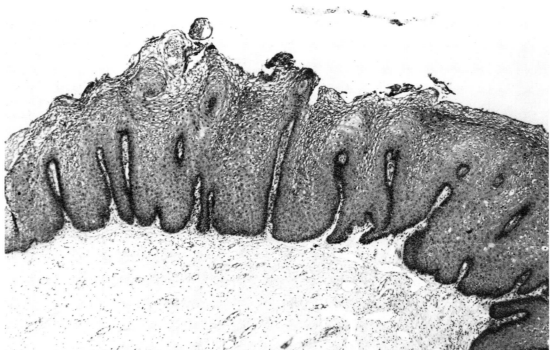

Fig. 3.**33** **A virtually flat con-dyloma** showing prominent epithelial pegs separated by tall stromal papillae. There is only slight cellular and nuclear pleomorphism

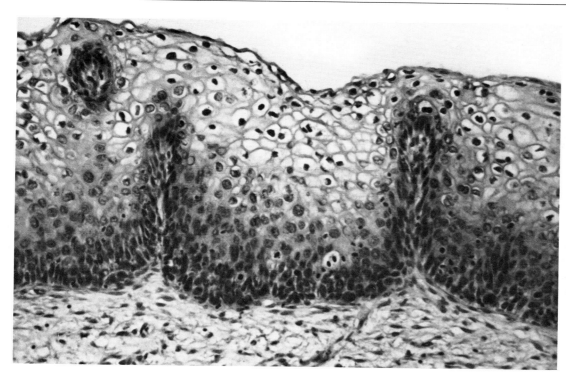

Fig. 3.34 Flat condyloma with tall stromal papillae and numerous koilocytes. The mildly atypical cells are mostly confined to the basal layers. This type of epithelial change could also be designated as mild dysplasia (CIN 1)

may contain glycogen (see p. 177). As in other condylomas, the stromal papillae are elongated. The frequent occurrence of warty lesions outside the glandular field, in original squamous epithelium, provides good evidence that lesions with papillary contours do not necessarily arise in the undulating matrix of the endocervical mucosa (see p. 80).

Meisels et al. (77) have described a variant of the flat condyloma designated as *condylomatous cervicitis and vaginitis.* The typical colposcopic appearances (see p. 178) have been misinterpreted in the past. Histologically, the epithelium appears normal at first, but a more detailed examination reveals tall stromal papillae or an undulating surface (Figs. 3.35 and 3.36). The normal honeycomb arrangement of the epithelium is disturbed, but the cells do contain glycogen. The spikes over the papillae may show keratinization. In contrast to flat condyloma, which is well circumscribed, condylomatous cervicitis and vaginitis is a diffuse lesion with a poorly defined margin.

Inverted condyloma (Fig. 3.37) also produces surface excrescences that may be distinctly keratinized. Characteristically, portions of the endocervical crypts, especially those of an ectopy, are involved. Such cases appear to be due to infection of metaplastic squamous epithelium. Cytologically, the epithelium resembles the flat type.

Atypical condyloma (Figs. 3.38 and 3.39) was first described by Meisels and associates (78). There is a mixed cell population in the middle and superficial zones of the epithelium, consisting of moderately to severely dysplastic cells admixed with cells showing perinuclear haloes. Tall stromal papillae, however, are often absent. Some koilocytes still retain pyknotic but irregular nuclei, but others show pronounced atypia, with enlarged and irregular nuclei containing coarse chromatin clumps. There is also cellular pleomorphism; cytoplasmic borders, however, are distinct. Stratification is relatively well preserved, with basal, middle, and superficial zones being recognizable. The atypical basal layers show increased cellularity and are rich in nuclei, reflecting their high turnover.

Condylomatous lesions may arise in the metaplastic squamous epithelium of the transformation zone or in original squamous epithelium. Condylomatous lesions are more common than noncondylomatous atypias at the latter site. Flat condylomas, like atypical epithelia, develop in clearly defined fields (78). The border between an exophytic condyloma and normal squamous epithelium is also sharp, and gradual transitions are not seen. This observation supports the development of epithelial lesions in areas whose boundaries are set by foregoing metaplasia (see p. 32), while the reason for their circumscription in original squamous epithelium is not so easy to explain.

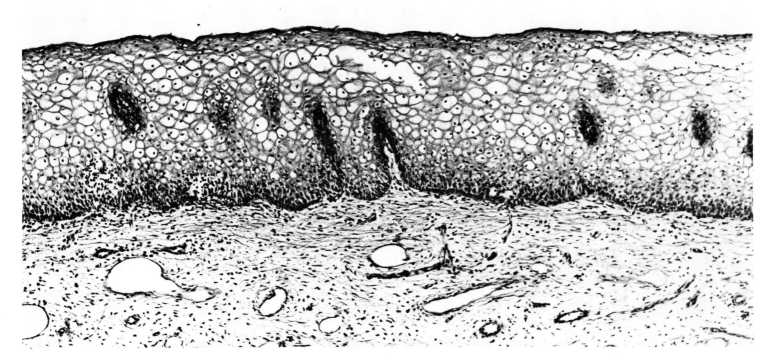

Fig. 3.35 Biopsy from a case of condylomatous cervicitis. The normal architecture of the squamous epithelium is disturbed, and the enlarged glycogenized cells show some pleomorphism, but no true atypia. Some of the elongated stromal papillae have been tangentially cut

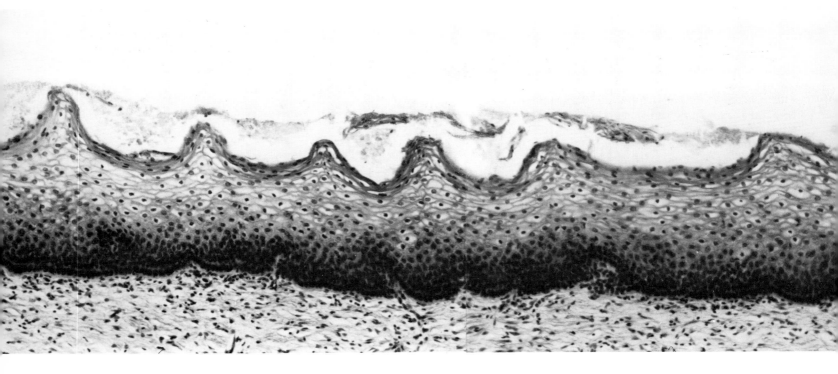

Fig. 3.36 Papillary epithelium from a case of condylomatous cervicitis. The colposcopic appearance rests on the undulating tissue surface. Apart from mild thickening of the basal layers and an occasional koilocyte, there is no disturbance of the epithelial architecture

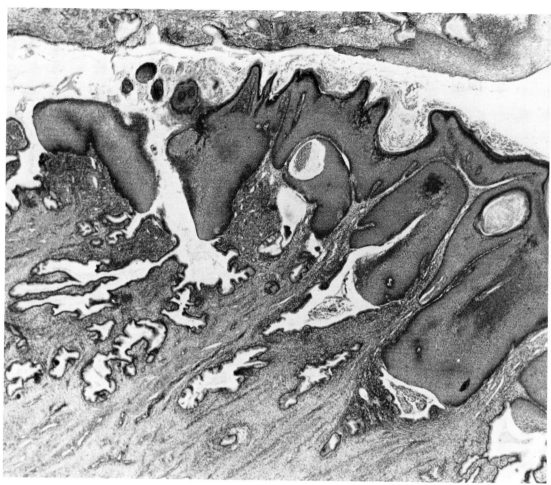

Fig. 3.**37 Inverted condyloma** arising in the region of the external os. The keratinizing papillary squamous epithelium involves not only the surface but also the endocervical crypts, parts of which, however, are intact

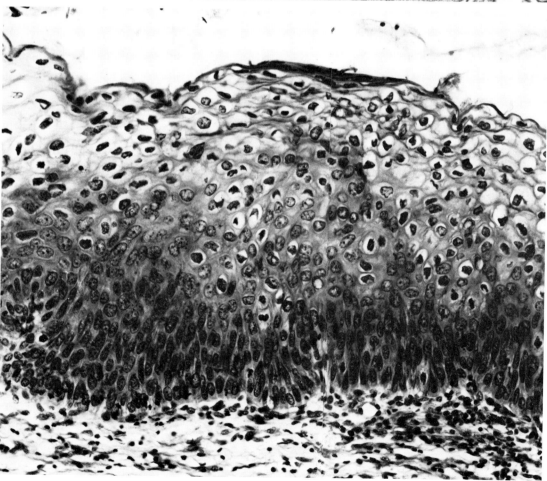

Fig. 3.**38 Markedly atypical epithelium,** with koilocytes distributed mostly in the superficial and middle layers (atypical condyloma)

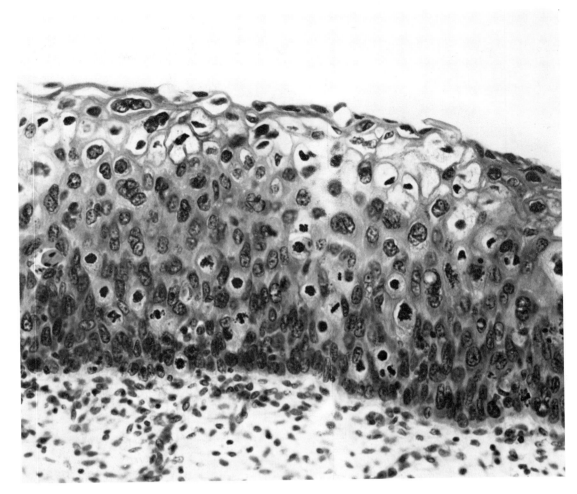

Fig. 3.**39   Atypical condyloma.** The superficial and middle layers contain multinucleated cells and koilocytes. Mitotic figures abound in the basal layers. No tall stromal papillae are present

HPV Infection

The viral etiology of condylomata is not in doubt. Intranuclear viral particles can be demonstrated electron-microscopically, immunohistochemically, and by molecular biology (94). The sexual transmission of condylomatous lesions is well known, the putative agent being the human papillomavirus (HPV).

These long-accepted or suspected relationships took on a new dimension when it was established that not only full-blown condylomata but also the flat lesions described above, which at times can only be identified colposcopically and are consequently also referred to as "subclinical lesions" (102, 109) are related to HPV infection. Finally, it was repeatedly shown that signs of HPV infection could be demonstrated with varying frequency in the various forms of CIN (27, 58, 66, 69, 79, 102, 115, 117). Indeed, condylomatous and CIN lesions may be found in close proximity to each other (Fig. 3.40; see also Fig. 11.84).

The papillomavirus is not a single agent, but comprises a whole family of subtypes (89). Those of significance for the genital tract include HPV genotypes 6, 11, 16, 18, 31, 33, 35, 39, 42, 43, 45 and others. There is a close relationship between the viral subtype and the type of histologic change. Mundane condylomata are mostly associated with types 6 and 11. These subtypes are also found in mild CIN, whereas types 16 and 18 are more often found in high grades of CIN and invasive carci-

nomas (36, 44, 50, 71). The assertion that the DNA of HPV is integrated into the cell genome only in invasive tumors (45) was not confirmed in our material.

Using the highly specific technique of Southern blot hybridization, it has been shown the the viral DNA of types 6 and 11 is found in a proportion of mild dysplasia (CIN 1), but more rarely in cases of severe dysplasia, carcinoma in situ (CIN 3) and invasive cancer. Type 16 is found especially in cases of high-grade CIN and invasive carcinoma but also in normal squamous and acanthotic epithelium (Table 3.2). Type 18 is encountered in cases of CIN 1, as well as in CIN 3 and invasive carcinoma (Table 3.1). Recently, type 31 has been linked to CIN 3, whereas type 33 is found especially in cases of CIN 3 and invasive carcinoma (43, 44). As can be seen in Table 3.1, combinations of viral types occur more often in CIN and invasive carcinomas. Finally, the same viral DNA found in primary tumors has been demonstrated in their metastases (45).

Most HPV-associated lesions have the potential to regress. The regression rate for CIN shows a wide range, between 30% (117) and 70% (79, 117). It must be pointed out, however, that there is no difference between the regression rates of HPV-associated CIN and non-HPV-associated CIN (6). However, regressing HPV-induced lesions do have a tendency to recur (36). A close relationship exists between regression, persistence and progression, on the one hand, and HPV types on the other; le-

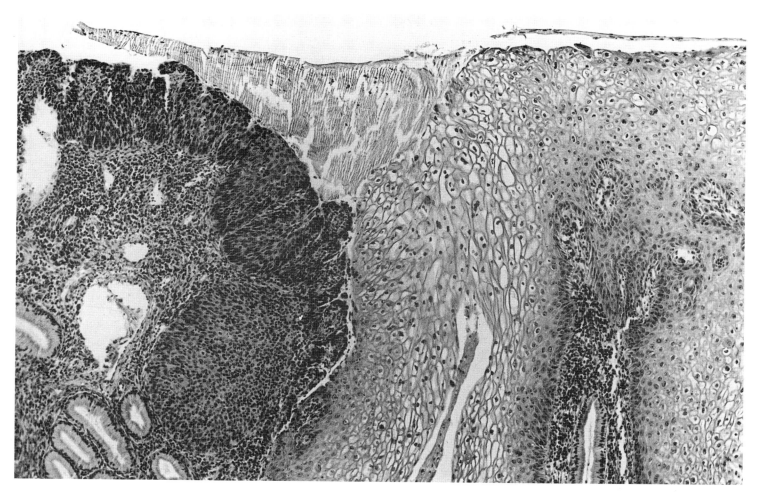

Fig. 3.**40**   **Carcinoma in situ**
immediately next to a typical
condyloma with tall stromal
papillae and marked koilocytosis

sions associated with types 6 and 11 are much more likely to
regress than those associated with types 16 and 18 (27, 44,
105, 110). On the other hand, the transformation of HPV-16 infected but otherwise normal squamous epithelium into atypical
epithelium has not as yet been documented.

Similar data from epidemiological studies and animal ex-
periments, linking HPV infection to the stepwise development
of preinvasive and invasive carcinoma, have been known for
some time (58, 59, 101). Considering the above, and the unpredictable behavior of the putative HPV-induced lesions, more accurate prognostic criteria are highly desirable. The best of these
is the spectrophotometric estimation of the DNA content of individual nuclei: using this technique, it has been demonstrated
that reversible lesions are mostly euploid or tetraploid, whereas
those which persist or progress are almost always aneuploid
(45, 101).

The viral etiology of carcinoma does not completely mesh
with the known steps in the morphogenesis of cervical carcinoma. Integration of viral DNA into the cell's genome is sup-
posed to result in a mutation of a single cell, this mutant stem
cell leading to the development of carcinoma. This would account for the observed monoclonality of most carcinomas. In
contrast, morphologic studies support the simultaneous development of carcinomatous atypia from the underlying subcolumnar or basal cells of entire fields. The possibility that during
induction of the process of squamous metaplasia, the sum total

Table 3.**1**   Human papillomavirus (HPV) in cervical intraepithelial
neoplasia (CIN) and invasive cancer; n = 459

HPV	CIN 1		CIN 2		CIN 3		Carcinoma	
	n	%	n	%	n	%	n	%
Negative	40	67.8	50	47.1	76	45.8	44	34.4
6, 11	7	11.9	6	5.7	12	7.2	6	4.7
16	7	11.9	44	41.5	72	43.4	52	40.6
18	2	3.4	0		4	2.4	6	4.7
6, 11 + 16	3	5.0	6	5.7	2	1.2	4	3.1
16 related	–		–		–		16	12.5
Total	59		106		166		128	

Table 3.**2**   HPV in benign cervical epithelium; n = 187

HPV	Normal epithelium		Acanthotic epithelium	
	n	%	n	%
Negative	46	90.2	113	83.1
6, 11	1	2.0	6	4.4
16	4	7.8	14	10.3
18	0	–	2	1.5
6, 11 + 16	–	–	1	0.7
Total	51		136	

of the subcolumnar cells becomes infected cannot be entirely excluded. Such an occurrence would be a lot more difficult to explain in original squamous epithelium, in which viral DNA can only be demonstrated in the superficial layers. The sharp borders, which are such distinctive histologic and colposcopic features, would also militate against the spread of infection from cell to cell.

In view of the above, various mechanism for the role of HPV infection may be envisaged.

a) The presence of the virus may be purely coincidental, playing no role in the pathogenesis of the epithelial alterations. Atypical epithelium may be more prone to viral infection than healthy epithelium.

b) The virus brings about an epithelial atypia, such as koilocytotic atypia, which, however, has no relation to carcinogenesis, and which returns to normal after the viral infection has subsided.

c) Certain viral types do produce cancer-specific atypia. They may be at least one factor in the multifactorial process of carcinogenesis. The fact that virus-related DNA cannot be demonstrated in all cancer-specific atypias may be explained by a "masking" of the viral DNA.

Columnar Epithelium and Its Pathology

Normal Columnar Epithelium (Endocervical Mucosa)

Normal columnar epithelium is single-layered, and consists of tall mucin-secreting cells with basal nuclei; it is synonymous with endocervical mucosa. Its junction with original squamous epithelium—the "original squamocolumnar junction"—is situated ideally at the external os (Fig. 3.41). Columnar epithelium not only covers the endocervical mucosa but also lines the "glands". These are not true glands, but merely invaginations of the mucosa, the surface of which is thereby greatly increased (41, 46). The surface of the mucosa in the canal is only gently undulating, and parts of it may be smooth. If the original squamocolumnar junction is situated on the ectocervix, the surface of the resulting *ectopy* is markedly papillary. The characteristic step-like squamocolumnar junction is due to the great difference between the respective epithelial heights (Fig. 3.41).

Squamous Metaplasia (Indirect Metaplasia)

The term *squamous metaplasia* is misleading. Literally, it means that columnar epithelium changes to squamous. Such *direct metaplasia*, however, does not occur. The replacement of columnar epithelium by squamous epithelium depends on the appearance of the so-called *subcolumnar cells* situated under the columnar epithelium (Fig. 3.42). The squamous epithelium, which results from the multiplication of these cells, eventually lifts off the preexistent columnar epithelium (Fig. 3.43). This process is best referred to as *indirect metaplasia* (39).

A number of theories have been proposed to explain the origin of the subcolumnar cells (39, 40). The best known postulates that these cells stem from the columnar epithelium. As the reserve cells of this layer, the subcolumnar cells would have the capacity to develop into either columnar epithelium or squamous epithelium (40). Other authors favor a derivation of the subcolumnar cells from the stroma (32, 112). However, recent studies showing that the subcolumnar cells express cytokeratins but do not react with vimentin indicate that the subcolumnar cells are of epithelial origin (95a, 111a).

To understand the metaplastic process, it is essential to bear in mind the following:

1. Subcolumnar cells are not found in normal unaltered columnar epithelium.
2. When they appear, subcolumnar cells form a discrete row (Fig. 3.44), or well-circumscribed *fields* when seen in three dimensions.
3. Different fields of subcolumnar cells may arise at the same time, and may be isolated or adjacent to each other.
4. Proliferation of subcolumnar cells results in formation of squamous epithelium only. Thus it is a misconception to refer to them as *reserve cells*.

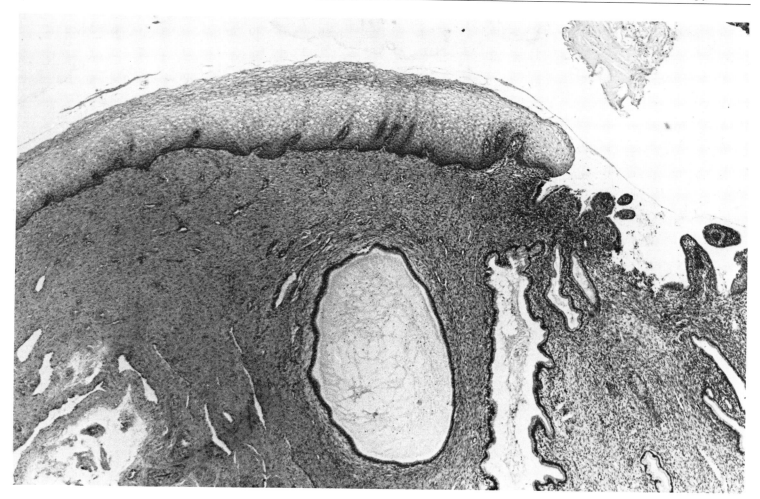

Fig. 3.**41** The squamocolumnar junction is situated at
the external os. The irregular
contour of the base of the right
half of the squamous epithelium, and the presence of the
last gland beneath, indicate
metaplastic origin

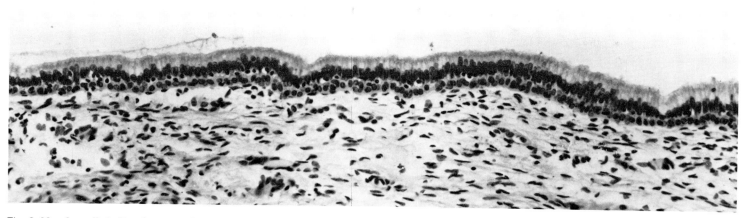

Fig. 3.**42** **A well-defined row
of subcolumnar (reserve)
cells,** lying under otherwise
normal columnar epithelium

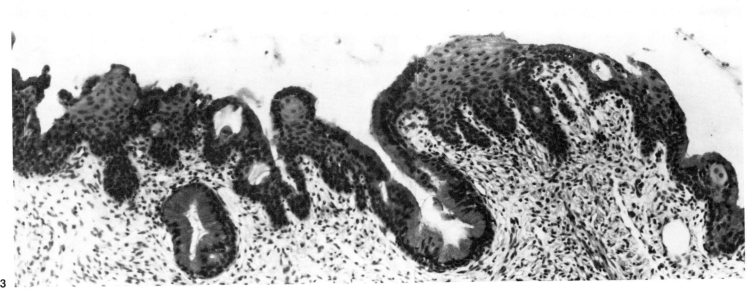

3.43

Fig. 3.**43** The process of squamous metaplasia begins with proliferation of the subcolumnar cells, which results in separation and eventual shedding of the columnar epithelium

Fig. 3.**44** A discrete row or field of subcolumnar cells

3.44

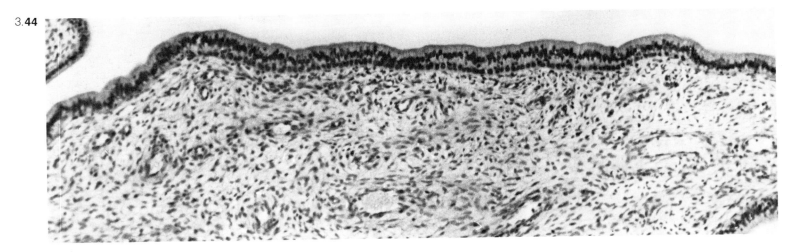

Further development of they newly formed metaplastic squamous epithelium may take one of three directions, as represented schematically in Figure 3.45.

In the vast majority of cases, the squamous epithelium that results is hardly different from the normal glycogen-containing original epithelium of the ectocervix, and can be distinguished from it only be *karyometry* (28) and by its undulating border with the stroma (Fig. 3.50).

Less frequently, metaplasia results in the formation of *acanthotic epithelium*. It is erroneous to deduce that acanthotic epithelium always arises on the papillary framework of an ectopy because of its tall stromal papillae and baggy-pants appearance, as if molded by the crypts. Indeed, the epithelial-stromal junction of acanthotic epithelium covering an ectopy may be quite regular, and the stromal papillae of normal height. On the other hand, regenerating squamous epithelium may form prominent epithelial pegs during its early stages,

without being related to papillary glandular structures (see p. 84). Finally, the tall papillary architecture of some condylomata which develop from original squamous epithelium is independent of the configuration of its tissue of origin.

The same applies to the third contingency, the production of *atypical epithelium* in its many forms, that is, cervical intraepithelial neoplasia (CIN). Epithelial bud formation and prominent stromal papillae may be features of CIN, but the base of the epithelium may be straight, even in an ectopy.

As the reserve cells appear in well-defined rows and fields, any squamous epithelium resulting from metaplasia must have *sharp borders* (Figs. 3.46 and 3.47; see also Figs. 3.61–3.65). Distinct epithelial borders imply *true epithelial transformation* rather than reactive changes due to inflammation or regeneration.

Metaplastic epithelium may exhibit *cellular atypia* at a very early stage of its development (Fig. 3.47). It is proper, therefore, to designate such a change as *atypical squamous metaplasia,* as distinct from simple squamous metaplasia (Figs. 3.43, 3.46). Although it may be difficult to distinguish between them, it appears that *simple metaplasia* results in either normal or acanthotic epithelium, whereas *atypical metaplasia may also give rise to atypical epithelium.*

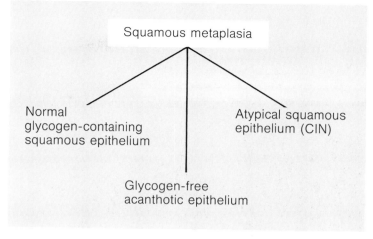

Fig. 3.**45 The fate of squamous metaplasia**

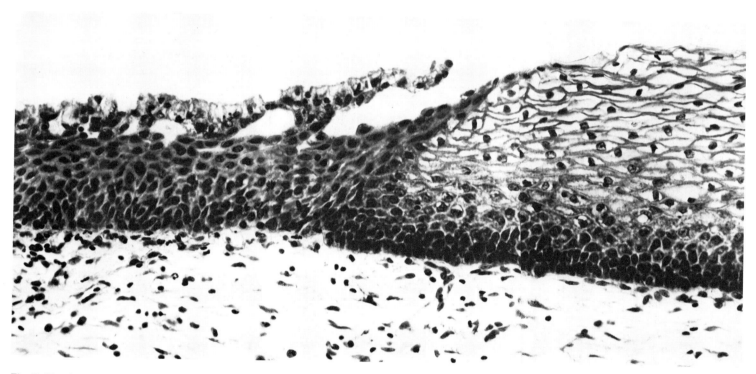

Fig. 3.**46 A sharp border separates metaplastic and original glycogen-containing squamous epithelium.** The columnar epithelium that once covered the metaplastic epithelium has been shed

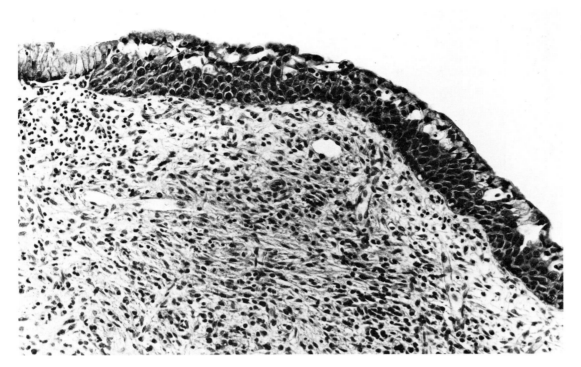

Fig. 3.**47** **Atypical squamous metaplasia.** The epithelium, which shows definite cellular and nuclear atypia, is still partly covered by columnar epithelium

Adenocarcinoma in Situ

Adenocarcinoma in situ may be defined as non-invading but highly atypical columnar epithelium (7, 9, 16, 90). Both the surface and the crypts may be involved (Fig. 3.48). The atypical glands are hypercellular. The enlarged pleomorphic nuclei, have clumped chromatin, and are disposed at various levels within the cells appearing pseudostratified. Mitoses are characteristically found in the scanty cytoplasmic seam above the compact, densely nuclear layer. It is noteworthy that the transition between the atypical and normal columnar epithelium is *abrupt*.

Adenocarcinoma in situ is frequently associated with atypia of the squamous epithelium, the incidence varying between 33 and 77% (5, 65, 86, 118). In our experience, it is usually an incidental finding in conization specimens carried out for CIN, although it is increasingly detected by cytology (85).

Microinvasive Adenocarcinoma

Histologically, it is extremely difficult, if not impossible, to determine where adenocarcinoma in situ stops and early invasion begins (7, 9, 16). The well-established criteria for early invasive squamous carcinoma do not apply. The often bizarre ramifications of the atypical glands may mimic invasion. Nevertheless, if the stroma investing the glandular outpouchings is completely normal, it is unlikely that microinvasion has begun.

Nevertheless, the glands of small invasive adenocarcinomas (microcarcinomas) are closely grouped, with many being back to back (Fig. 3.49); their upper volume may be set at the same figure as for the squamous variety (see p. 19).

3.**48**

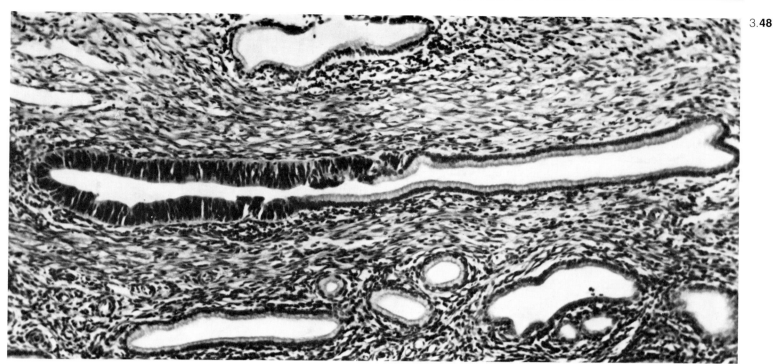

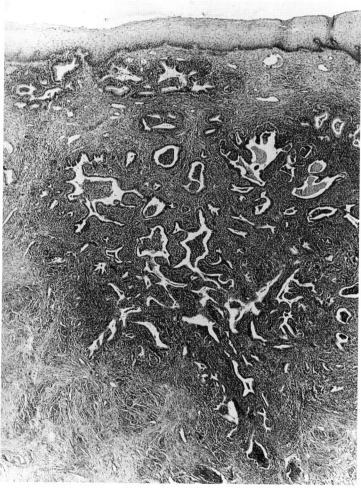

Fig. 3.**48** **Adenocarcinoma in situ involving a cervical gland.** Note that only part of the gland shows neoplastic transformation, the transition between normal and neoplastic tissue being abrupt

Fig. 3.**49** **Microinvasive adenocarcinoma.** The neoplastic glands, and the stromal reaction to them, form a small invasive tumor with 4 mm depth of invasion and 3 mm lateral spread. Normal cervical glands are present just under the surface

3.**49**

Topography and Extension of Pathologic Squamous Epithelia

The location of atypical epithelia was determined by the study of representative sections from 152 conization specimens, the details of which have been fully described elsewhere (9, 18). The various epithelial segments were measured and recorded schematically, using the external os and the last gland on the ectocervix as reference points. The last gland was used as the main reference point, because of its unique biologic significance and because the exact position of the external os cannot always be determined with certainty in fixed specimens.

The Last Gland

The concept of the last gland was introduced by Hamperl and co-workers (57, 84), who studied epithelial shifts (see also p. 70). They noticed that the endocervical mucosa often extended onto the ectocervix (ectopy) during reproductive life, but retracted back into the canal in postmenopausal women, its distal extent being marked by the last gland. The last gland is also the focal point for the distribution of the stromal connective tissue and blood vessels of the outer area of the cervix. These structures accompany any change in location of the last gland, and serve as permanent indicators of its position from intrauterine life to the postmenopausal period.

The significance of the last gland lies not only in its constant position, but also in the fact that it is a biologic landmark separating endocervical mucosa (columnar epithelium) proximally and original squamous epithelium distally (Fig. 3.50 a). Ideally, this squamocolumnar junction lies at the external os. When it is located at some distance outside the external os, the appearances are those of ectopy. The columnar epithelium of an ectopy is often replaced by metaplastic squamous epithelium that is in continuity with and at first glance indistinguishable from the original squamous epithelium. The squamo-co-

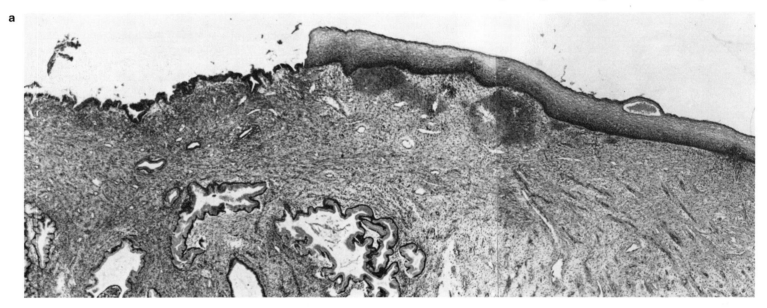

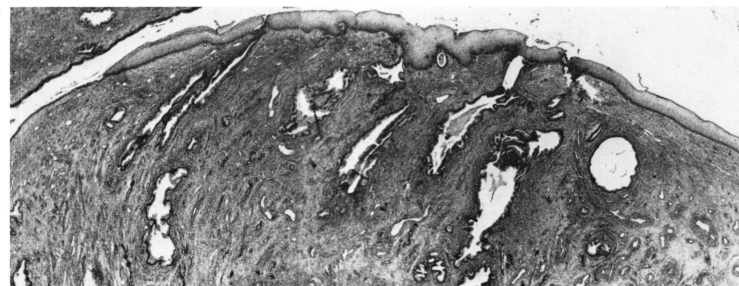

3.**50**

Fig. 3.**50 a   The original squamocolumnar junction,** located at the last endocervical gland (from Obstet Gynecol 1983;60:117)

Fig. 3.**50 b   The new squamocolumnar junction.** Note that it lies proximal to the last gland. The segment of epithelium lying between the new and the original squamocolumnar junction (the position of which is indicated by the last gland) is metaplastic, as it covers preexistent columnar epithelium. The general architecture of this metaplastic epithelium is somewhat disordered when compared with that of the original (from Obstet Gynecol 1983;60:117)

Fig. 3.**51**   The border between normal original and atypical squamous epithelium (showing increased cellularity) is sharp and perpendicular

Fig. 3.**52   Sharp borders between different types of metaplastic epithelia.** On the left is a thin, normally maturing metaplastic epithelium, still covered in part by columnar epithelium. In the middle, the metaplastic epithelium is thick, mature, and shows a suggestion of epithelial peg formation. On the right, the metaplastic epithelium is thin and is covered by columnar epithelium

lumnar junction is thus shifted proximally to some distance away from the last gland, resulting in what Pixley has called the *new squamocolumnar junction* (93). Thus, there are three biologically different epithelia in the cervix: the original squamous epithelium, the columnar epithelium, and the squamous epithelium admixed with and covering the glandular field (Fig. 3.50 b). Beato and associates (4) refer to the latter as the *third mucosa*, which of course corresponds to the *transformation zone* of colposcopy, being situated between the new squamocolumnar junction and the last gland (original squamocolumnar junction). Accordingly, every type of squamous epithelium, normal or pathologic, proximal to the last gland, must arise via squamous metaplasia. Conversely, original squamous epithelium must be the soil on which epithelial abnormalities distal to the last gland evolve. This concept would be invalid if pathologic epithelium could spread along the surface, an event dictated by the theory that states that neoplasia begins in a single cell or clone of cells (87, 103, 104). We shall now consider whether there is any histologic support for either of these theories.

3.**51**

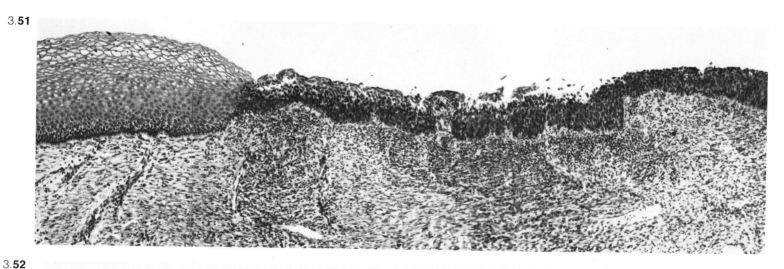

3.**52**

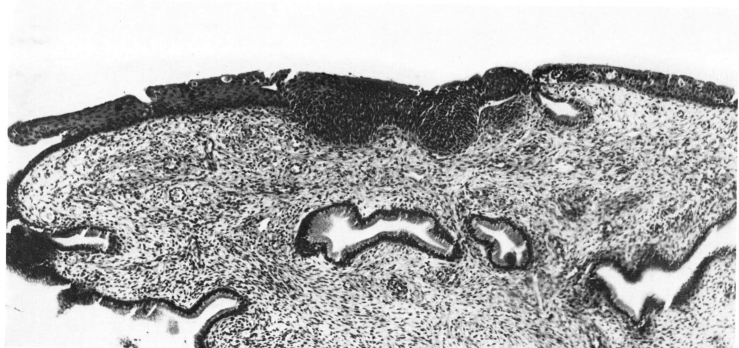

Surface Spread of Pathologic Epithelium

There is absolutely no histologic evidence to support the growth of intraepithelial neoplasia from a single focus of cells. Such an occurrence would be expected to cause, ipso facto, either invasion of the neighboring epithelia or peeling of the undermined epithelia. However, the existence of sharp and often perpendicular borders between adjacent but different epithelia militates against such events (2, 9, 11, 22). Epithelial borders come about because the ordered arrangement of subcolumnar cells in discrete fields results in a similar disposition of the metaplastic epithelium and its products, that proliferate simultaneously to cover the entire surface of each field. The sharp border with original squamous epithelium can be clearly seen (Fig. 3.51). Similar borders are also found between adjacent but different metaplastic epithelia (Fig. 3.52; see also Fig. 3.61). When atypical epithelial transformations involve the original squamous epithelium, these also appear in well-defined fields and arise via basal hyperplasia, a vertical rather than a horizontal growth pattern (see Fig. 3.9).

Lastly, if atypical epithelium or invasive carcinoma displayed aggressive intraepithelial spread, the last gland would not play the significant role that it does (see below).

Glandular Involvement

The poorly differentiated forms of carcinoma in situ (CIN 3) frequently involve not only the surface but also the endocervical glands, whether forming part of an ectopy or located within the endocervical canal. This involvement may be focal, seen only in a few glands (Fig. 19.2) or more generalized, involving most of the glandular field (Fig. 3.15). Endocervical crypts may be replaced completely by the atypical squamous epithelium, resulting in solid epithelial buds lying within the stroma (Fig. 3.53), or only in part, leaving segments of columnar epithelium intact (Figs. 3.53 and 3.54).

In the past, glandular involvement was differently interpreted. Under the influence of Meyer's theory of the healing of an erosion (see p. 70), one talked of active downgrowth of surface epithelium into the crypts, with undermining and peeling of the columnar epithelium; illustrations were shown to depict these events. Glandular involvement came to be regarded later as a more advanced stage of carcinoma in situ (52). It was of gravest therapeutic import to mistake glandular involvement for invasion.

As active surface extension of epithelium cannot take place (see above), the presence of atypical squamous epithelium in endocervical glands, which are merely invaginations of the surface columnar epithelium, must be explained by metaplasia (9, 35, 113, 119). This is supported by the similar genesis of normal (Fig. 3.54) and acanthotic epithelium in glands. The mistaken interpretation of the replacement of columnar epithelium by a "squamous epithelial plough" rests on the observation that columnar epithelium is often preserved at the outer margins of metaplastic squamous epithelium, but has completely disappeared from the surface.

However, when various forms of atypical epithelium involve endocervical crypts, the borders between them are sharp. Furthermore, squamous metaplasia may be found isolated within the crypts (Fig. 3.55). As the mild epithelial atypias (well-differentiated forms of CIN) often arise in original squamous epithelium, glandular involvement by such epithelium is infrequent.

Fig. 3.**53 Carcinoma in situ** (CIN 3) showing glandular involvement. The gland on the right is completely replaced and filled by carcinoma in situ, whereas parts of the gland on the left remain unaltered

Fig. 3.**54 Normal squamous epithelium** partly replaces an endocervical gland; the lumen is not completely filled

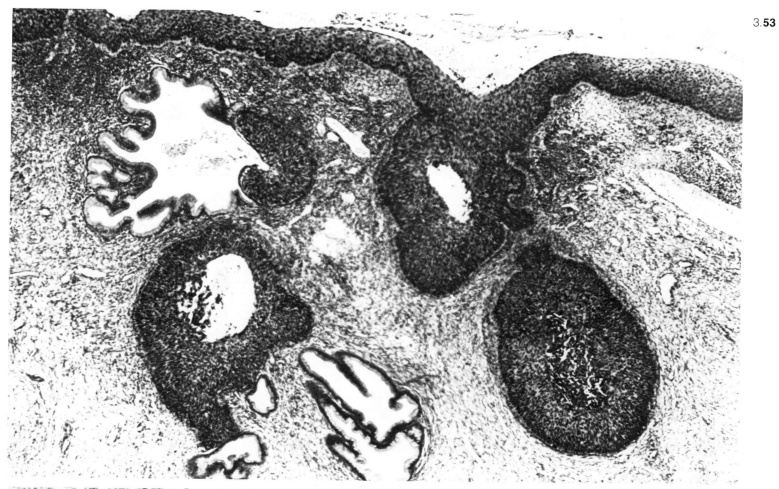

3.**53**

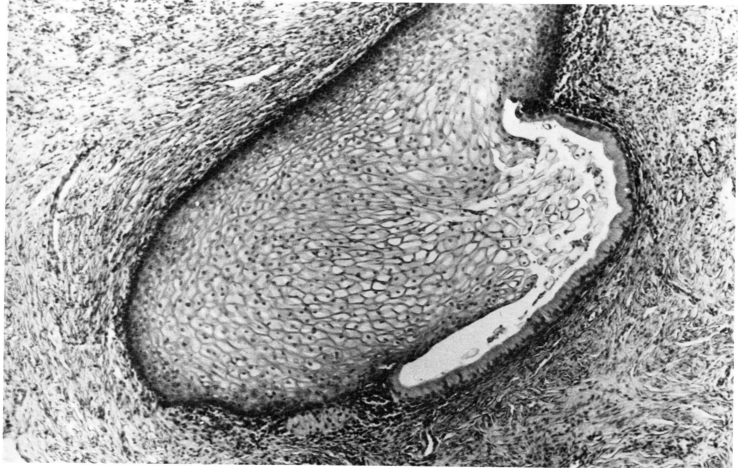

3.**54**

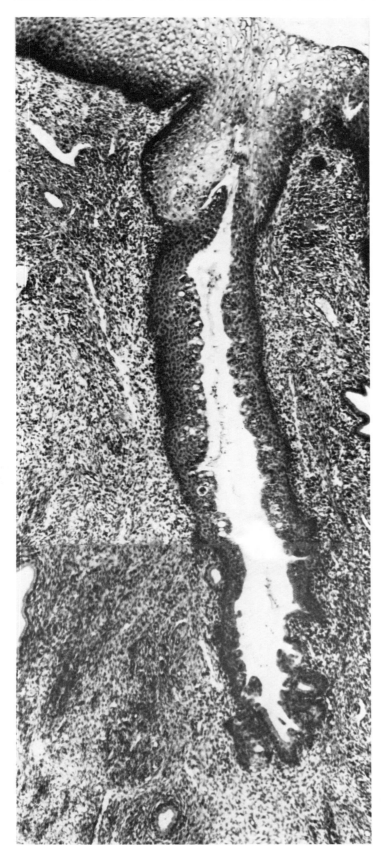

Fig. 3.**55 Focal involvement of a gland by squamous metaplasia**. The immature metaplastic epithelium is clearly demarcated from the fully differentiated squamous epithelium seen both on the surface and at the gland opening

Location of Atypical Epithelium

Careful examination of serial-step sections from conization specimens reveals that atypical epithelia frequently end at the last gland (Fig. 3.56 a–d) whether arising in the glandular field (Fig. 3.56 b–d) or in original squamous epithelium (Fig. 3.56 a).

A study of 152 conization specimens showed that atypical epithelium was located exclusively on one or the other side of the last gland in 96.9% of cases (Fig. 3.57). In 80.6%, the columnar epithelium was involved, and in 33.1% the lesions ended at the last gland. In 16.3% of cases, atypical epithelium was situated distal to the last gland, and in 13.2% the proximal portion ended at the last gland. Thus the last gland frequently (46%) represented either the distal or proximal border of CIN. Only in 3.1% of cases did atypical epithelium extend beyond the last gland (10, 11, 14). This may be due to the simultaneous generation of two identical epithelia at either side of the last gland, or to preceding ascending healing (see p. 75) with subsequent atypical transformation (see p. 56).

The relationship of the various atypical epithelia to the last gland is illustrated in Figure 3.58. The bars representing each epithelial type include all the areas involved by 95% of the respective epithelia. That some of these overlap and extend beyond the last gland is not due to active spread, but to the fact that similar epithelia are found on either side of the last gland.

Detailed study of Figure 3.58 is invaluable for understanding the morphogenesis of pathologic cervical squamous epithelia (see also p. 56). First, we may note that the more distal (beyond the last gland, on the ectocervix) the location of atypical epithelium, the higher its differentiation. Mild dysplasia behaves in this respect like well-differentiated carcinoma in situ. Undifferentiated carcinoma in situ [3] is exclusively situated within the glandular field, whereas moderately differentiated carcinoma in situ [4] and moderate dysplasia [6] are also located mostly in the glandular field, but may sometimes be found distal to the last gland. Undifferentiated carcinoma in situ [3] is often situated high in the endocervical canal, where dysplasia is never seen. Thus, carcinoma in situ is situated proximal to dysplasia as a rule, an observation also made by others (29, 96).

It is noteworthy that simple metaplastic epithelium [1] reaches farther up the canal than atypical metaplasia [2], the upper border of which coincides with that of carcinoma in situ. The same applies to the distal borders of atypical basal hyperplasia [8] and well-differentiated carcinoma in situ [5] and mild dysplasia [7]. While, by definition, metaplastic squamous epithelium cannot exist outside the last gland, basal hyperplasia may extend for short distances up the endocervical canal, in which case it must have arisen in metaplastic squamous epithelium. Moderately differentiated carcinoma in situ [4] and moderate dysplasia [6] are infrequently found distal to the last gland (in original squamous epithelium), where mild dysplasia and well-differentiated carcinoma in situ are more common. Acanthotic [9] epithelium – of great colposcopic significance may be found in the glandular field or in original squamous epithelium, the latter site being somewhat favored.

Considering the above facts, it becomes clear that undifferentiated carcinoma in situ arises mostly via atypical squamous metaplasia (circles), atypical basal hyperplasia (crosses) playing only a minor role in its genesis. As carcinoma in situ may occur in areas where dysplasia does not, the latter cannot be the precursor of the former. The location of moderately dif-

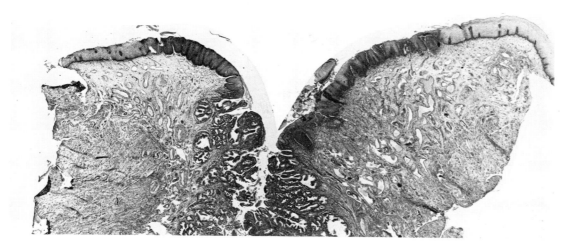

Fig. 3.**56 a   Dysplastic epithelium** (CIN 2) with a "baggy pants" appearance, in the area of original squamous epithelium of the ectocervix, outside the last gland. Note the abrupt junctions with normal squamous epithelium on both lips (from Obstet Gynecol 1983;62:117)

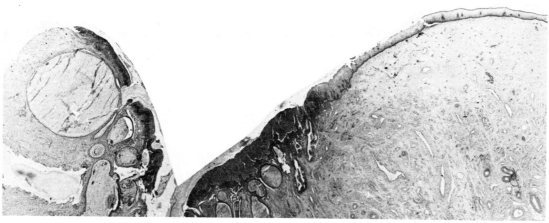

Fig. 3.**56 b   Carcinoma in situ** (CIN 3) involving the glandular field. Note its abrupt junction with normal original squamous epithelium at the last gland (from Obstet Gynecol 1983;62:117)

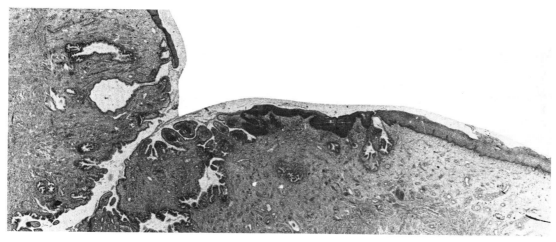

Fig. 3.**56 c   Carcinoma in situ** (CIN 3) occupying the area between the external os and the last gland, the latter indicating the junction with original squamous epithelium (from Obstet Gynecol 1983;62:117)

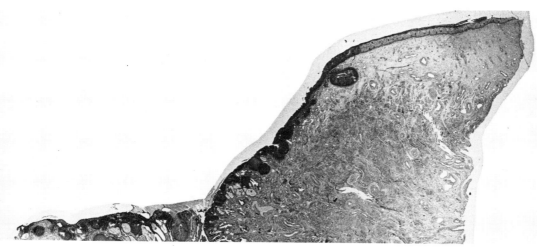

Fig. 3.**56 d   Carcinoma in situ** (CIN 3) involving both cervical lips. The abrupt junction with normal squamous epithelium is well shown. The last gland underneath the junction is also involved by carcinoma in situ (from Obstet Gynecol 1983;62:117)

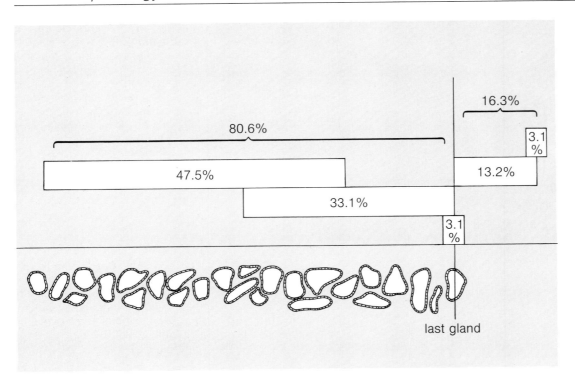

80.6%

16.3%

47.5%

3.1 %

13.2%

33.1%

3.1 %

last gland

Fig. 3.**57** **The topographic relationship between the last gland and atypical epithelia** (CIN). In only 3.1% of cases do atypical epithelia of uniform appearance exist on either side of the last gland in continuity. The last gland indicates either the distal or proximal border of atypical epithelia in 46.3% of cases (from Obstet Gynecol Surv 1979;34:862)

ferentiated carcinomas in situ and higher-grade dysplasias mostly coincides with that of atypical metaplasia, and overlaps to some extent that of atypical basal hyperplasia. Less frequently, they may arise in original squamous epithelium by way of atypical basal hyperplasia, as indeed does most well-differentiated carcinoma in situ and low grade dysplasia. In some cases it may be impossible to determine the exact mode of morphogenesis. Finally, it can be seen that acanthothic epithelium also has a dual origin—from metaplastic or from original squamous epithelium.

Location of Early Stromal Invasion

Ninety-three individual foci of early stromal invasion were studied in eighty-one conization specimens (91), again using the external os and the last gland as reference points. The first observation to emerge was that early stromal invasion originated from atypical epithelium situated within endocervical glands in 70% of cases. Consequently, only 30% of cases originated from the surface epithelium. Topographically, there were four different groups (Fig. 3.59). The mode of origin of the invasive foci, from carcinoma in situ or dysplasia, was also determined. The carcinomas were divided into poorly differentiated, moderately differentiated, and well-differentiated types.

In the majority (72%), the early invasive foci arose in an ectopy, on the ectocervix. In only 18% of cases were such foci situated in the endocervical canal, in the neighborhood of the external os. In the remaining 10% of cases, invasion began in atypical epithelium, outside the glandular field.

The parent epithelia were most often undifferentiated (37.6%) or moderately differentiated carcinoma in situ (38.7%), and in only 10.7% of cases was well-differentiated carcinoma in situ the precursor. In the rest (12.9%), dysplasia was the point of origin. From these figures it appears at first that the frequency of invasion from undifferentiated and moderately differentiated carcinoma in situ is the same. Considering, however, that moderately differentiated carcinoma in situ is three times as common as the undifferentiated variety (9, 18), the latter is more likely to become invasive.

When arising from well-differentiated carcinoma in situ or dysplasia, the invasive foci were located on the ectocervix, with a good number outside the glandular field. In 43% of early invasive tumors originating from the surface, the parent epithelium was dysplastic, or showed well-differentiated carcinoma in situ.

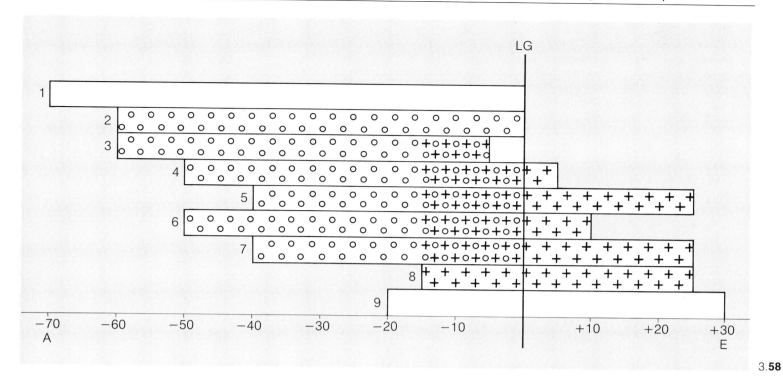

3.**58**

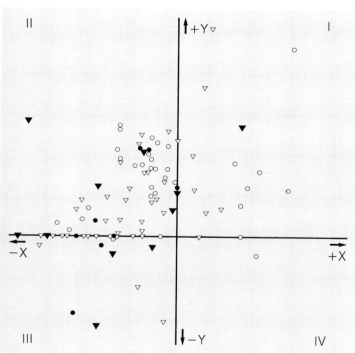

3.**59**

Fig. 3.58 The topography of 95% of all the various epithelia. The location of least-differentiated CIN coincides with that of atypical metaplasia in the canal (A), whereas the topography of well differentiated CIN is similar to that of basal hyperplasia on the ectocervix (E). [1] Simple squamous metaplasia. [2] Atypical squamous metaplasia. [3] Undifferentiated carcinoma in situ. [4] Moderately differentiated carcinoma in situ. [5] Well differentiated carcinoma in situ. [6] Moderate dysplasia (CIN2). [7] Mild dysplasia (CIN1). [8] Atypical basal hyperplasia. [9] Acanthotic epithelium.

LG = last cervical gland
E = peripheral (vaginal) edge of resection of conization specimen
A = endocervical (apical) edge of resection of conization specimen
○ = squamous metaplasia
+ = basal hyperplasia
⊕ = area where both kinds of epithelia are found
(from Arch Gynäkol 1972;212:130)

Fig. 3.59 Topography of early stromal invasion. The abscissa represents the last gland; the ordinate, the external os. The negative sides of the X and Y axes point in a vaginal direction, whereas the positive sides point into the canal. Quadrant I indicates entirely endocervical location, quadrant II foci between the external os and the last gland, quadrant III the ectocervix outside the last gland, and quadrant IV a focus lying outside the last gland which has been retracted back into the canal. The lesions along the X axis have arisen from or above the last gland. The lesions along the Y axis lie at the external os. The following symbols indicate the type of parent epithelium that has become invasive: ○ undifferentiated carcinoma in situ, ▽ moderately differentiated carcinoma in situ, ● well differentiated carcinoma in situ, ▼ moderate dysplasia (from Arch Gynäkol 1973;215:187)

Epithelial Borders

When large-surfaced panoramic sections from conization specimens are examined, it becomes apparent that different pathologic epithelia frequently coexist in the same cervix (Fig. 3.60). This may be explained by the simultaneous or subsequent appearance of squamous metaplasia in different fields (Figs. 3.52 and 3.61) or involvement of both the glandular field and original squamous epithelium (Fig. 3.62). When 657 conization specimens were examined, it was found that in 45.8% of cases two different types of intraepithelial neoplasia were present in the same cervix and in 30.1% of cases there were three (Table 3.3). Acanthotic epithelium was not recorded in this study. When various epithelia are adjacent, they are well demarcated from each other by sharp borders that are often perpendicular. Occasionally the junctions are less distinct, being irregular or wavy (2, 9). Abrupt borders are clearly seen between normal or atypical metaplastic and original squamous epithelium (Fig. 3.46 and 3.51) and are especially pronounced when the different epithelia are thick (Figs. 3.62 to 3.64). Again the more highly differentiated epithelium lies distal to the less differentiated (Figs. 3.58 and 3.75).

Table 3.**3** Percentage frequency of different forms of atypical epithelium coexisting in the cervix (n = 657)

One epithelial type	Two epithelial types	Three or more epithelial types
24.1%	45.8%	30.1%

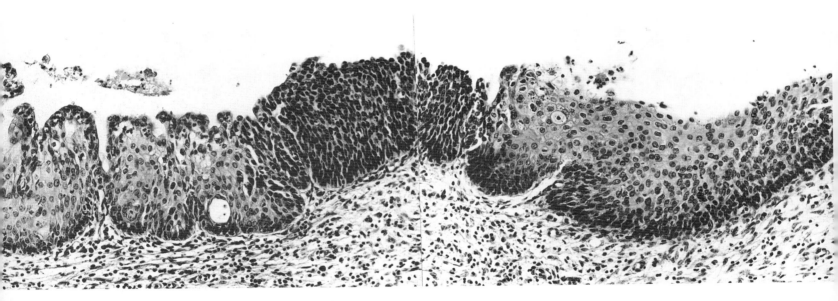

Fig. 3.**60** **Three types of epithelium on the surface of the cervix.** The metaplastic epithelium on the left shows tall stromal papillae, slight nuclear atypia, and residual columnar epithelium. In the middle, there is a completely undifferentiated carcinoma in situ (CIN 3). On the right, there is moderate dysplasia, with nuclear proliferation in the basal layer. The borders between the different types of epithelium are sharp

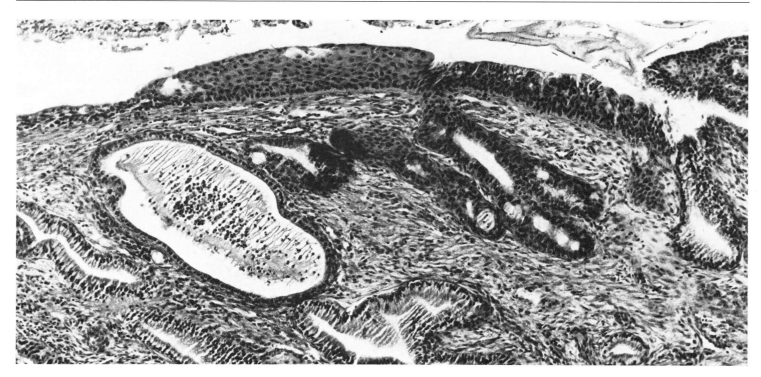

Fig. 3.61 Various fields of metaplastic epithelium sharply demarcated from each other

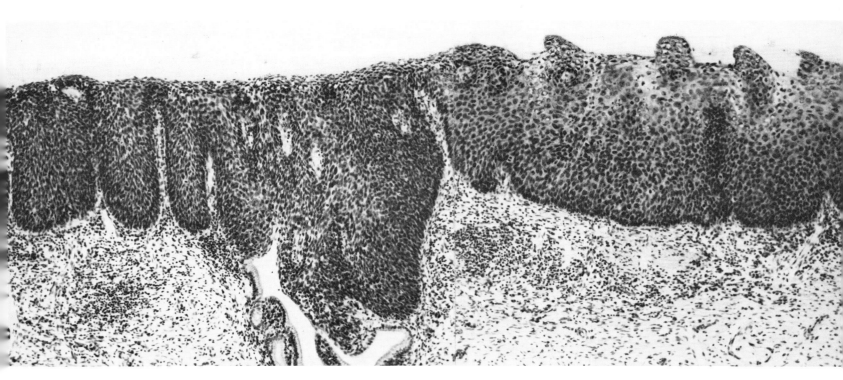

Fig. 3.62 The last gland indicates the boundary between carcinoma in situ showing prominent epithelial peg formation (CIN3), and dysplasia (CIN2) showing papillary excrescences. The dysplastic epithelium is situated outside the glandular field (from Obstet Gynecol 1983;62:117)

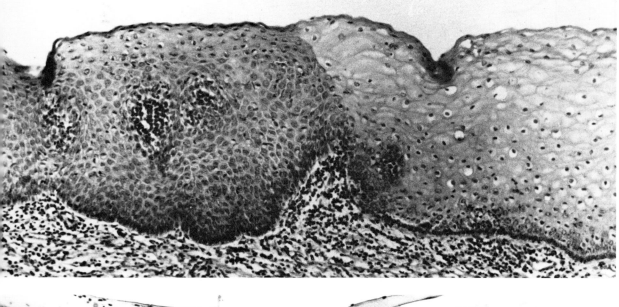

Fig. 3.63 a   Discrete margin between neighboring acanthotic epithelium (left) and normal squamous epithelium (from Obstet Gynecol 1983;62:117)

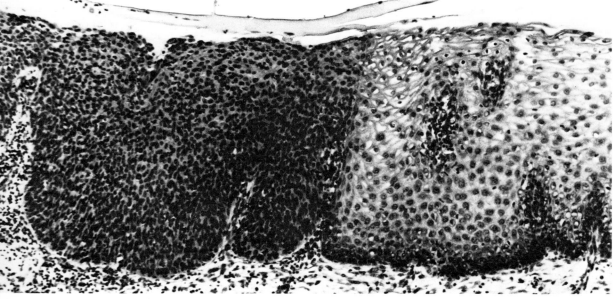

Fig. 3.63 b   Sharp border between carcinoma in situ (CIN 3) and adjacent normal squamous epithelium (from Obstet Gynecol 1983;62:177)

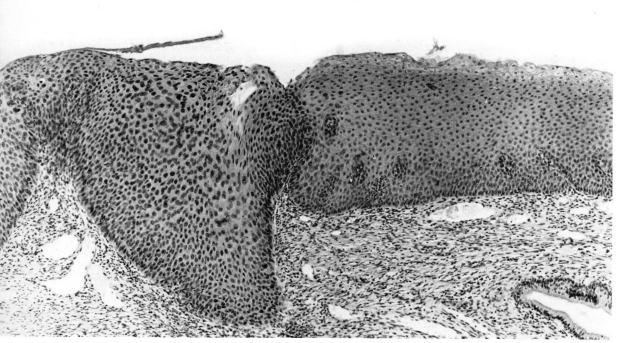

Fig. 3.64   Sharp border between moderately dysplastic epithelium (CIN 2) and acanthotic epithelium (right)

Fig. 3.65 a–c   Sharp borders between various forms of atypical epithelia

Fig. 3.65 a   Different types of carcinoma in situ (CIN 3) (from Obstet Gynecol 1983;62:117)

Fig. 3.65 b   Carcinoma in situ (CIN 3) and moderate dysplasia (CIN 2) (left)

Fig. 3.65 c   Two different kinds of carcinoma in situ (CIN 3) (from Clin Obstet Gynecol 1982;25:849)

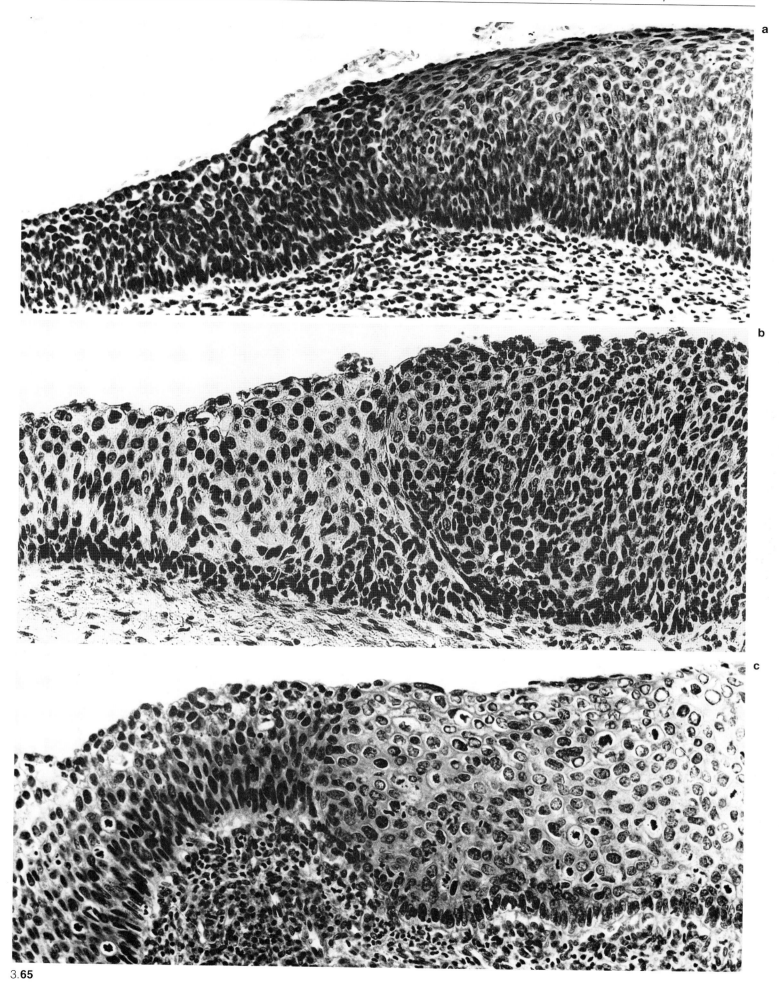

3.**65**

Size and Extent
of Pathologic Epithelial Fields

Examination of conization specimens showed that dysplastic lesions were completely excised more frequently than those showing carcinoma in situ, incomplete excision being most common in cases of early stromal invasion (see Table 19.9, p. 263). The actual surface area of involvement increased in the same order (Fig. 3.**66**).

These observations might be seen as supporting the concept of stepwise evolution of intraepithelial neoplasia, beginning with dysplasia that increases in atypia and enlarges in size as it progresses to carcinoma in situ and eventually to invasive cancer. On the contrary, however, it can be demonstrated that enlargement of lesions is due to recruitment and apposition of new fields showing a higher degree of atypicality (Figs. 3.**67**–3.**70**). This interpretation is particularly plausible when comparing carcinoma in situ and early stromal invasion. The increase in extent of carcinoma in situ is not due to its active spread, but to coalescence with adjacent dysplastic fields that have arisen independently (63).

The above investigations also confirmed the theory of development of pathologic atypia in well-circumscribed fields. It also became apparent that the likelihood of invasion was directly related to the size of the lesion. Whether the disturbance of the normal relationship between epithelium and stroma depends on the mass of atypical cells or some other factor is not clear. For the proper evaluation of colposcopic findings we must bear in mind the following: *the smaller the area of a lesion, the more likely that it is preinvasive; the larger it is, the greater the likelihood of invasion.*

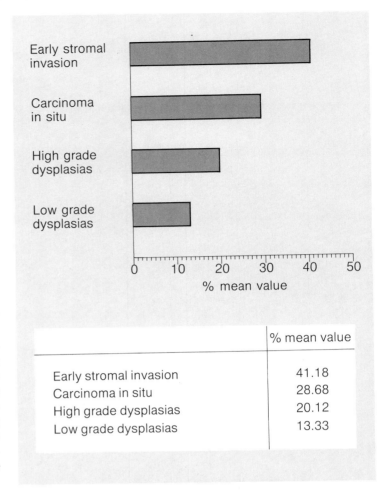

	% mean value
Early stromal invasion	41.18
Carcinoma in situ	28.68
High grade dysplasias	20.12
Low grade dysplasias	13.33

Fig. 3.**66** **Surface involvement by the various forms of atypical epithelium** with and without early stromal invasion

Fig. 3.**67** **Extent of atypical epithelium with mild dysplasia as the sole lesion.** The bars above and below indicate anterior and posterior cervical lip

Fig. 3.**68** **Extent of atypical epithelia with moderate dysplasia as the most advanced lesion** (see also the legend to Fig. 3.**67**)

Fig. 3.**69** **The extent of atypical epithelia with carcinoma in situ as the most advanced lesion** (see also the legend to Fig. 3.**67**)

Fig. 3.**70** **The extent of involvement by atypical epithelia** associated with early stromal invasion (see also the legend to Fig. 3.**67**)

3.**67**

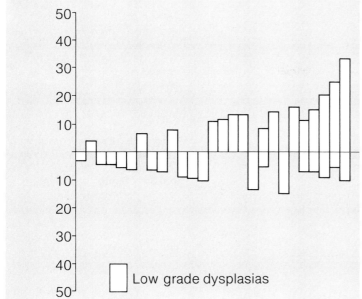

Low grade dysplasias

3.**68**

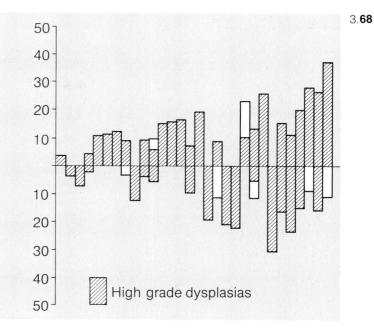

High grade dysplasias

3.**69**

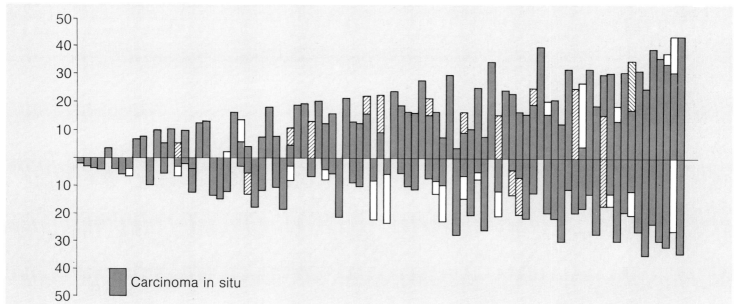

Carcinoma in situ

3.**70**

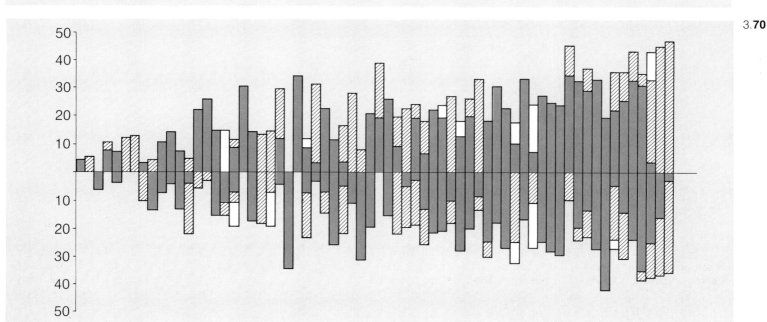

Evaluation of Atypical Epithelia

In examining atypical epithelium, the surgical pathologist's aim is to assess its *invasive potential*. The appearances have been variously interpreted in the past. Among the first observers, Williams (121) and Schauenstein (107) believed that atypical epithelia resembled invasive carcinoma. Since these epithelia were still confined to the surface, they were regarded as the *precursors* of invasive carcinoma. Later it was recognized that these epithelia could display a whole spectrum of appearances, the degree of atypia ranging from mild to severe. Although mildly atypical epithelium could be compared to well-differentiated carcinoma, the idea developed that atypical epithelium shows a sliding scale of increasing atypia (51), eventually acquiring invasive potential. This ideology resulted in the two-tier, two-disease terminology of "dysplasia" and "carcinoma in situ."

The observations, however, that dysplasia and carcinoma in situ are differently located (Fig. 3.75) are inconsistent with the concept of a stepwise progression from one to another. Furthermore, the location of undifferentiated small-cell carcinoma coincides with that of carcinoma in situ, while the topography of keratinizing squamous cell carcinoma is similar to that of dysplasia (96), which is frequently seen at the periphery of these carcinomas (1, 96). Invasive carcinomas not infrequently originate from "dysplastic" epithelium (8, 9, 16, 30, 68, 97), either as early stromal invasion (Fig. 3.72) or microcarcinoma (Figs. 3.71 and 3.73), even if the dysplasia is of a mild degree. In these circumstances, the invasive buds are characteristically surrounded by a basal layer (Figs. 3.16, 3.72 and 3.73), while such a pattern is not seen when carcinoma in situ is the parent

Fig. 3.**71 Biphasic microcarcinoma.** The well-differentiated tumor on the right arises from dysplastic epithelium (CIN 2), while the undifferentiated type on the left arises from a surface epithelium showing carcinoma in situ (CIN 3)

Fig. 3.**72 Early stromal invasion** arising from mild dysplasia (CIN 1). The margins of the well-differentiated invasive nests consist of basal-type cells. Distinctive stromal changes are in evidence. Note the abrupt junction with carcinoma in situ (CIN 3) on the right

Fig. 3.**73 Well-differentiated microcarcinoma,** originating from mild dysplasia (CIN 1). Note the basal cells at the margins of the tumor and signs of differentiation in the center

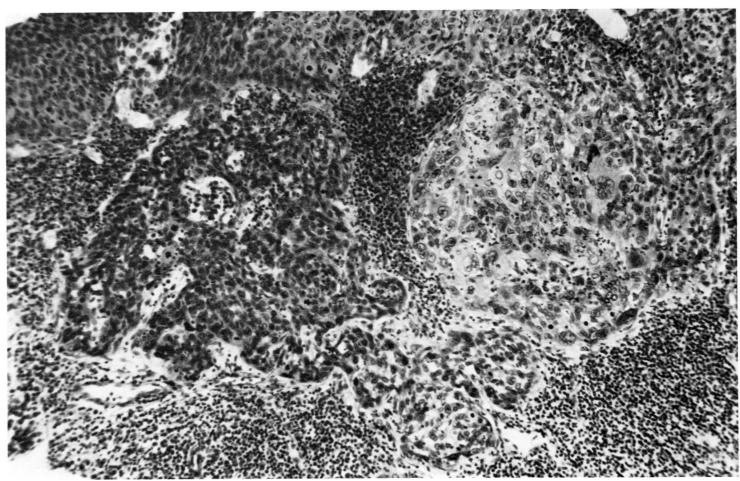

3.**71**

3.**72**

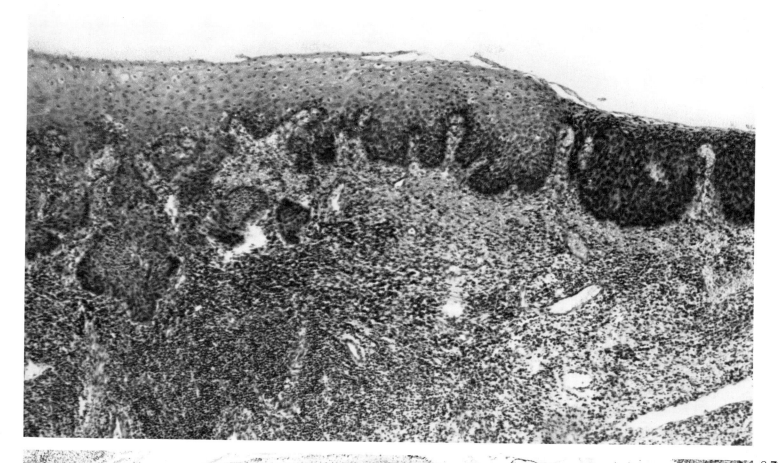

3.**73**

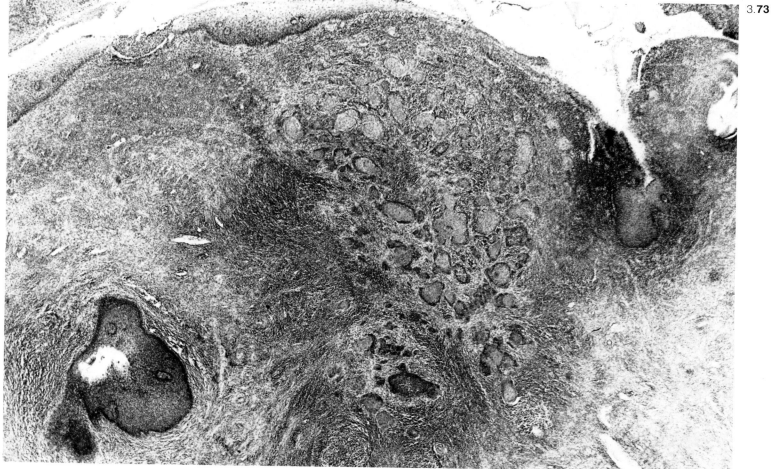

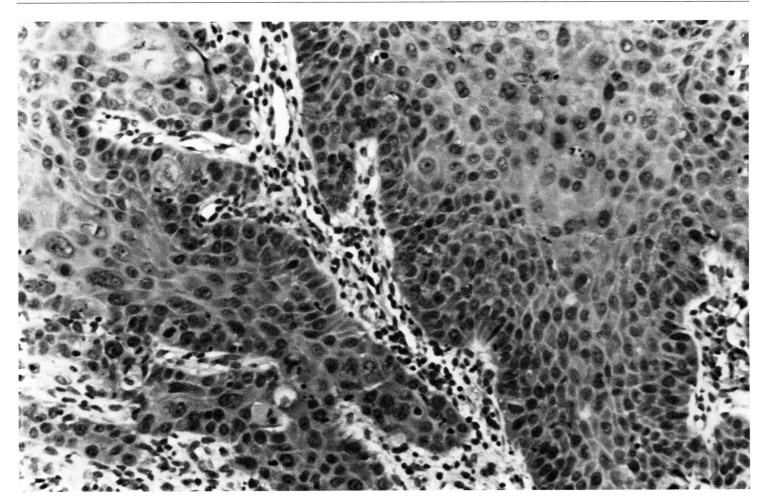

Fig. 3.74 Biopsy from a well-differentiated invasive squamous cell carcinoma.
There is little in the way of cellular and nuclear atypia; note, however, the definite stromal reaction. Similar changes in an intraepithelial situation would be interpreted as those of mild dysplasia only

epithelium (Fig. 3.13). In well-differentiated carcinomas, the actively proliferating cells are at the periphery of the invasive nests, those in the central portions being only a product of differentiation.

The way in which dysplasia and well-differentiated carcinoma in situ are situated distal (vaginal) to undifferentiated carcinoma in situ has already been described (Fig. 3.58). This is to be expected, as poorly differentiated carcinoma in situ arises from metaplastic epithelium in the endocervical mucosa, whereas better-differentiated lesions arise primarily from original squamous epithelium.

The more differentiated a carcinoma is, the more it resembles the epithelium from which it originates. Well-differentiated squamous cell carcinoma shows rather distinct layering and only moderate cellular and nuclear enlargement, corresponding to lower grades of CIN (dysplasia); the latter may therefore be regarded as a well-differentiated form of carcinoma in situ. Indeed, many invasive carcinomas closely mimic the features of dysplasia (Fig. 3.74).

At variance, however, with this interpretation is the fact that dysplasia may be reversible, the incidence of apparent regression being inversely proportional to its severity (46, 51, 55,

88, 103). Accordingly, unequivocal carcinoma in situ should not revert to normal. Based on cytologic studies, it has also been assumed that *dysplasia* can *progress* to carcinoma in situ. There are, however, simple and satisfactory explanations for such observations:

Even now there are no *infallible criteria for cancer-specific* atypia. Some nonspecific *hyperplastic epithelial proliferations* are difficult to distinguish from intraepithelial neoplasia, especially when the latter is well differentiated, and pose problems in routine pathologic diagnosis. If the former are designated as dysplasia, then dysplasia must on occasion be reversible. Nevertheless, the more pronounced the criteria for atypia in a particular epithelium are, the greater the likelihood of it being neoplastic in nature. It is for this reason that "classical" carcinoma in situ almost always persists.

The "reversibility" of dysplasia has been clarified by the recent recognition of flat condylomas. These are characterized by only a mild or moderate degree of cellular and nuclear pleomorphism, and have been misinterpreted in the past as dysplastic changes; no doubt these lesions account for cases of "dysplasia" that regress.

The progression of dysplasia to carcinoma in situ may be

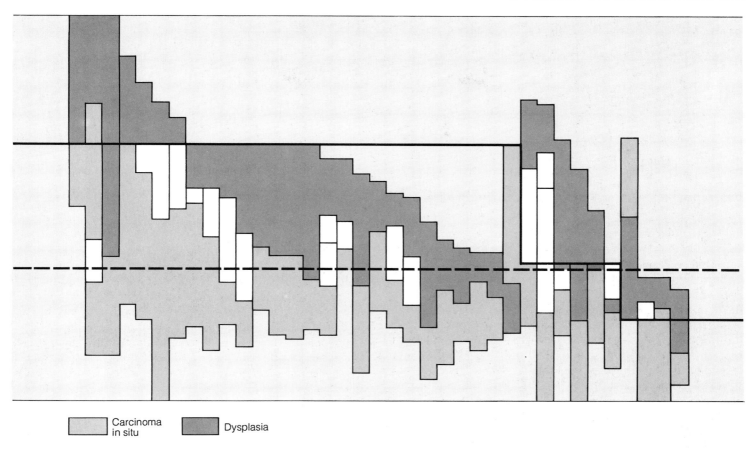

Carcinoma in situ   Dysplasia

Fig. 3.**75** **The topographic relationship between co-existing carcinoma in situ and dysplasia,** based on 33 cases. With 2 exceptions, the dysplastic epithelium is distal to carcinoma in situ

explained by the subsequent development of carcinoma in situ elsewhere in the cervix. Systematic histologic studies reveal that carcinoma in situ and dysplasia coexist in the same cervix in approximately 40% of cases (see Table 14.2, p. 228) with the dysplastic fields located almost always distal to those showing carcinoma in situ (Fig. 3.75).

It is impossible to determine morphologically whether a given instance of dysplasia is biologically a nonspecific prolifer-

ation or a premalignant lesion; its neoplastic nature is suggested, however, by such features as pronounced cellular and nuclear atypia, and, above all, by its *persistence.*

Well-circumscribed atypical epithelia that persist while under observation, or in spite of local treatment, are most likely premalignant, irrespective of the degree of atypia.

Synopsis of the Morphogenesis of Cervical Squamous Carcinoma

General Considerations

On the basis of the above considerations, we are in a position to formulate a theory of the development of intraepithelial neoplasia, embracing its topography, extension, and progression.

Other hypotheses that ignore these data are misleading.

1. Intraepithelial neoplasia arises in clearly circumscribed fields simultaneously, from the base of a whole segment of pre-existent epithelium. This process cannot be explained by proliferation a single cell or a single clone of cells.
2. Intraepithelial neoplasia remains within its original boundaries and does not enlarge its size by active surface spread. Different forms of intraepithelial neoplasia coexist, and may be adjacent to or removed from each other (see Fig. 3.65). The location of the various types conforms to a regular pattern, with the more highly differentiated forms lying distally, even extending to the region of the original squamous epithelium (see Fig. 3.58).
3. Poorly differentiated carcinoma in situ arises exclusively in columnar epithelium and often involves "glands" (Fig. 3.56). Original squamous epithelium is usually the matrix of dysplasia and well-differentiated carcinoma in situ (see Fig. 3.58).

According to its mode of origin, intraepithelial neoplasia lies either proximal to the last gland, in columnar epithelium, or distal to the last gland, in original squamous epithelium (see Figs. 3.56 and 3.58). As surface spread of atypical epithelium does not take place, epithelium with a uniform appearance cannot cross the domain of the last gland.
4. There is no stepwise progression of dysplasia (low-grade CIN) to carcinoma in situ (high-grade CIN) by acquisition of an increasing degree of atypia by the same epithelium. Persistent dysplasia, even of mild degree, represents biologically well differentiated carcinoma in situ and may become invasive per se.
5. Enlargement and extensions of intraepithelial neoplasia take place by recruitment and apposition of new fields of varying appearance (see Figs. 3.60–3.62, 3.64, 3.65).
6. The larger the area of the atypical epithelium, the greater the likelihood of invasion (Fig. 3.66).
7. Invasion proceeds from the base of the epithelium, with a small nest of cells penetrating the stroma. Should invasion occur at a single focus only, one may speak of a monoclonal tumor. The early invasive buds may, however, be destroyed by the body's immune response. When several invasive foci arise simultaneously, a more advanced tumor develops from only one of them. Less commonly, a carcinoma may arise synchronously from two or more invasive foci. It is in this way that polyclonal tumours of varying histologic types and differentiation develop (Fig. 3.71).

Morphogenesis within Columnar Epithelium

Squamous carcinoma develops in the glandular field via the process of squamous metaplasia, which begins with the appearance of subcolumnar reserve cells, the origin of which is not known. These lie under the columnar epithelium, but are not identifiable as single cells. When they appear, they do so in well-defined rows or fields when seen in two dimensions. The squamous epithelium that is subsequently formed must also be restricted to such fields.

These fields of metaplastic squamous epithelium may be unicentric or multicentric, and may have a different appearance in the latter case (Figs. 3.52 and 3.61). The subcolumnar cells in some areas remain unchanged, but in others they assume markedly atypical features; the different types may coexist in the same cervix. The atypia may appear at the very beginning of the metaplastic process. When more advanced and multifocal, the appearance of atypical metaplasia may vary surprisingly from field to field (see Fig. 4.20). When adjacent, they are separated from each other by sharp borders.

It can no longer be doubted that the first morphologically detectable step in carcinogenesis in columnar epithelium is atypical squamous metaplasia. It is, of course, not possible to predict which cases of atypical metaplasia will progress to fully developed CIN. What we do know, however, is that when CIN develops in the proximal portion of the glandular field, it always does so via atypical squamous metaplasia. As it is possible to distinguish between simple and atypical metaplasia right from the outset, the further development of metaplastic epithelium is predestined ab initio. Nevertheless, a number of questions remain to be answered.

First of all, what triggers squamous metaplasia? Metamorphosis of columnar epithelium in an ectopy may be due to the different milieu and pH to which it is exposed. Both Hinselmann (62) and Meyer (80, 81) have alluded to the different environments in the vagina and endocervical canal. It appears that the metaplastic process is initiated by the acid milieu of the vagina. This theory, however, fails to explain the occurrence of squamous metaplasia in the alkaline environment of the upper reaches of the endocervical canal. In addition, squamous metaplasia is also seen in organs (e.g., the bronchial tree) in which differences in pH do not play a role.

Hormonal factors during different epochs of a woman's life, e.g., the fetal period, pregnancy, and the beginning of menopause, may also influence the timing of squamous metaplasia (60, 106). This is supported by the induction of metaplasia by estrogens in experimental animals (17, 28, 32, 34, 83).

There are, however, no satisfactory explanations of why squamous metaplasia is a focal process arising in clearly defined fields, since large areas or even the whole organ must be exposed simultaneously to environmental stimuli. It may be that as yet unknown local factors are involved.

The exact point in time at which the metaplastic process is determined as simple or atypical is not known. A formerly fashionable theory stated that the young, delicate reserve cell tended to imbibe carcinogenic material, such as sperm DNA, which then induced malignant transformation (28, 98). This theory has now largely been discounted in favor of one of viral genesis of cervical cancer which postulates that viral DNA acts at least as a cofactor in the transformation of normal cells into neoplastic cells. The belief that only single or small clones of cells undergo neoplastic transformation is contrary to the established steps of morphogenesis.

There is no basis for the assertion that tissue changes that give rise to the colposcopic pictures of punctation and mosaic are invariably the first morphologically detectable change in carcinogenesis. To designate every type of epithelium leading to punctation or mosaic as being due to atypical metaplasia is therefore also incorrect.

The development of squamous metaplasia in uniform discrete fields, with early expression and frequent coexistence of simple metaplasia and atypical metaplasia, leads to the following conclusions:

The nature of the metaplastic process, whether simple or atypical, is determined very early, perhaps from its very moment of conception.

Atypical cells arise simultaneously from whole fields of metaplastic epithelium. Atypical transformation therefore concerns epithelial fields in toto, and not single cells in an initial focus.

Only fields with intrinsic malignant potential can therefore sustain "hits" by external carcinogens.

in so far as normal differentiation is concerned. In this way, an epithelium will develop from undifferentiated or maldifferentiated cells, which may be distinguished from normal "basal cells" by their atypia. It is significant that this occurs in discrete fields which, in the case of the metaplastic process, are preformed. The fundamental question is which factors are responsible for the disruption of these control mechanisms. Various mechanisms may be envisaged. They must, however, be compatible with the fact that a whole field or fields must sustain the oncogenic "hit" simultaneously. It is this last contingency, the synchronous development of atypia in various epithelial fields, that should play a particularly vital role in the understanding of carcinogenesis.

Morphogenesis in Original Squamous Epithelium

A certain percentage of CIN is known to occur in original squamous epithelium (9, 18, 20, 29). This is not due to active spread of CIN across the last gland. In analogy with atypical epithelium stemming from subcolumnar cells, CIN arises by proliferation of the basal and parabasal layers of the original squamous epithelium, from the same cells involved in normal day-to-day regeneration. This results in a compact layer of atypical cells with increased mitoses, confined to the lower quarter or third of the epithelium, characteristically clearly demarcated from the overlying layers (Fig. 3.9). Eventually there is fullchickness replacement by the atypical epithelium. There is evidence that acanthotic epithelium also arises from original squamous epithelium in this way (9).

As to the mechanism of carcinogenesis at this site, external irritants or chemical factors in the vagina should be even less relevant than for squamous metaplasia. The cause of cancerous transformation of fully developed squamous epithelium is therefore more difficult to understand than that of metaplastic squamous epithelium, even if condylomatous lesions of viral origin provide a clue. On the other hand, it must be acknowledged that squamous carcinoma can arise in organs in which viral origin has not as yet been postulated.

Final Considerations

Bearing in mind all the known morphologic observations, we can hardly avoid the conclusion that carcinogenesis must be linked to epithelial regeneration. By the 1920s, Fischer-Wasels (39) had already formulated a theory which emphasized the role of epithelial regeneration, in which he also included the so-called indirect metaplasia. The ongoing regeneration of epithelial tissues is subject to various influences which are still poorly understood. These bring about multiplication of cells from the germinal layers or the "reserve cells", as well as increasing differentiation of the new cell population pari passu with control and limitation of their growth. Carcinogenesis may therefore be simply due to failure of these mechanisms to come into play

References

1   Bajardi F. Les zones transitionelles de bordure des carcinomes épidermoïdes du col utérin. Rev Fr Gynécol 1961;56:633.

2   Bajardi F. Über Wachstumsbeschränkungen des Collumcarcinoms in seinem invasiven und auch präinvasiven Stadium. Arch Gynäkol 1962;197:407.

3   Bajardi F. Burghardt E. Ergebnisse von histologischen Serienschnittuntersuchungen beim Carcinoma colli. Arch Gynäkol 1957;189:392.

4   Beato M, Castano-Almendral J, Barcellos M. Die Frühstadien des Plattenepithelcarcinoms des Collum uteri, 1: Histotopographische Untersuchungen. Arch Gynäkol 1968;205:410.

5   Bertrand M. Lickrish GM, Colgan TJ. The anatomic distribution of cervical adenocarcinoma in situ: implications for treatment. Am J Obstet Gynecol 1987;157:21.

6   Boon ME, Fox C. Simultaneous condyloma acuminatum and dysplasia of uterine cervix. Acta Cytol 1981;25:393.

7   Burghardt E. Das Adenocarcinoma in situ der Cervix. Arch Gynäkol 1966;203:57.

8   Burghardt E. Besonders Epithelbilder als Ausgangspunkt beginnend invasiven Krebswachstums an der Portio. Geburtshilfe Frauenheilkd 1967;27:1170.

9   Burghardt E. Early histological diagnosis of cervical cancer. Stuttgart: Thieme; Philadelphia: Saunders, 1973.

10   Burghardt E. Gibt es ein Flächenwachstum des intraepithelialen Carcinoms an der Cervix? Arch Gynäkol 1973;215:1.

11   Burghardt E. Premalignant conditions of the cervix. Clin Obstet Gynecol 1976;3:257.

12   Burghardt E. Das Mikrokarzinom der Cervix uteri. Wien Klin Wochenschr 1978;90:477.

13   Burghardt E. Histological terminology. In: Burghardt E, Holzer E, Jordan JA, eds. Cervical pathology and colposcopy. Stuttgart: Thieme, 1978:131.

14   Burghardt E. Cancer intra-épithélial du col utérin: conduite à tenir. Bull Cancer 1979;66:425.

15   Burghardt E. Precancerous lesions in the cervix. Acta Endoscop 1980;10:151.

16   Burghardt E. Pathology of preclinical invasive carcinoma of the cervix (microinvasive and occult invasive carcinoma). In: Coppleson M, ed. Gynecologic oncology. Edinburgh: Churchill Livingstone, 1981:434.

17   Burghardt E. Diagnostic and prognostic criteria in cervical microcarcinoma. In: Burghardt E, Holzer E, eds. Minimal invasive cancer (microcarcinoma). Clin Oncol 1982; 1:323.

18   Burghardt E, Holzer E. Die Lokalisation des pathologischen Cervixepithels, 1: Carcinoma in situ, Dysplasien und abnormes Plattenepithel. Arch Gynäkol 1970;209:305.

19   Burghardt E, Holzer E. Die Lokalisation des pathologischen Cervixepithels, 4: Epithelgrenzen, letzte Cervixdruse, Schlußfolgerungen. Arch Gynäkol 1972;212:130.

20   Burghardt E, Holzer E. Diagnosis and treatment of microinvasive carcinoma of the cervix uteri. Obstet Gynecol 1977;49:641.

21   Burghardt E, Mestwerdt K, Ober G. Der Unterschied zwischen der Einstufung Zervixkrebs des Stadiums Ia und dem Begriff Mikrokarzinom. Geburtshilfe Frauenheilkd 1973;33:168.

22   Burghardt E, Östör AG. Site of origin and growth pattern of cervical cancer: a histomorphological study. Obstet Gynecol 1973;62:117.

23   Burghardt E, Pickel H. Die Entwicklung zum Zervixkarzinom. In: Käser O, Friedberg V, Ober KG, Thomsen K, Zander J. eds. Gynäkologie und Geburtshilfe. Stuttgart: Thieme, 1988:14.

24   Burghardt E, Pickel H. Local spread and lymph node involvement in cervical cancer. Obstet Gynec. 1978;52:138.

25   Burrows H. The localisation of response to oestrogenic compounds in the organs of male mice. J Pathol 1935;41:423.

26   Buscema J, Woodruff JD, Parmley TH, Genadry R. Carcinoma in situ of the vulva. Obstet Gynecol 1980;55:225.

27   Campion MJ, McCance DJ, Cuzick J, Singer A. Progressive potential of mild cervical atypia: prospective cytological, colposcopic, and virological study. Lancet 1986;II:237.

28   Castano-Almendral A, Beato M. Die Frühstadien des Plattenepithelcarcinoms des Collum uteri, 2: Histometrische Untersuchungen. Arch Gynäkol 1968;205:428.

29   Castano-Almendral A, Müller H, Naujoks H, Castano-Almendral JL. Topographical and histological localization of dysplasias, carcinomata in situ, microinvasions, and microcarcinomata. Gynecol Oncol 1973;1:320.

30   Christopherson WM, Parker JE. Microinvasive carcinoma of the uterine cervix. Cancer 1964;17:1123.

31   Coppleson M, Reid B. Preclinical carcinoma of the cervix uteri. Oxford: Pergamon Press, 1967.

32   Coppleson M, Reid B. Aetiology of squamous carcinoma of the cervix. Obstet Gynecol 1968;32:432.

33   Dunn AEG, Ogilvie MM. Intranuclear virus particles in human genital wart tissue: observations on the ultrastructure of the epidermal layer. J Ultrastruct Res 1968;22:282.

34   Fennel RH Jr. Carcinoma in situ of the cervix with early invasive changes. Cancer 1955;8:302.

35   Fennel RH Jr. Carcinoma in situ of uterine cervix. Cancer 1956;9:374.

36   Ferenczy A, Mitao M, Nagai N, Silverstein SJ, Crum CP. Latent papillomavirus and recurring genital warts. N Engl J Med 1985;313:784.

37   Fidler HK, Boyd JR. Occult invasive squamous carcinoma of the cervix. Cancer 1960;13:764.

38   FIGO news: changes of the 1985 FIGO report on the result of treatment in gynecological cancer. Int J Gynaecol Obstet 1987;25:87.

39   Fischer-Wasels B. Metaplasie und Gewebsmißbildung. In: Bethe N, ed. Handbuch der normalen und pathologischen Physiologie, vol. 14:2. Berlin: Springer, 1927:1211.

40   Fluhmann CF. Comparative studies of squamous metaplasia of the cervix uteri and endometrium. Am J Obstet Gynecol 1954;68:1447.

41   Fluhmann CF. The cervix uteri and its diseases. Philadelphia: Saunders, 1961.

42   Fu YS, Reagan JW, Richart RM. Definition of precursors. Gynecol Oncol 1981;12:220.

43   Fuchs PG, Girardi F, Pfister H. Papillomavirus infections in cervical tumors of Austrian patients. In: P, ed. Cancer cells 5: Cold Spring Harbor Laboratory Meeting. Cold Spring Harbor: L, 1987:297.

44   Fuchs PG, Girardi F, Pfister H. Human papillomavirus DNA in normal, metaplastic, preneoplastic and neoplastic epithelia of the cervix uteri. Int J. Cancer 1988;41:41.

45 Fuchs PG, Girardi F, Pfister H. Human papillomavirus 16 DNA in cervical cancers and in lymph nodes of cervical cancer patients: a diagnostic marker for early metastases? Int J Cancer 1989;43:41.

46 Galvin GA, Jones HW, TeLinde RW. The significance of basal cell hyperactivity incervival biopsies. Am J Obstet Gynecol 1955;70:808.

47 de Girolami E. Perinuclear halo versus koilocytotic atypia. Obstet Gynecol 1967;29:479.

48 Gissmann L. Papillomaviruses and their association with cancer in animals and in man. Cancer Surv 1984;3:161.

49 Gissmann L, zur Hausen H. Partial characterization of viral DNA from human genital warts (condylomata acuminata). Int J Cancer 1980;25:605.

50 Gissmann L, Dürst M. Oltersdorf T, von Knebel Doeberitz M. Human papillomaviruses and cervical cancer. In: P, ed. Cancer cells 5: Cold Spring Harbor Laboratory Meeting. Cold Spring Harbor: L, 1987:134.

51 Glatthaar E. Studien über die Morphogenese des Plattenepithelkarzinoms der Portio vaginalis uteri. Basle: Karger, 1950.

52 Glücksmann A, Cherry CP. Microinvasive carcinoma of the cervix: histopathological aspects. In: Gray LA, ed. Dysplasia, carcinoma in situ and microinvasive carcinoma of the cervix uteri. Springfield, IL: Thomas, 1964:351.

53 Gosch J. Bilder des klimakterischen und senilen Korpusendometriums bei starken hormonellen und entzündlichen Reizen. Geburtshilfe Frauenheilkd 1949;9:201.

54 von Haam E, Old JW. Reserve cell hyperplasia, squamous metaplasia and epidermization. In: Gray LA, ed. Dysplasia, carcinoma in situ and microinvasive carcinoma of the cervix uteri. Springfield, IL: Thomas, 1964:41.

55 Hall JE, Walton L. Dysplasia of the cervix. Am J Obstet Gynecol 1968;100:662.

56 Hamperl H, Kaufmann C. The cervix uteri at different ages. Obstet Gynecol 1959;14:621.

57 Hamperl H, Kaufmann C, Ober KG, Schneppenheim P. Die "Erosion" der Portio (die Entstehung der Pseudoerosion, das Ektropion und die Plattenepithelüberhäutung der Cervixdrüsen auf der Portiooberfläche). Virchows Arch [A] 1958;331:51.

58 zur Hausen H. Human papillomaviruses and their possible role in squamous cell carcinomas. Curr Top Microbiol Immunol 1977;78:1.

59 zur Hausen H, Gissmann L. Papillomaviruses. In: Klein G, ed. Viral oncology. New York: Raven Press, 1980.

60 Hellmann L, Rosenthal AH, Kistner RW, Gordon R. Some factors influencing the proliferation of the reserve cells in the human cervix. Am J Obstet Gynecol 1954;67:899.

61 Hills E, Laverty CR. Electron-microscopic detection of papillomavirus particles in selected koilocytotic cells in a routine cervical smear. Acta Cytol 1979;23:53.

62 Hinselmann H. Das klinische Bild der indirekten Metaplasie der ektopischen Zylinderzellenschleimhaut der Portio. Arch Gynäkol 1928;133:64.

63 Holzer E, Pickel H. Die Ausdehnung des atypischen Plattenepithels an der Zervix. Arch Geschwulstforsch 1975;45:79.

64 Jagella HP, Stegner HE. Zur Dignität der Condylomata acuminata. Arch Gynäkol 1974;216:119.

65 Jaworski RC, Pacey NF, Greenberg ML, Osborn RA. The histologic diagnosis of adenocarcinoma in situ and related lesions of the cervix uteri. Cancer 1988;61:1171.

66 Jenkins D, Tay SK, Maddox PH. Routine papillomavirus antigen staining of cervical punch biopsy specimens. J Clin Pathol 1987;40:1212.

67 Josey WE, Nahmias AJ, Naib ZM. Viruses and cancer of lower genital tract. Cancer 1976;38;526.

68 Koss LG. Diagnostic cytology and its histopathologic bases. 3rd ed. Philadelphia: Lippincott, 1979.

69 Koss LG. Carcinogenesis in the uterine cervix and human papillomavirus infection. In: Syrjänen K, Gissmann L, Koss LG, eds. Papillomaviruses and human disease. Berlin: Springer, 1987:235.

70 Koss LG, Durfee GR. Unusual patterns of squamous epithelium of the uterine cervix: cytologic and pathologic study of koilocytotic atypia. Ann NY Acad Sci 1956;63:1245.

71 Laverty CR, Russell P, Hills E, Booth N. The significance of noncondylomatous wart virus infection of the cervical transformation zone: a review with discussion of two illustrative cases. Acta Cytol 1978;22:195.

72 Linhartová A, Stafl A. Zur Morphologie des Ectropiums an der Portio vaginalis uteri. Arch Gynäkol 1964;200:131.

73 Meanwell CA, Blackledge G, Cox MF, Maitland NJ. HPV 16 DNA in normal and malignant cell epithelium: implications for the aetiology and behaviour of cervical neoplasia. Lancet 1987;I/87:703.

74 Meisels A. Is condyloma virus a potential human oncogen? Contemp Obstet Gynecol 1980;16:99.

75 Meisels A, Fortin R, Roy M. Condylomatous lesions of the cervix, 2: cytologic, colposcopic and histopathologic study. Acta Cytol 1977;21:379.

76 Meisels A, Roy M, Fortier M, Morin C. Condylomatous lesions of the cervix: morphologic and colposcopic diagnosis. Am J Diagn Gynecol Obstet 1979;1:109.

77 Meisels A, Morin C, Casas-Cordero M, Roy M, Fortier M. Condylomatöse Veränderungen der Vervix, Vagina und Vulva. Gynäkologe 1981;14:254.

78 Meisels A, Roy M, Fortier M, et al. Human papillomavirus infection of the cervix: the atypical condyloma. Acta Cytol 1981;25:7.

79 Meisels A, Morin C, Casas-Cordero M. Lesions of the uterine cervix associated with papillomavirus, and their clinical consquences. In: Koss LG, Coleman DV, eds. Advances in clinical cytology. New York: Masson, 1984, vol. 2.

80 Meyer R. Die Epithelentwicklung der Cervix and Portio vaginalis uteri und die Pseudoerosio congenita. Arch Gynäkol 1910;91:579.

81 Meyer R. Die Erosion und Pseudoerosion des Erwachsenen. Arch Gynäkol 1910;91:658.

82 Morin C, Braun L, Casas-Cordero M, et al. Confirmation of the papillomavirus etiology of condylomatous cervix lesions by the peroxidase-antiperoxidase technique. Natl Cancer Inst Monogr 1981;66:831.

83 Ober KG, Huhn FO. Die Ausbreitung des Cervixkrebses auf die Parametrien und die Lymphknoten der Beckenwand. Arch Gynäkol 1962;197:269.

84 Ober KG, Schneppenheim P, Hamperl H, Kaufmann C. Die Epithelgrenzen im Bereich des Isthmus uteri. Arch Gynäkol 1958;190:346.

85 Oriel JD, Almeida JD. Demonstration of virus particles in human genital warts. Br J Venereal Dis 1970;46:37.

86 Östör AG, Pagano R, Davoren RAM, Fortune DW, Cha-

nen W, Rome R. Adenocarcinoma in situ of the cervix. Int J Gynecol Pathol 1984;3:179.

87 Park J, Jones HW Jr. Glucose-6-phosphate dehydrogenase and the histogenesis of epidermoid carcinoma of the cervix. Am J Obstet Gynecol 1968;102:106.

88 Peckham B, Greene RR. Follow-up on cervical epithelial abnormalities. Am J Obstet Gynecol 1957;74:106.

89 Pfister H, Fuchs PG. Papillomavirus: particles, genome organisation and proteins. In: Syrjänen K, Gissmann L, Koss LG, eds. Papillomaviruses and human disease. Berlin: Springer, 1987:1.

90 Pickel H. Die Lokalisation des Adenocarcinoma in situ der Cervix uteri. Arch Gynäkol 1978;225:247.

91 Pickel H, Burghardt E. Die Lokalisation des beginnenden invasiven Krebswachstums an der Cervix. Arch Gynäkol 1973;215:187.

92 Pickel H, Haas H, Lahousen M. Prognostic factors in cervical cancer on the basis of morphometric evaluation. Baillière's Clin Obstet Gynecol 1988;2:805.

93 Pixley E. Morphology of the fetal and prepubertal cervicalvaginal epithelium. In: Jordan JA, Singer A, eds. The cervix. Philadelphia: Saunders, 1976:75.

94 Pixley EC. Colposcopic appearances of human papillomavirus of the uterine cervix. In: Syrjänen K, Gissmann L, Koss LG, eds. Papillomaviruses and human disease. Berlin: Springer, 1987:268.

95 Powell LC Jr. Condyloma acuminata: recent advances in development, carcinogenesis and treatment. Clin Obstet Gynecol 1978;21:1061.

95a Puts J, Moesker O, Kenemans P, Vooijs G, Ramaekers F. Expression of cytokeratins in early neoplastic epithelial lesions of the uterine cervix. Int J Gynecol Pathol 1985;4:300.

96 Reagan JW, Patten F Jr. Dysplasia: a basic reaction to injury in the uterine cervix. Ann N Y Acad Sci 1962;97:662.

97 Reagan JW, Wentz WB. Genesis of carcinoma of the uterine cervix. Clin Obstet Gynecol 1967;10:883.

98 Reid B, Coppleson M. Natural history: recent advances. In: Jordan JA, Singer A, eds. The cervix. Philadelphia: Saunders, 1976:317.

99 Reid R, Laverty CR, Coppleson M, Isarangkul W, Hills E. Noncondylomatous cervical wart virus infection. Obstet Gynecol 1980;55:476.

100 Reid R, Stanhope CR, Herschman BR, Booth E, Phibbs GD, Smith JP. Genital warts and cervical cancer. Cancer 1982;50:377.

101 Reid R, Crum C, Herschman BR, et al. Genital warts and cervical cancer, 3: subclinical papillomavirus infection and cervical neoplasia are linked by a spectrum of continuous morphologic and biologic change. Cancer 1984;53:843.

102 Reid R, Stanhope CR, Herschman BR, Crum CP, Agronow SJ. Genital warts and cervical cancer, 4: a colposcopic index for differentiating subclinical papillomaviral infection from cervical intraepithelial neoplasia. Am J Obstet Gynecol 1984;149:815.

103 Richart RM. Natural history of cervical intraepithelial neoplasia. Clin Obstet Gynecol 1967;10:748.

104 Richart RM. A theory of cervical carcinogenesis. Obstet Gynecol Surv 1967;24:874.

105 Richart RM. Causes and management of cervical intraepithelial neoplasia. Cancer 1987;60:1951.

106 Rosenthal AH, Hellmann LM. Epithelial changes in fetal cervix, including the role of the reserve cell. Am J Obstet Gynecol 1967;64:260.

107 Schauenstein W. Histologische Untersuchungen über atypisches Plattenepithel an der Portio und an der Innenfläche der Cervix uteri. Arch Gynäkol 1908;85:576.

108 Schernecks S, Rudolph M, Geissler E, et al. Isolation of an SV$_{40}$-like papovavirus from a human glioblastoma. Int J Cancer 1979;24:523.

109 Schneider A. Methods of identification of human papillomaviruses. In: Syrjänen K, Gissmann L, Koss LG, eds. Papillomaviruses and human disease. Berlin: Springer 1987:235.

110 Schneider A, Schuhmann R, De Villiers EM, Knauf W, Gissmann L. Klinische Bedeutung von humanen Papilloma-Virus-(HPV)-Infektionen im unteren Genitaltrakt. Geburtshilfe Frauenheilkd 1986;46:261.

111 Selye H, Thomson DL, Collip JB. Metaplasia of uterine epithelium produced by chronic oestrin administration. Nature 1935;135:65.

111a Serra V, Lara C, Ramirez AA, Marzo MC, Valcuende F, Castells A, Bonilla-Musoles F. Precocious appearance of markes of squamous differentiation in metaplastic cells of human endocervix. Arch Gynecol Obstet 1989;246:233.

112 Song J. The human uterus. Springfield, IL: Thomas, 1964.

113 Stoddard LD. The problem of carcinoma in situ, with reference to the human cervix uteri. In: McManus N, ed. Progress in fundamental medicine. Philadelphia: Lea and Febiger, 1952.

114 Stoddard LD, Erickson CC, Howard HL. Further studies on the histogenesis of intraepithelial carcinoma and early invasive carcinoma of the cervix uteri. Am J Pathol 1950;26:679.

115 Syrjänen KJ. Morphologic survey of the condylomatous lesions in dysplastic and neoplastic epithelium of the uterine cervix. Arch Gynäkol 1979;227:153.

116 Syrjänen KJ, Heinone UM, Karanienis T. Cytologic evidence of the association of condylomatous lesions with dysplastic and neoplastic changes in the uterine cervix. Acta Cytol 1981;25:17.

117 Syrjänen KJ, Väyrynen M, Saarikoski S, et al. Natural history of cervical human papillomavirus (HPV) infections based on prospective follow-up. Br J Obstet Gynaecol 1985;92:1086.

118 Teshima S, Shimosato Y, Kishi K, Kasamatsu T, Ohmi K, Uei Y. Early stage adenocarcinoma of the uterine cervix: histopathologic analysis with consideration of histogenesis. Cancer 1985;56:167.

119 Thornton WN Jr, Fox CH, Smith DE. The relationship of the squamocolumnar junction and the endocervical glands to the site of origin of carcinoma of the cervix. Am J Obstet Gynecol 1959;78:1060.

120 Tidy JA, Parry GCN, Ward P, et al. High rate of human papillomavirus type 16 infection in cytologically normal cervices. Lancet 1989;I 89:434.

121 Williams J. Cancer of the uterus. London: Lewis, 1888. (Harveian lectures for 1886.)

122 Woodruff JD, Braun L, Cavalieri R, Gupta P, Pass F, Shah KV. Immunologic identification of papillomavirus antigen in condyloma tissue from the female genital tract. Obstet Gynecol 1980;56:727.

123 Woodruff JD, Peterson WF. Condylomata acuminata of the cervix. Am J Obstet Gynecol 1958:75:1354.

124 Zander JJ, Baltzer J, Lohe KJ, Ober KG, Kaufmann C. Carcinoma of the cervix: an attempt to individualize treatment. Am J Obstet Gynecol 1981;139:752.

4

Histopathologic Basis of Colposcopy

Introduction

Meaningful interpretation of colposcopic appearances is impossible without a firm grasp of the histopathologic changes that take place in the cervix. One must understand how the fixed and stained tissue artifact seen under the microscope can be translated into the living biologic image afforded by direct magnification. One must also learn which histomorphologic alteration gives rise to which colposcopic pattern. In the first instance, it must be recognized that the colposcopic appearance is determined by the architecture of the epithelium and of the underlying stroma. Variation in the thickness of, or peg formation by, the surface epithelium and a heavy inflammatory infiltrate in the stroma are obvious features. By means of numerous microphotographs, it will be shown here how colposcopy is based on histology.

The sequence of the changes to be described follows their temporal appearance. The first to appear is ectopy (eversion), which is defined as the presence of columnar epithelium on the ectocervix. The columnar epithelium of an ectopy is usually replaced, at least in part, by newly formed squamous epithelium. This is the crucial step in the dynamics of cervical epithelia: whether the new squamous epithelium becomes normal, acanthotic (but benign), or neoplastic. In short, this is the scenario the colposcopist can observe and evaluate in terms of biologic behavior and significance.

Microscopic versus Colposcopic Morphology

The magnified image of the colposcope is based on the reciprocal relationship between the epithelium and the stroma. The epithelium acts as a *filter* through which both the incident and reflected light must pass.

The epithelium itself is colorless. The stroma is red, because it contains blood vessels. The redness of the stroma will be transmitted to a certain extent through the epithelium, and will be visible with the colposcope.

The nature and intensity of this coloration depend on
(a) the thickness of the epithelium,
(b) the optical density of the epithelium, i.e., its architecture,
(c) the nature of the stroma.
A further characteristic of colposcopic lesions is their clear demarcation from their normal surroundings and from each other. It is important to appreciate that practically all colposcopically suspicious lesions have *sharp borders*.

Role of the Epithelium in the Genesis of Colposcopic Morphology

The *normal glycogen-containing squamous epithelium* during reproductive life is thick and multilayered, and acts as a fairly effective filter (Fig. 4.1 a). A surface covered by such epithelium will appear *pink to reddish* (see Fig. 11.1).

Acanthotic epithelium is somewhat thinner than fully differentiated normal squamous epithelium, and is composed almost entirely of prickle cells which do not contain glycogen. It always displays some degree of parakeratosis or keratosis, or both (Fig. 4.1 b). The end result is somewhat higher optical density than that of normal squamous epithelium. Colposcopically, it appears pale red (see Fig. 11.30 a), but it may be gray or grayish white (see Fig. 11.25), depending on the degree of keratinization. Occasionally, it may be difficult to distinguish from normal squamous epithelium, but it does not stain with iodine (see p. 117).

Atypical epithelium differs from normal in that it is often thinner, does not contain glycogen, and, most importantly, is more cellular with a higher nuclear content (Fig. 4.1 c). The end result is deep red admixed with a dirty gray or whitish discoloration (see Figs. 11.27 and 11.41).

Atrophic postmenopausal and prepubertal squamous epithelium is thinner than normal squamous epithelium, and does not contain glycogen (Fig. 4.1 d). The stromal blood supply is reduced. The cervicovaginal mucosa appears pale red (see Fig. 11.2).

Columnar epithelium is rather thin, contains mucin, and is therefore highly transparent (Fig. 4.2 a). The part of the cervix covered by columnar epithelium looks *intensely red* (see Fig. 11.8 a).

The thickness of *regenerating epithelium* in the transformation zone varies according to its stage of development, but it is thinner than the normal squamous epithelium (Fig. 4.2 b) and devoid of glycogen. Consequently, it is relatively transparent and therefore appears *intensely red* (see Fig. 11.11).

Both acanthotic and atypical squamous epithelia may display *distinct keratinization* (Fig. 4.3) and may appear colposcopically as keratosis. The keratotic layer is opaque, white, and grainy. The underlying epithelium is hidden, and cannot be evaluated (see Fig. 11.23).

In *true erosion* the stroma is exposed (Fig. 4.4), and its surface is rough, red, and raw (see Fig. 11.47).

Fig. 4.**1 a–d The squamous epithelium of the cervix displays variable thickness** at the same magnification

Fig. 4.**1 a Normal squamous epithelium**

Fig. 4.**1 b Acanthotic epithelium** forming epithelial buds and parakeratosis

Fig. 4.**1 c Peg-forming carcinoma in situ** (CIN 3)

Fig. 4.**1 d Atrophic, postmenopausal squamous epithelium**

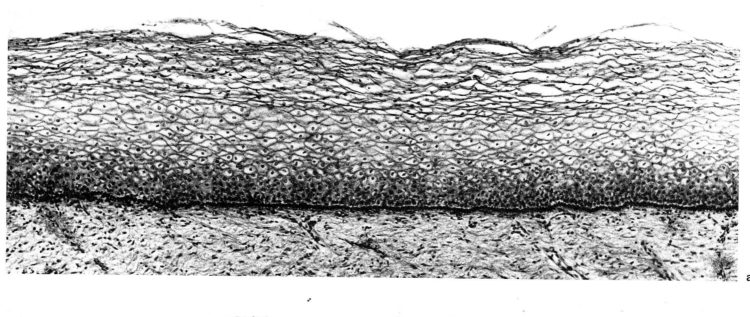

a

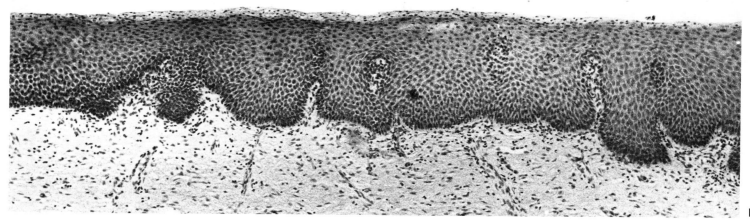

b

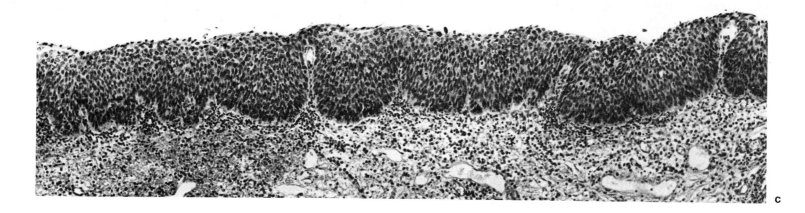

c

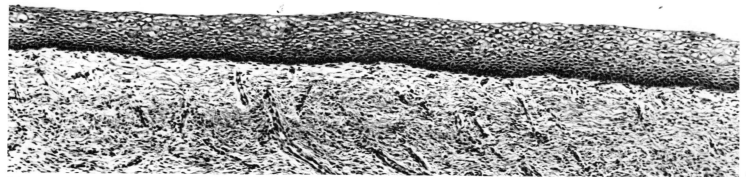

d

4.**1**

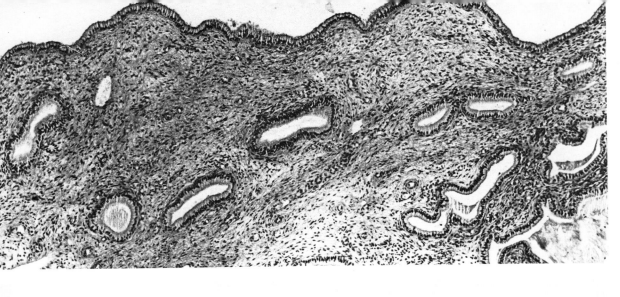

Fig. 4.**2 a**, **b** **Cervical epithelium** of varying thickness

Fig. 4.**2 a** **Columnar epithelium** of the endocervical mucosa

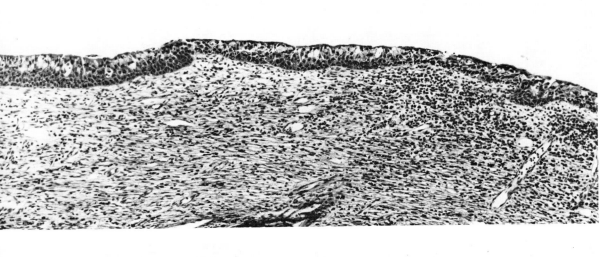

Fig. 4.**2 b** **Regenerating metaplastic squamous epithelium**

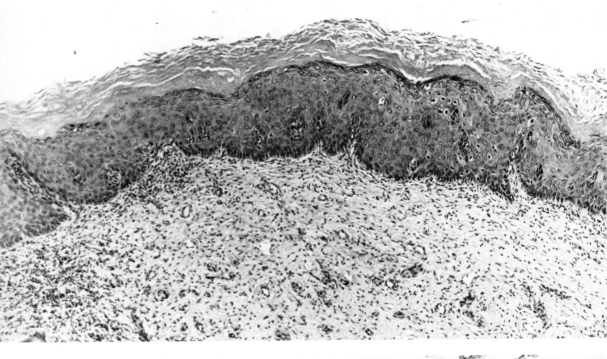

Fig. 4.**3** **Well-differentiated, keratinizing carcinoma in situ** (CIN 3)

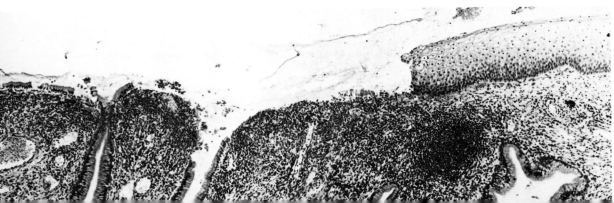

Fig. 4.**4** **True erosion (ulceration) of the cervical mucosa.** Most of the columnar epithelium adjoining the squamous has been lost. The stroma shows an inflammatory reaction

Role of the Stroma in the Genesis of Colposcopic Morphology

The colposcopically evident hues also depend on the composition of the stroma.

Normal stroma (Fig. 4.5). The closer to normal the stroma is, the more it assumes the color of blood.

Abnormal stroma (Fig. 4.6). When the stroma is inflamed, the reddish hue will be muted to a gray-white or yellow, depending on the degree of inflammatory infiltrate.

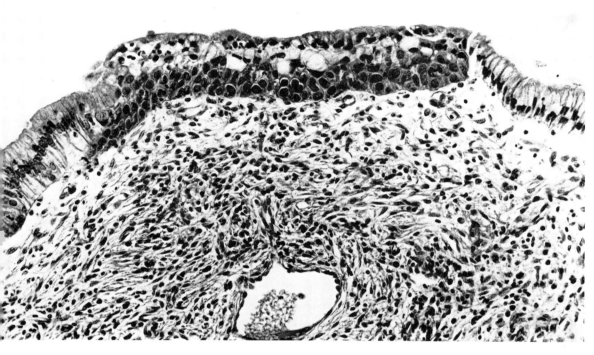

Fig. 4.**5** **Normal cervical stroma.** Deep down is a large venous channel. The metaplastic epithelium arose in a clearly defined area

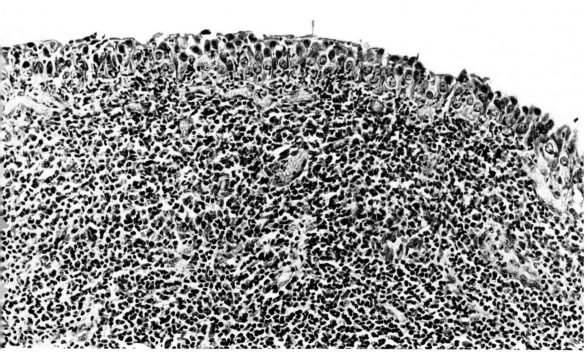

Fig. 4.**6** **Heavy round cell infiltrate in the stroma** obscures the epithelial-stromal junction. Irritated columnar epithelium and immature squamous metaplasia cover the surface

Colposcopic Surface Configuration

This is determined by the interplay of the following factors: the surface relief of the cervix, the planes between different epithelia, and the thickness of the epithelium.

The *surface relief* is either smooth or papillary; in the latter case, the mucosa appears colposcopically as grapelike villi. This appearance is most pronounced in an ectopy (see Fig. 11.9 and 11.10). The papillae are usually covered by columnar epithelium (Fig. 4.7).

Differences in epithelial planes are most pronounced between normal squamous and columnar epithelium, especially in an ectopy. Because the epithelial-stromal interface is normally at the same level, the junction between the thick stratified squamous epithelium and the relatively thin, single-layered columnar epithelium is steplike (Fig. 4.8) and most pronounced in ectopy with no transformation zone (see Figs. 11.7 and 11.9). The effect of *variation in thickness of the squamous epithelium* is most marked when the stromal papillae are elongated. The thin epithelial covering of the papillae will allow the rich capillary network to shine through, whereas the thick rete pegs between them will be less translucent (Fig. 4.9).

The resulting colposcopic appearance depends on the spatial arrangement of the papillae. There are two possibilities. They may form isolated *columns* (Fig. 4.10); the capillaries then shine through the attenuated epithelium covering the tips, and give rise to red dots, referred to as *punctation* (see Fig. 11.27). Alternatively, the arborizing network of stromal *ridges* subdivides the surface epithelium into discrete *fields* (Fig. 4.11), producing a *mosaic* pattern (see Fig. 11.37).

Gland openings. The replacement of columnar epithelium by squamous epithelium takes place mostly on the exposed surfaces, leaving the recesses of the glands or crypts intact and their mouths open. The margins of the squamous epithelium reach just to the gland openings. Should the metaplasia also involve the lower portions of the duct, the gland openings may be lined by the squamous epithelium (Fig. 4.13). The circular gland openings are easily seen colposcopically (see Fig. 11.17),

Fig. 4.**7** **The papillae of an ectopy are covered by columnar epithelium**

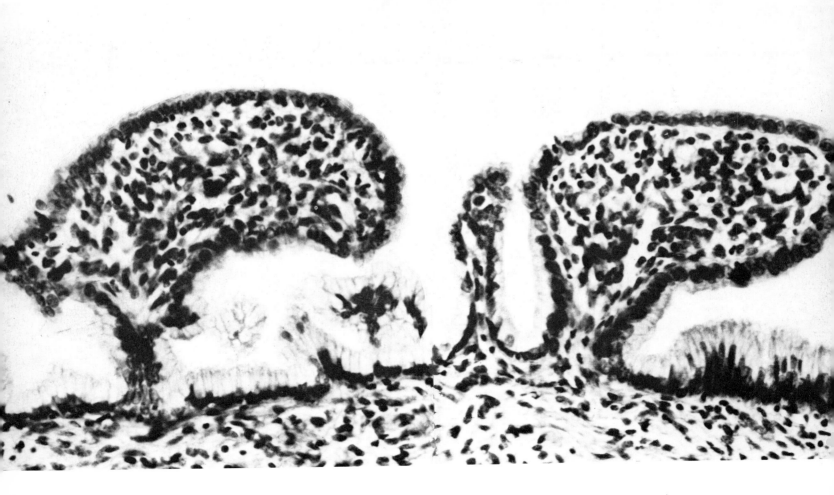

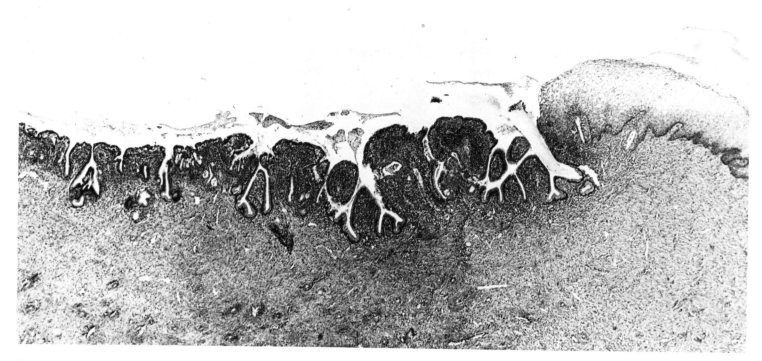

Fig. 4.**8** **The junction between original squamous
epithelium** *(right)* **and the
columnar epithelium** of an
ectopy is distinctly step-like.
The stroma underlying the
ectopy contains a definite
round-cell infiltrate

Fig. 4.**9** **Acanthotic epithelium** with markedly elongated
stromal papillae. The epithelium capping the vascular papillae is attenuated in comparison with the thick pegs between them

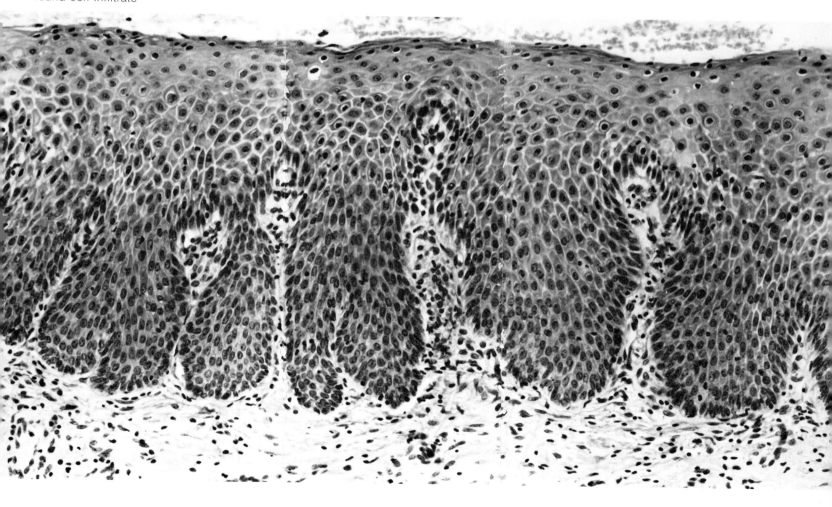

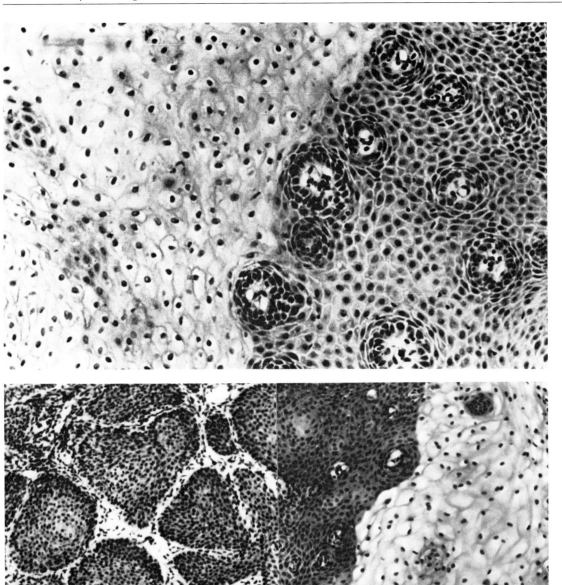

Fig. 4.**10 Punctation as seen in histologic sections.** The tangential cut shows the elongated stromal papillae of acanthotic epithelium *(right)* and their absence in normal epithelium *(left)*. The border between the two is sharp

Fig. 4.**11 The histologic appearance of mosaic.** The stroma supporting the acanthotic epithelium forms interlacing, net-like ridges *(left)*, which subdivide the epithelium into discrete fields. The junction with normal squamous epithelium *(right)* is sharp

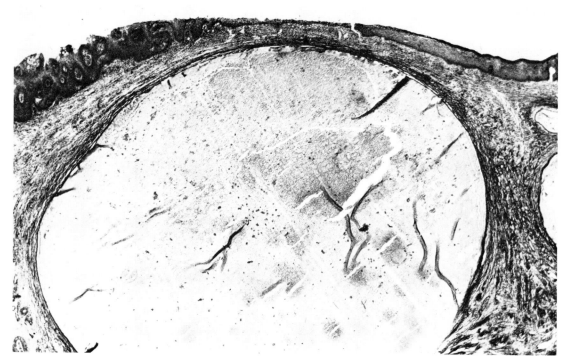

Fig. 4.**12 Nabothian follicle** at the junction between acanthotic epithelium *(right)* and carcinoma in situ (CIN 3). The squamous epithelium is attenuated over the dome of the distended gland

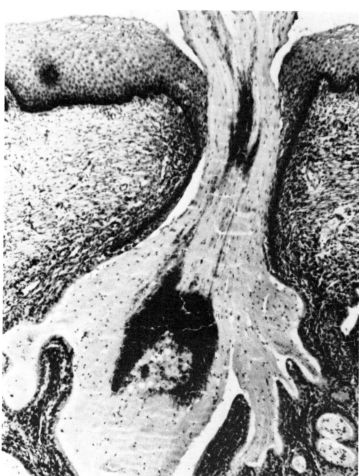

Fig. 4.**13 Gland opening amid normal squamous epithelium;** the latter must have arisen secondarily in an ectopy. The wedge shaped epithelium produces the colposcopically visible white rings around the gland openings

the characteristic white rings around them being due to the tangential view of the wedge-shaped squamous epithelium (Fig. 4.13). Their presence may be the only indication that the squamous epithelium is metaplastic and not original, i.e., that one is dealing with a "healed" transformation zone.

Retention cysts (nabothian follicles) form under the surface when the outlets of crypts are occluded by squamous metaplasia. The buried columnar epithelium continues to secrete mucus, which eventually fills and distends the gland. The cysts so formed indent the overlying squamous epithelium, which becomes attenuated because of stretching (Fig. 4.12). A branching network of vessels characteristically courses over their surface (see Figs. 11.18 and 11.19). The entrapped mucus gives the cyst an ivory-yellow tinge. The latter feature allows recognition of a more deeply situated cyst, even when the surface is flat.

Obliteration of the outlets of glands by squamous metaplasia does not always result in cyst formation. This explains the discrepancy between the number of glands and outflow tracts demonstrable by examination of serial sections.

The *columnar epithelium lining crypts* may also undergo metaplasia; the end result is usually acanthotic epithelium, but may also be normal glycogen-containing epithelium (see Fig. 3.54). The impression of active downgrowth of squamous epithelium is wrong (see p. 40). The columnar epithelium may be either partly or completely replaced by squamous metaplasia, producing in the latter case more or less well defined squamous balls lying beneath the surface, which may be visible colposcopically. If numerous, a mosaic appearance (see Fig. 11.38) may be simulated. The prominent network of the capillary-rich stromal ridges, however, will be lacking (see also Pathogenesis of Mosaic and Punctation, p. 80).

Tissue Basis of Special Colposcopic Appearances

Ectopy (Columnar Epithelium)

Histology

Ectopy is defined as the presence of columnar epithelium (mucosa) on the ectocervix. In the "ideal" situation, the squamocolumnar junction is situated at the external os. In the case of ectopy, the squamocolumnar junction is situated outside the external os, on the ectocervix. Occasionally, the columnar epithelium extends to the vaginal fornix. In *vaginal adenosis*, columnar epithelium may appear isolated in the fornices as well as in the midst of the vaginal epithelium.

Not only the surface columnar epithelium but the whole mucosa, including glands and supporting stroma, is displaced in an ectopy (Fig. 4.14). It is not always possible to see the original squamocolumnar junction on the surface; however, its true position is permanently marked histologically by the *last gland* (see Fig. 3.50).

The surface of the ectopy is usually highly papillary (Fig. 4.14). The stroma usually contains a light inflammatory infiltrate, but occasionally this is dense and is associated with a prominent capillary network (Fig. 4.15).

Pathogenesis of Ectopy

In the past, ectopy was regarded erroneously as *erosion*. Concepts of its pathogenesis have been dominated by Robert Meyer's time-sanctioned *theory of healing of an erosion* (22, 23). He viewed the squamocolumnar junction as a battlefront contested by the two rival epithelial types. According to this theory, a true traumatic erosion of squamous epithelium during pregnancy, and especially during childbirth, was healed by a dressing of columnar epithelium. The columnar epithelium was believed to creep over the denuded area from the adjacent mucosa, as well as from heterotopic endocervical glands that had migrated to the inflamed area. According to Meyer, the surface columnar epithelium could even form glandular crypts. Meyer's theory was difficult to reconcile with the papillary architecture of ectopy (which one would have expected to be flat and smooth) and its close resemblance to the endocervical mucosa, with its crypts and stromal framework.

The modern concepts of the pathogenesis of ectopy are based on the work of a group from Cologne (17, 26). They have shown that the distance between the isthmus of the uterus and the *last gland* is constant throughout life. During the various epochs of a woman's life, the whole length of the columnar mucosa tends to be displaced, distally in the late fetal period and during reproductive life, while retracting after menopause. Thus ectopy is due to shifting of the cervical mucosa as a whole. In fact, ectopy is really an *eversion*.

The pathogenesis of vaginal adenosis (the presence of columnar mucosa in the vagina) is entirely different, and is mostly brought about by the teratogenic effect of intrauterine exposure to diethylstilbestrol (DES) (see page 190). This results in a shift of the squamocolumnar junction distally onto the vagina or in the development of ectopic columnar epithelium in the vagina during organogenesis. It may be noted, however, that vaginal adenosis may occur in the absence of known teratogens.

Fig. 4.**14   The surface configuration of an ectopy is papillary.** Ectopy is brought about not by simple displacement of the surface columnar epithelium but by a shift of the whole mucosa, including the crypts

Fig. 4.**15   Ectopy has a markedly papillary surface.** The stroma contains a fairly dense round-cell infiltrate and dilated capillaries

4.**14**

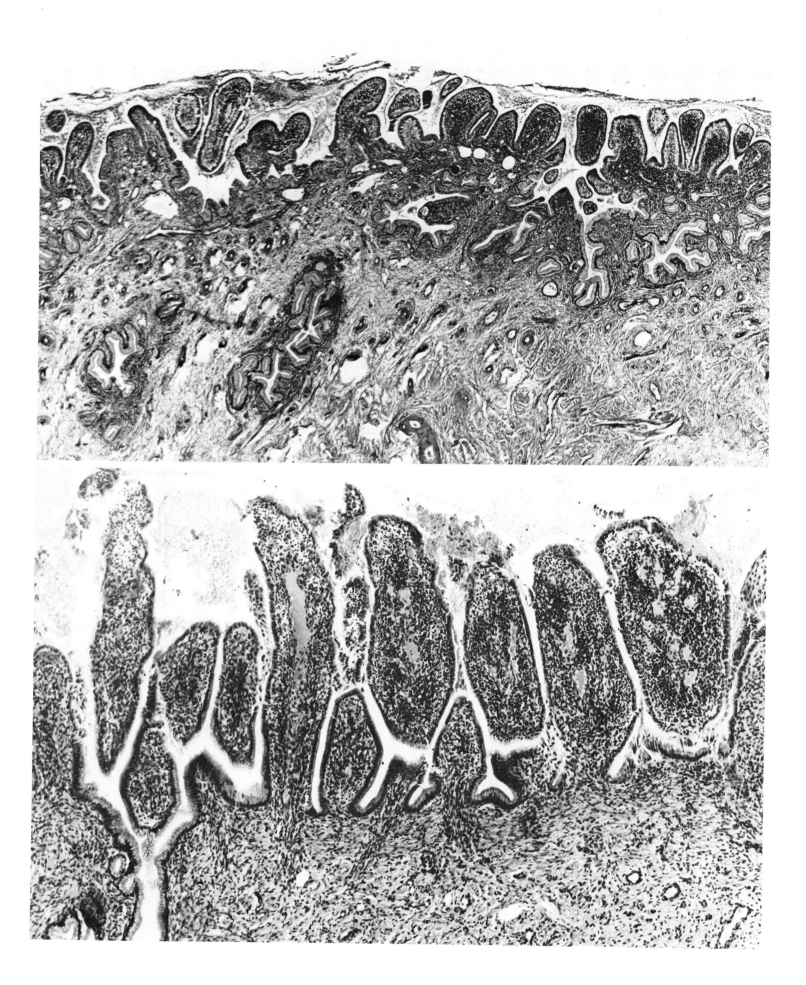

The Normal Transformation Zone

Histology

The transformation zone comes about when columnar epithelium on the ectocervix is replaced by squamous epithelium. It must be realized, however, that such transformation may involve normally situated columnar epithelium in the endocervical canal as well.

As a rule, transformation begins at the squamocolumnar junction (Fig. 4.16; see also Figs. 11.12 a and 12.8). Less commonly, it begins amid columnar epithelium (Figs. 4.5 and 4.17) near this junction (see Fig. 12.8). The epithelium that appears first is thin and multicellular, but lacks stratification (Fig. 4.18). The histologic appearance resembles the various stages of evolution of "regenerating" epithelium (see Figs. 3.51 and 3.61). The epithelium becomes gradually thicker (Fig. 4.19) and stratified, and finally becomes scarcely distinguishable from normal glycogen-containing squamous epithelium. Only the underlying columnar mucosa indicates its true origin (Fig. 4.13; see also Fig. 3.50 b).

Castano-Almendral and Beato (5) found that karyometry can detect differences between the two types of squamous epithelia, the relative nuclear area of original squamous cells being $26.24 \pm 0.3\%$, while that of metaplastic squamous cells is $31.14 \pm 0.3\%$. These differences are statistically significant ($P < 0.001$).

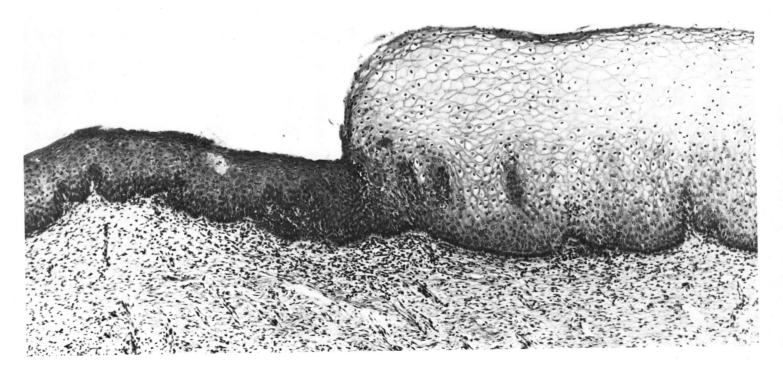

Fig. 4.**16** **The sharp border between original and metaplastic squamous epithelia** indicates the metaplastic origin of the thinner epithelium

Fig. 4.**19** **More advanced stage of immature metaplasia.** Columnar epithelium still covers the relatively orderly squamous epithelium

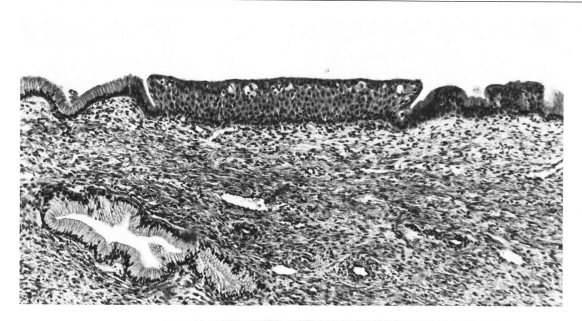

Fig. 4.**17** **An island of squamous metaplasia in a sea of columnar epithelium.** The metaplastic epithelium is still covered by columnar epithelium, although this has degenerated

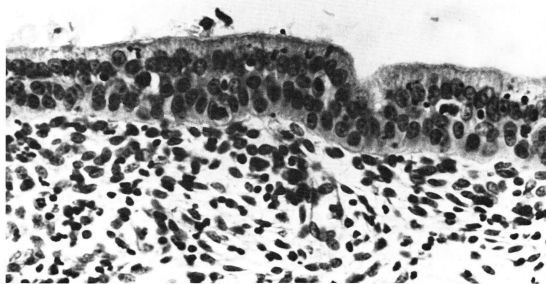

Fig. 4.**18** **The initial proliferation of subcolumnar cells produces a multilayered metaplastic epithelium**

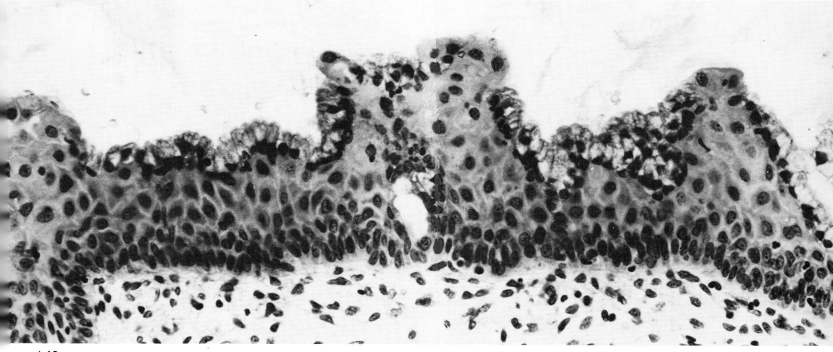

The Mechanism of "Transformation"

The explanation of the mechanism by which columnar epithelium is replaced by squamous epithelium has been dominated for decades by Meyer's theory of healing of erosion (see p. 70). According to this hypothesis, wedge-shaped offshoots from the surrounding original squamous epithelium undermine, lift off, and eventually detach, the columnar epithelium, uprooting it from its base "rather like a plough". It is difficult to understand today how Meyer's authority went unchallenged by a generation of surgical pathologists. Meyer did not believe in the existence of squamous metaplasia, and formulated a theory of his own. Although this theory should now be of only historical interest, its influence is still seen when one speaks of active epithelial spread at the cost of neighboring epithelium, and especially of its downward extension or penetration into the endocervical crypts.

According to modern concepts, there are two different mechanisms involved in the morphogenesis of the transformation zone: squamous metaplasia and ascending healing.

Squamous metaplasia plays the pivotal role in the replacement of columnar epithelium. It does not mean, however, that columnar epithelium simply changes to squamous epithelium.

Rather, the process of squamous metaplasia is heralded by the appearance of a new cell type under the columnar epithelium, the so-called subcolumnar cells (see Fig. 3.42). These cells multiply and mount up, form layers, and eventually produce normally differentiating squamous epithelium. The columnar epithelium may remain sitting on top of the squamous for some time, but is eventually shed (Fig. 4.19).

It has been suggested that the process of squamous metaplasia progresses through several stages. Staging, however, is not important, histologic description of the thickness and stratification of the epithelium being all that is required for its definition.

The origin of the subcolumnar cells is poorly understood. They are often referred to as *reserve cells* (1, 14, 19), which are believed to be pluripotential cells native to the endocervical mucosa and which bring about not only the day-to-day regeneration of columnar cells but also initiate the metaplastic process. The difficulty with this theory is the observation that subcolumnar cells are not seen normally in the cervix. When they appear, they form neat rows in well-defined segments of the mucosa (see Figs. 3.42 and 3.44) and correspond three-dimensionally to discrete *fields* of varying size. One or several of these may be present at the same time, either isolated or closely

Fig. 4.20 Sharp border between two quite different forms of atypical metaplasia. Both are quite thin, and cannot as yet be designated as either dysplastic or showing carcinoma in situ

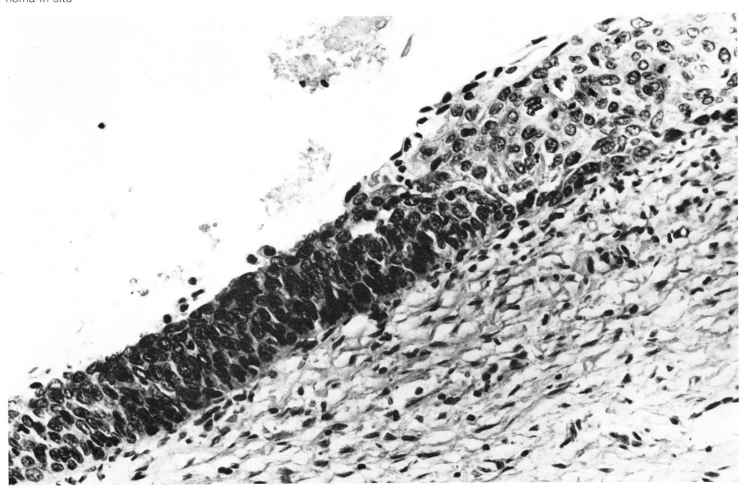

joined together, like patchwork. Only in the latter case is it possible to observe the different stages of maturation of the metaplastic epithelium (Fig. 4.20).

Some authorities believe that subcolumnar cells originate from stromal cells (27), but this has not been conclusively proven. It must be admitted that the nature of the metaplastic process is not known. The solution of this problem will be a milestone in the understanding of carcinogenesis.

The crucial question concerns the fate of the evolving metaplastic epithelium: whether the end result is normal glycogen-containing squamous epithelium, acanthotic epithelium, or atypical epithelium characteristic of malignancy (see Fig. 3.45). Within the normal transformation zone, the developing squamous epithelium is cytologically benign, so it may be expected that the epithelium that is eventually formed will also lack atypia. The question remains whether atypical epithelium develops only when a carcinogen interferes with the normal transformation process. From histologic evidence it appears that atypical transformation commences at the initiation of the metaplastic process, with the eventual development of atypical epithelium. We distinguish, therefore, between *normal* and *atypical squamous metaplasia* (see p. 34).

In the colposcopic literature (9), the concept of atypical metaplasia is invoked to explain the morphogenesis of the various components of the atypical transformation zone (see p. 85), that is, punctation, mosaic, and keratosis. The fact that in many cases the same appearance may be produced by benign epithelia showing abnormal maturation only (see p. 12) has led to complicated hypothetical explanations. One of these stated that the colposcopic findings do not represent false positives in such cases, but in fact biologically predate the histologic changes (30). Appreciation of the existence and nature of acanthotic epithelium provides a simple solution of this problem.

As noted also by others (15), the term *atypical metaplasia* (atypical reserve cell hyperplasia) is restricted to a thin epithelium that shows *cellular atypia* ab initio. Such epithelium may be regarded as the earliest morphologic stage of development of CIN.

Ascending healing. The notion of ascending healing was first described by Hamperl and co-workers (16), who observed this process in the cervices of pregnant women. In complete contrast to Meyer's concept of the healing of an erosion (see p. 70), it is the columnar, not the squamous epithelium, that is likely to become traumatized and ulcerated (sustain true ero-

Fig. 4.**21 Ascending healing.**
A thin, wedge-shaped offshoot of the original squamous epithelium glides over the denuded surface of a true erosion of columnar epithelium. The duct of a cervical gland is apparently bypassed

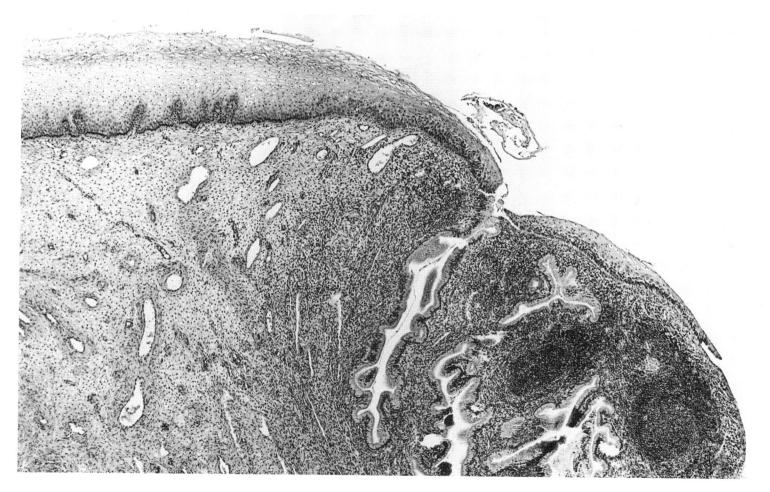

sions). The fate of erosions, if situated near the squamoco-lumnar junction, depends on several factors, including the pH (18, 22). In certain cases, the ulcerated surface will be covered by squamous epithelium in the same way that a skin wound heals. Tongues of squamous epithelium, in the shape of taper-ing or blunt wedges (Fig. 4.21), extend from the periphery to cover the denuded area. The fully regenerated epithelium is in-distinguishable from its parent.

When only a short segment of thin epithelium is available for histologic scrutiny, it is not always possible to distinguish be-tween ascending healing and metaplasia. In both cases, the epi-thelium is of the immature type, and is best referred to as *regen-erating*. When epithelium of this sort is seen in continuity with adjacent epithelium, it is almost always possible to determine its origin, because:

1. In ascending healing, the transition between the regenerat-ing epithelium and the thick stratified squamous epithelium is gradual (Fig. 4.21).
2. The border between original squamous epithelium and me-taplastic squamous epithelium in its various stages of devel-opment is always abrupt (Fig. 4.16; see also Figs. 3.46 and 3.51).
3. If squamous epithelium is found in the midst of columnar epithelium, its metaplastic origin cannot be doubted (Figs. 4.5 and 4.17).
4. The presence of columnar epithelium covering regenerating epithelium may be taken as evidence that the latter arose by metaplasia (Figs. 4.18, 4.19, and 3.47). The absence of co-lumnar epithelium, however, cannot be invoked to support either origin.
5. In contrast to metaplasia, ascending healing can occur only at the squamocolumnar junction. Although metaplasia is very common at this site, it can also arise as an island in a sea of columnar epithelium.

Sharp Epithelial Borders

As squamous metaplasia develops in well-defined fields and re-mains confined to these fields during the vertical growth phase (see p. 34), transformed metaplastic epithelium must also be-come sharply circumscribed. Such sharp borders can be seen colposcopically, especially in cases of suspicious findings. These margins, as well as those between different pathologic epithelia, can be accentuated by the application of iodine (Fig. 15.2) or acetic acid (Fig. 15.3). It is remarkable how the significance of these epithelial borders is ignored when theories of cervical carcinogenesis are formulated.

The colposcopic-histologic correlation is excellent in this respect (Figs. 15.1−4). The sharp border between normal and atypical squamous epithelia is well known (Fig. 3.63 b). From the foregoing discussion of acanthotic epithelium, it is apparent that its junction with normal squamous epithelium must also be clearly demarcated (Fig. 3.63 a). Since squamous metaplasia arises in various discrete fields either simultaneously or in se-quence, sharp borders must also exist between different forms of pathologic epithelia when they are adjacent to each other—hence the borders between various forms of carcinoma in situ (Fig. 3.65 a and c) and between carcinoma in situ and dysplasia (Fig. 3.65 b).

Leukoplakia

The histologic hallmark of leukoplakia is some degree of kera-tinization of the surface (Fig. 4.22 a−c) in the form of *parake-ratosis* or *hyperkeratosis*. Hyperkeratosis is classically seen in the skin, characterized by cornification without nuclei. Parake-ratosis implies retention of pyknotic nuclei in the horny layer (Fig. 4.22 b). Keratinization is associated only with pathologic epithelia; normal glycogen-containing squamous epithelium never displays it. The degree of keratinization does not depend on the type of underlying epithelium. In the same type of epi-thelium, the appearance may range from mild parakeratosis to full cornification (Fig. 4.22 b, c).

Keratosis may be produced by two fundamentally different kinds of epithelium:

(1) acanthotic (Fig. 4.22 a) and
(2) atypical (showing the features of CIN) (Fig. 4.22 b, c).

Parakeratosis or hyperkeratosis occur equally in both epithelial types. There are no differences as to the structure and the thick-ness of the keratotic layers, or the presence or absence of a stra-tum granulosum (Figs. 4.22 b, c). It is therefore impossible to predict the nature of the underlying epithelium from the type of cornification.

That keratosis is produced by two entirely different kinds of epithelium is of the utmost importance. Historically, and even today, leukoplakia has been regarded by many as precan-cerous, and not only by those in the field of gynecology. Biop-sies of leukoplakia may provide histologically harmless acan-thotic epithelium, atypical epithelium, or even invasive carci-noma. It was for this reason that the concept of malignant de-generation of leukoplakia arose and that leukoplakia came to be regarded as premalignant (see p. 4).

We now know that acanthotic epithelium plays no greater role in cervical carcinogenesis than normal glycogen-contain-ing epithelium (see p. 5) even if keratinized. It is therefore es-sential to qualify the company that keratosis keeps. Keratosis due to histologically acanthotic epithelium calls for neither the-rapeutic intervention nor careful follow-up. On the other hand, extensive leukoplakia may vary histologically from place to place. Furthermore, acanthotic epithelium may be combined with atypical epithelium in the same lesion (Figs. 15.1−15.4). A small biopsy specimen from such a large lesion may therefore be nonrepresentative and misleading.

Finally, keratosis may mask a *keratinizing invasive carci-noma* (see. Fig. 11.67).

Keratinizing epithelium may be found in the transforma-tion zone. Whether there is epithelial atypia or not, it must have arisen by way of squamous metaplasia. Hyperkeratotic epithelium, however, may be found well out on the ectocervix, as well as in the vagina, in the absence of columnar epithelium, indicating its development from original squamous epithelium. As already mentioned, normal glycogen-containing cervico-vaginal squamous epithelium may give rise to glycogen-free, keratinized, epidermis-like epithelium. This is especially com-mon in cases of prolapse. This reactive form of acanthotic epi-thelium is reversible. However, well-circumscribed keratosis is biologically irreversible, and is caused by acanthotic or atypical epithelia only.

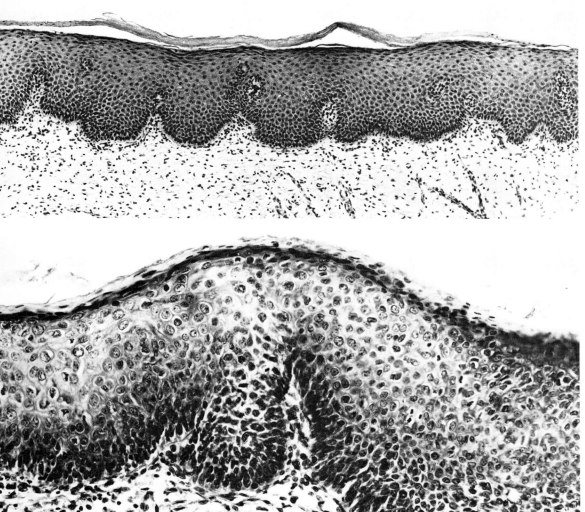

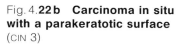

Fig. 4.**22 a−c** **Various types of keratosis**

Fig. 4.**22 a** **True hyperkeratosis** associated with acanthotic epithelium

Fig. 4.**22 b** **Carcinoma in situ with a parakeratotic surface** (CIN 3)

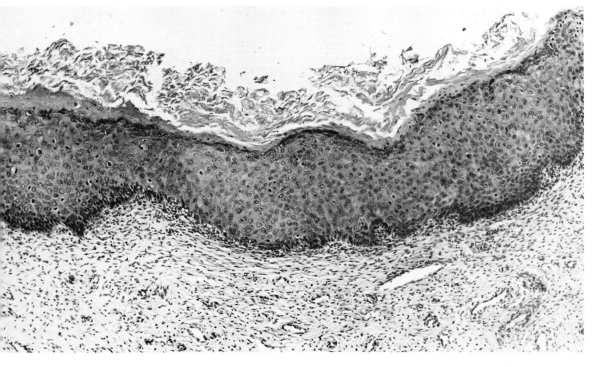

Fig. 4.**22 c** **Keratinizing carcinoma in situ** (CIN 3) with an undulating surface. Note the distinct stratum granulosum

Mosaic and Punctation

The colposcopic patterns of mosaic and punctation depend on certain architectural features of the squamous epithelium. The blood vessels in the elongated stromal papillae that perforate the squamous epithelium shine through the attenuated portion of the epithelium covering them (Figs. 11.26, 11.37). Punctation and mosaic are produced by isolated stromal papillae and interlacing stromal ridges, respectively (Figs. 4.10, 4.11).

It is absolutely essential to appreciate that these colposcopic patterns may be produced by two histologically entirely different epithelia: *acanthotic epithelium* may display extensive budding and branching, the epithelial pegs interdigitating with quite slender stromal papillae. The interpapillary distance varies, but is usually not excessive (Fig. 4.23).

In contrast, the epithelial pegs of *atypical epithelium* are heftier and regular, the stromal papillae are more robust, and the interpapillary distance is greater (Fig. 4.24).

Only rarely does peg-forming epithelium contain glycogen (Fig. 4.25). In such cases, the epithelial segments between the red dots or lines will stain brown with iodine (Figs. 11.83, 11.85). The histologic architecture of such epithelium, however, is disturbed. Such an appearance should nowadays raise the possibility of condylomatous change.

The stromal papillae supporting markedly hyperkeratotic epithelium are often elongated (Fig. 4.26). The expected colposcopic pattern, however, may be masked by the blanket of keratin, the removal of which may reveal punctation or mosaic colposcopically. The old term *ground* for punctation was merely short for *ground of leukoplakia*. When Hinselmann removed the keratin layer from an area of leukoplakia for the first time, the predominant pattern he uncovered was punctation.

Tall stromal papillae usually go conjointly with keratinization, especially when the squamous epithelium is acanthotic—hence the colposcopic white color. Thus, epithelial types that appear colposcopically as mosaic and punctation, and those showing distinct keratinization, differ only in their degree of keratinization and may in fact be the same. Initially, Hinselmann equated all these lesions with leukoplakia (see p. 4).

Peg-forming epithelium, whether acanthotic or atypical, is characterized by sharp borders with adjoining epithelia (Figs. 4.10, 4.11)—hence the sharp delineation of colposcopic areas of mosaic and punctation. Sharp circumscription is therefore a diagnostic criterion.

As acanthotic and atypical epithelia have the same architectural configuration, one cannot predict with certainty the histology of mosaic or punctation. Thus, the relationship between these characteristic colposcopic patterns and cervical carcinogenesis is tenuous. As Hinselmann was the first to see such appearances, it is understandable that he equated them with the matrix area of cancer (see p. 5). It has been shown subsequently that when such appearances are due to acanthotic epithelium, they are unrelated to the development of carcinoma (10). In spite of this, some still adhere to Hinselmann's original mistaken belief, and conclude that the "atypical transformation zone" is a discrete entity with malignant potential. Only experience will show that this is not always so (9). Actually, only 18% of cases of mosaic and punctation are due to atypical epithelium (see Table 14.1).

Fig. 4.24 **Dysplastic epithelium** (CIN 2) with a "baggy pants" appearance. The interpapillary (and aslo intercapillary) distance is increased

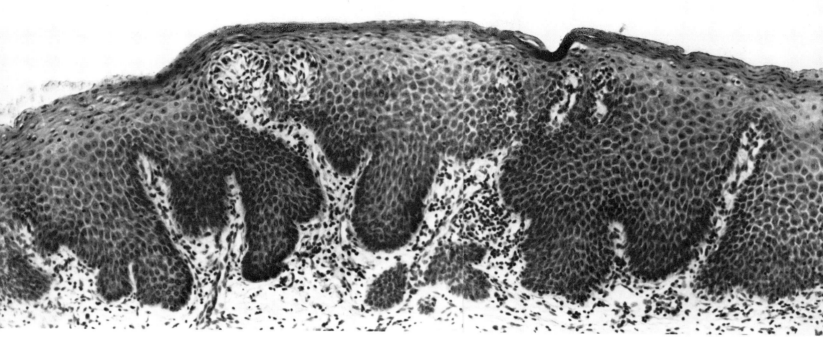

Fig. 4.**23** **Peg-forming acan-thotic epithelium** showing mild parakeratosis. The stromal papillae are elongated, and show some degree of branching

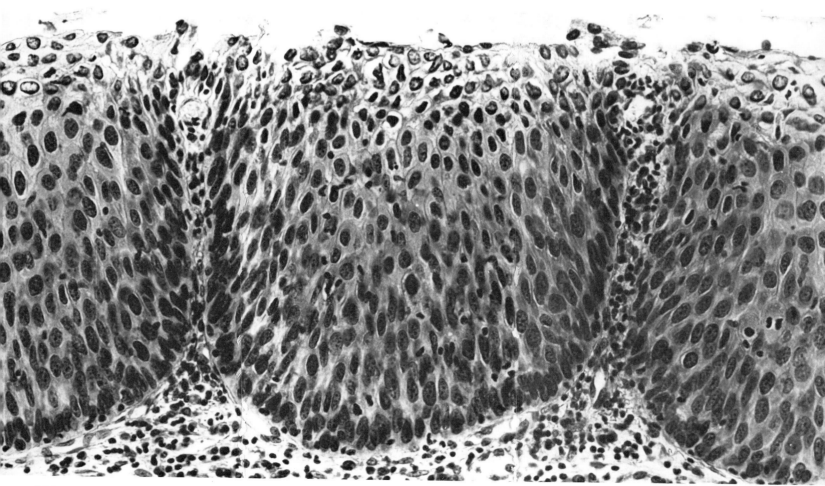

4.**24**

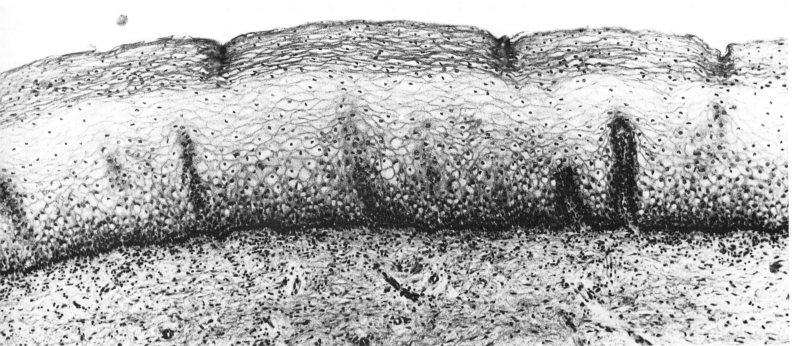

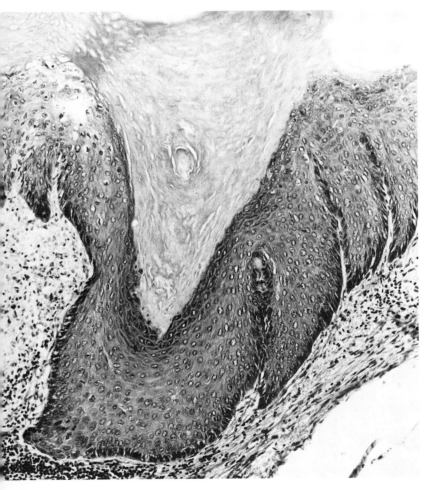

Fig. 4.**26** **Dysplastic epithelium** (CIN 2) with an essentially papillary architecture due to elongated stromal papillae. The thick keratin layer "irons out" the undulations, making the surface almost flat

Pathogenesis of Mosaic and Punctation

There are two theories of the evolution of mosaic and punctation, based on the development of corresponding epithelial architecture. According to the first theory, peg formation occurs during metaplasia, being molded by the papillary scaffolding of ectopy (9, 31). The crypts between the villi become filled with epithelial buds, while the epithelium is attenuated over the tall stromal papillae (Fig. 4.27 a, b). In some cases, the latter are compressed and may completely disappear, resulting in epithelium with normal architecture. Only when the elongated stromal papillae persist do the patterns of mosaic and punctation appear.

The angioarchitecture plays a vital role in this model (30), being regarded as the first morphologically recognizable sign of cervical neoplasia, even preceding the appearance of epithelial atypia. This concept can be traced to Hinselmann (see Chap. 2), who attributed greater significance to colposcopy than to histology.

This deceptively sound theory, however, cannot explain all aspects of the morphogenesis of mosaic and punctation. For instance, it is well known that squamous epithelium covering the papillary mucosa in ectopy may be completely flat (Fig. 4.28). It is also difficult to grasp how peg-forming epithelium with tall stromal papillae can arise outside the transformation zone, in original squamous epithelium (Figs. 3.3, 3.56 a and 3.62) and why one hardly ever sees gland openings or islands of columnar epithelium within a mosaic or punctation (Figs. 11.26, 11.30, and 11.35–11.37). The same applies to the squamous epithelium of the vulva (Fig. 4.29 a), where the identical appearance of sharply circumscribed mosaic or punctation

Fig. 4.**27 a**, **b** **Ongoing metaplasia in papillary endocervical mucosa.** It is feasible that the filling of crypts by epithelial pegs gives rise to the "baggy pants" appearance, while the stromal papillae remain intact

Fig. 4.**25 Glycogen-containing epithelium** with tall stromal papillae. Such epithelium can no longer be regarded as normal, and may be related to condylomas

Fig. 4.**28 Metaplastic epithelium** agglutinates the superficial papillae of an ectopy. In spite of the papillary scaffolding, the surface becomes flat. The stroma is infiltrated by numerous round cells

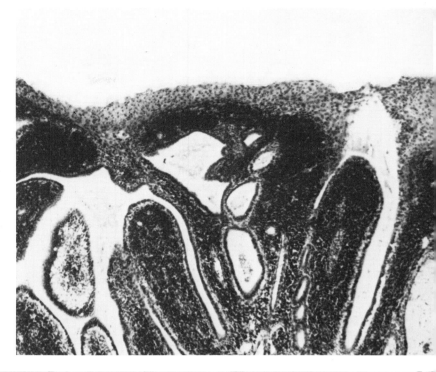

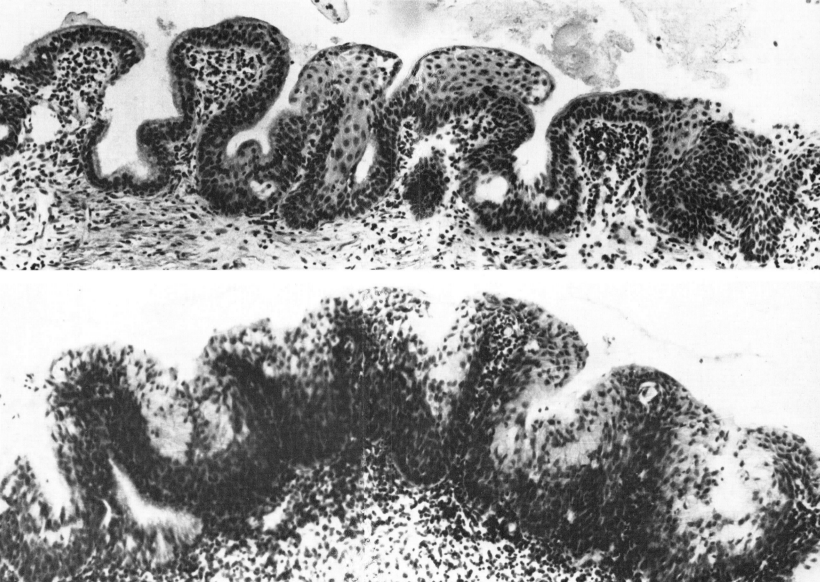

4.**27 a, b**

4.**29 a**

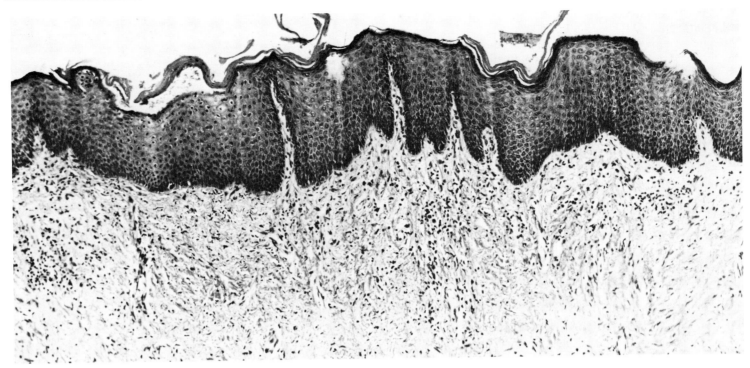

4.**29 b**

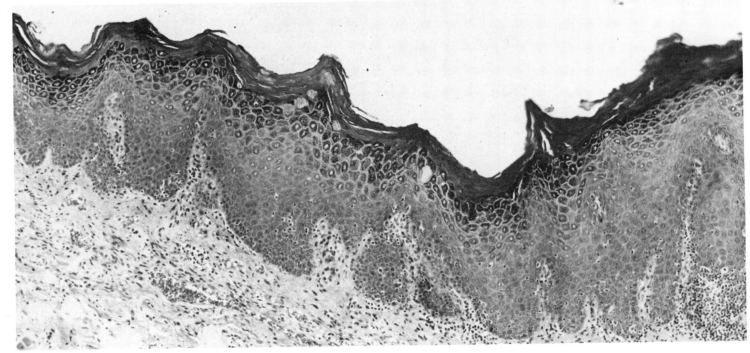

4.**30**

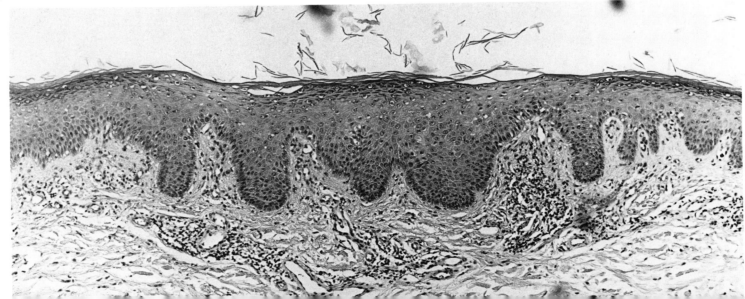

Fig. 4.**29 a**, **b** **Different epithelia supported by tall stromal papillae.** The biopsies were taken from parts of the body in which metaplasia does not take place

Fig. 4.**29 a** **Vulvar dysplasia**

Fig. 4.**29 b** **Epithelium from the buccal mucosa** showing acanthosis, a stratum granulosum, and hyperkeratosis

Fig. 4.**30** **Psoriasis.** The epithelium shows acanthosis, peg formation, and hyperkeratosis. The stromal papillae are accentuated

Fig. 4.**31** **De novo development of tall stromal papillae and elongated epithelial pegs** in the cervix

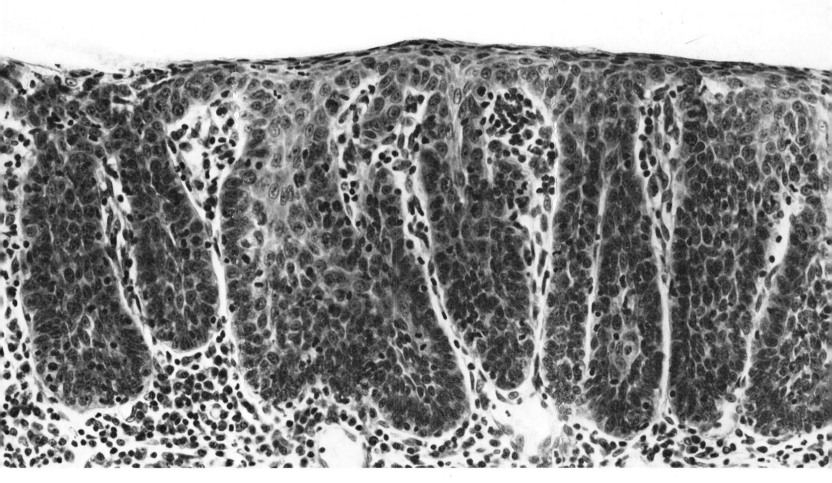

4.**31**

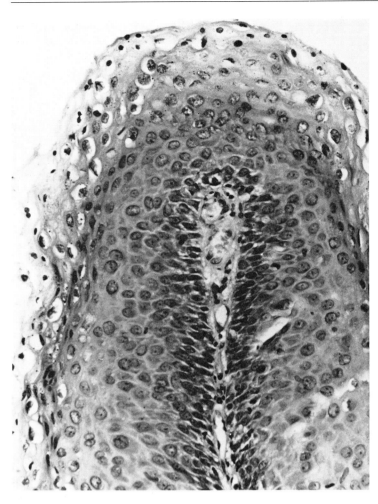

Fig. 4.**32** **Markedly elongated stromal papilla of a condyloma**

may be seen (31) and, so too, epithelial changes in other organs such as buccal mucosa (Fig. 4.29b) and esophagus. Furthermore, there are numerous dermatologic abnormalities that are characterized by acanthosis with parakeratosis or hyperkeratosis and papillomatosis (Fig. 4.30). Finally, it is not clear why disturbance of epithelial architecture goes hand in hand with disturbance of epithelial differentiation, the epithelia being either benign acanthotic or atypical. Completely normal squamous epithelium, which can also arise by the process of metaplasia (Fig. 3.45), is not associated with elongated stromal papillae.

According to the second theory, to which we subscribe, epithelial changes develop in clearly circumscribed fields pari passu with changes in the accompanying stroma and blood vessels. Every type of squamous epithelium, and especially that of the epidermis (Fig. 4.30), is capable of peg formation, quite independent of metaplasia or regeneration. In the cervix, the same change may occur in original squamous epithelium (see above). The fact that punctation and mosaic are always associated with epithelia showing changes in architecture and cellular differentiation supports their fundamental rather than adaptive nature. Finally, one can find examples of immature regenerating epithelium forming prominent pegs, quite independent of preexisting papillary endocervical scaffolding (Fig. 4.31).

Virus-induced papillary lesions of the cervix may also display the above histologic features (Fig. 4.32), and consequently may appear colposcopically as punctation or mosaic (Fig. 4.33). As they not uncommonly arise outside the transformation zone, their configuration cannot be influenced by glandular structures.

Fig. 4.**33** **Tangentially cut cervical condyloma.** The tall stromal papillae account for the punctation seen colposcopically. Moderate cellular and nuclear atypia indicates some degree of dysplasia

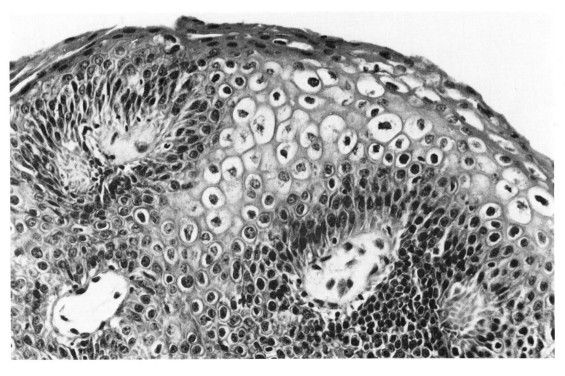

Unusual (Atypical) Transformation Zone

Problem of the Atypical Transformation Zone

Although this term has been used in colposcopy for a long time, problems have arisen because it has recently acquired new significance (8, 9). As it no longer corresponds to the original definition of the "transformation zone," the long-winded explanations that are necessary give rise to difficulties (7). The International Federation for Cervical Pathology and Colposcopy established a Standing Committee some time ago to tackle this problem.

It is now a matter of urgency to clarify the confusion. The normal transformation zone has, and always has had, a very precise definition. Transformation refers to the replacement of columnar by squamous epithelium through the process of metaplasia, including the partial or complete covering of an ectopy by a blanket of initially immature squamous epithelium (see p. 74). The completed transformation zone may still be recognized by the persistence of gland openings or retention cysts, or both (Figs. 11.17–11.19). The colposcopic appearance is therefore characteristic: gland openings, islands of columnar epithelium, retention cysts, and a sometimes prominent but regular network of vessels, are scattered in an intensely red but thin epithelial field. However, even within a normal-looking squamous cover, gland openings and retention cysts are evidence of this process of transformation (see p. 66). It is well known that squamous metaplasia may give rise to epithelia of differing types (Fig. 3.45). According to whether the end-product is normal squamous epithelium, glycogen-free acanthotic epithelium, or atypical epithelium (i.e. showing features of CIN), the colposcopic appearance will also vary: in both acanthotic and atypical epithelium, there are distinct color differences compared with normal epithelium. Using Schiller's test, acanthotic and atypical epithelia can be sharply demarcated from normal epithelium, at least at parts of the circumference. Acanthotic epithelium is not as aceto-white as atypical epithelium. The basic components of the transformation zone are nevertheless preserved in all types, but increased vascularity, atypical blood vessels, and cuffed gland openings may indicate that the process has become atypical (Figs. 11.39–11.46). Thus, we are dealing with a typical transformation zone on the one hand, and a non-typical, atypical, abnormal or unusual transformation zone on the other.

The confusion arose because, according to recent colposcopic literature, all atypical changes—including punctation, mosaic, and leukoplakia—can occur only in the atypical transformation zone. In this way, the concept arose that CIN (and indeed invasive carcinoma) always develops in the atypical transformation zone through the process of squamous metaplasia (6, 9, 27). However, this view ignores the fact that the usual signs of transformation, such as gland openings, columnar epithelial rests, or Nabothian follicles, are mostly absent in otherwise typical fields of punctation or mosaic (Figs. 11.25–11.38). The possibility that these changes might arise in original squamous epithelium, as in acanthotic skin disease, is summarily dismissed. Since the term "atypical transformation zone" had acquired a new meaning, the pattern of this lesion in its original sense, as described by Treite (32) and Glatthaar (13), and, with respect to its histologic basis, by Burghardt (2), had to be described in a different way. Terms like "white epithelium," "aceto-white epithelium," and "atypical vessels" were introduced into colposcopic terminology (p. 135), although these did not represent specific colposcopic patterns but were only diagnostic features also occurring in punctation, mosaic and suspected invasion. This "new" terminology was based on restricting the use of colposcopy to an evaluation of the abnormal smear, an evaluation therefore mostly concerned with atypical changes. Wider experience shows, however, that the pattern of mosaic and punctation is often also found in benign conditions, such as acanthotic epithelium. This fact demanded lengthy explanation, and it was necessary to subdivide the "atypical transformation zone" into the following groups (7):

Atypical transformation zone consistent with CIN.
Atypical transformation zone of doubtful significance.
Atypical transformation zone of physiological significance.

The weakness of the concept of the atypical transformation zone—that all atypical lesions must arise within the framework of columnar cell metaplasia—is exposed by recent knowledge gained from viral lesions. We have learned that many viral changes not only involve original squamous epithelium, but also produce the concomitant colposcopic patterns of mosaic, punctation and leukoplakia. For all these reasons, it is still better to define the classical colposcopic appearances of mosaic, punctation and leukoplakia as such. On the other hand, an area recognized as originating from ectopic columnar epithelium, and which exhibits the reaction to acetic acid and iodine expected from an atypical epithelium, should be designated as a non-typical transformation zone.

Since the concept of the "atypical transformation zone" has long been misused, it is more reasonable to designate the relevant changes as "unusual transformation zone" until such time as the misleading use of the term "atypical transformation zone" has been discontinued.

Colposcopic Diagnosis of the Unusual (Atypical) Transformation Zone

The colposcopic appearances described so far depend on a papillary surface configuration (ectopy) or thin regenerating epithelium (transformation zone), on pronounced surface keratinization (leukoplakia), or epithelium supported by elongated stromal papillae (mosaic and punctation). There are, however, smooth-surfaced but altered epithelia within the transformation zone that, although they have a certain thickness, are not keratinized and do not rest on tall stromal papillae (Figs. 4.34 and 4.35). In the light of the foregoing discussion, the question must arise as to how such an epithelium looks like colposcopically. This depends entirely on the nature of the epithelium itself, whether it is acanthotic or atypical. The difference from normal glycogen-containing epithelium is merely due to the variable translucency of the glycogen-free acanthotic epithelium, on the one hand, and the nuclear and cellular density of the atypical epithelium on the other. These circumstances may result in colposcopic lesions having a color scarcely different from that of normal squamous epithelium. The color change is more pronounced when there is increased vascularity or round-cell infiltration of the stroma; this is likely to be the case when the epithelium is atypical. Finally, acanthotic and atypical epithelia generated by metaplasia are always sharply demarcated from normal epithelium.

The differences between the typical and the unusual transformation zone depend on:

1 Color of the colposcopic lesion

Acanthotic epithelium appears whitish because of the almost constant parakeratosis or hyperkeratosis (Fig. 15.1 a). If keratinization is very mild, acanthotic epithelium may be overlooked colposcopically, especially if flat; it stands out, however, with the Schiller test, being iodine-negative. Atypical epithelium is intensely red to yellowish red, and turns white after the application of acetic acid (Fig. 11.41). The latter phenomenon is regarded as particularly suspicious, and is due to epithelial swelling (see p. 114).

2 Sharpness of demarcation between the transformation zone and the original squamous epithelium

The changes may be heightened by the application of iodine (Fig. 11.46). The transition between the normal transformation zone and the surrounding original epithelium is indistinct and gradual (Figs. 11.12, 11.16).

3 Vascularity

The vascularity of the normal transformation zone is not pronounced, the vessels are fine, nontortuous, and show a regular, tree-like branching. Marked vascularity with a haphazard and irregular disposition of the blood vessels is a hallmark of the unusual transformation zone (Fig. 11.42).

4 Cuffed gland openings

When atypical epithelium involves both the surface and the outer portion of an endocervical crypt (Fig. 3.14), it often produces a thick rim around the gland opening which, after the application of acetic acid (see p. 114) appears as a white cuff colposcopically (Fig. 3.43). This is less pronounced in the case of acanthotic epithelium.

Fig. 4.**34 Acanthotic epithelium**, devoid of stromal papillae; the epithelial-stromal junction is therefore flat. Note the absence of keratinization

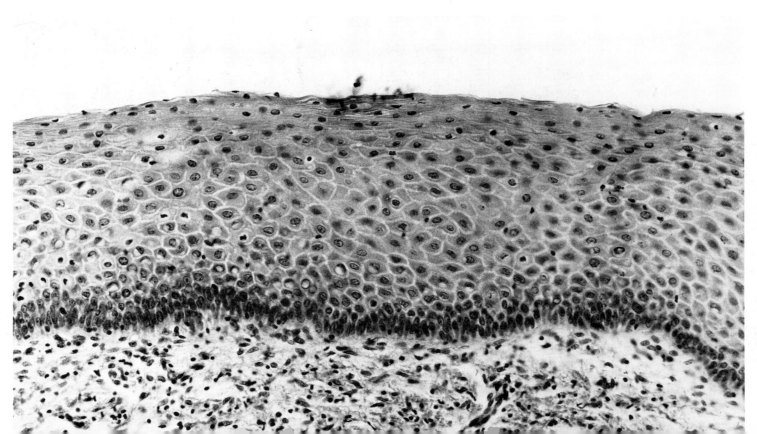

4.35

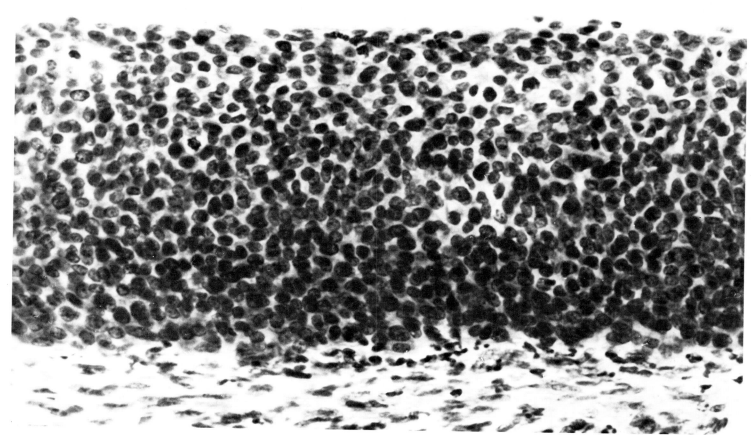

Fig. 4.**35 Undifferentiated carcinoma in situ** (CIN 3) with a flat surface and straight base: stromal papillae are absent

Fig. 4.**36 Regenerating squamous epithelium;** the stroma shows a definite round-cell infiltrate

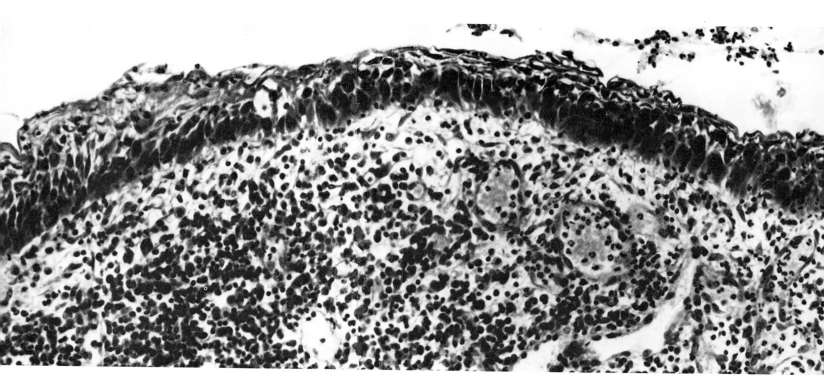

4.36

Fig. 4.**37** **"Fractures" between different epithelia.**
A dysplastic epithelial segment (CIN 2) has detached
from the underlying stroma.
It is obvious that there is no
unity with the normal squamous epithelium on the right
and carcinoma in situ (CIN 3)
on the left

is obvious that there is no unity with the normal squamous
epithelium on the right and
carcinoma in situ (CIN 3) on
the left

The colposcopic changes therefore depend on

(1) epithelial and
(2) stromal changes.

Stromal changes are, of course, not unique to atypical epithelium. Thin regenerating epithelium in the transformation zone
may be associated with a dense cellular infiltrate (Fig. 4.36)
that imparts to it a discoloration distinctly different from normal. Indeed there is a host of combinations between the epithelium and the stroma. The tissue basis of the unusual transformation zone may therefore be quite different from case to
case:

1. Atypical squamous epithelium without segmentation and
    keratinization (Fig. 4.35).
2. Acanthotic epithelium without segmentation and with mini-
    mal keratinization (Fig. 4.34).
3. Thin regenerating epithelium without atypia, supported by
    a markedly vascular and inflamed stroma (Fig. 4.36).

In spite of these differential diagnostic possibilities, we will see
that the unusual transformation zone, through its specific colposcopic appearance, nevertheless plays a most important part
in the detection of histologically atypical epithelia (see
Chap. 8).

Erosion — Ulcer

Traumatic Erosion

Traumatic erosions occur either in thin, nonestrogenized atrophic squamous epithelium or in the columnar epithelium of ectopy (see Fig. 4.4). They are difficult to study histologically, because of their short duration. The epithelial defect is poorly
circumscribed, and its margin is irregular. In the acute lesion
there is little alteration of the stroma. The surface may be covered by a fibrinous exsudate.

Erosion within a Colposcopic Lesion

Ulcers here may arise spontaneously. Atypical epithelium is
more friable and shows less intercellular cohesion than normal
or atrophic squamous epithelium. This accounts for the ease
with which the cells are exfoliated and for the success of cytologic examination. As its attachment to the underlying stroma
is also less tenacious, spontaneous detachment may occur.
Whole epithelial segments or fields may be lost. The "fracture
sites," well seen at epithelial junctions (Fig. 4.37), also show
that epithelia do not merge with each other and that their borders are real. The stroma underlying an epithelial detachment
displays reactive changes (Fig. 4.37; se also Fig. 4.4). The surface of an erosion is usually flat, although covered by fibrin.
Even if the epithelium encircling the erosion is normal, one
must bear in mind that the denuded epithelium may have been
atypical.

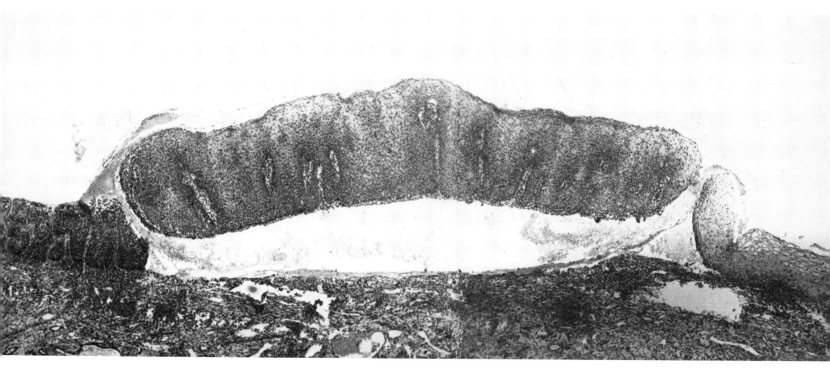

Microinvasive Carcinoma (Stage Ia)

The most recently published FIGO terminology divides microinvasive carcinoma (Stage Ia) into Stage Ia1, or early stromal invasion, and stage Ia2, or microcarcinoma (12). Early stromal invasion is a clear histological entity consisting of the first invasive expansion of atypical epithelium into the stroma. In contrast, a microcarcinoma is a frank, albeit small, tumor, and as such is a number of orders of magnitude larger than the lesions of early stromal invasion.

Early Stromal Invasion (Stage Ia1)

Early stromal invasion arises from carcinoma in situ or dysplasia (3). In this context it is easy to see that dysplasia may really be a well-differentiated form of intraepithelial carcinoma. The invasive foci form typical round, club-shaped, or finger-like processes extending from the base of the epithelium (Fig. 4.38). The less differentiated the parent epithelium is, the greater the contrast between it and the invasive buds. The latter show decreased cellularity; the cells and nuclei are enlarged, and the cytoplasm displays distinct eosinophilia. The cellular arrangement may be reminiscent of squamous pearls. One gains the impression that the invasive foci are better differentiated. The invasive buds usually measure only a fraction of a millimeter. The surrounding stroma shows characteristic changes, being loose, edematous, and infiltrated by round cells. The colposcopist must realize that early stromal invasion does not have the typical colposcopic pattern of frank invasion, and that the tiny invasive buds are not colposcopically visible (Fig. 4.39); see also Figs. 3.14 and 3.72). The more extensive an atypical colposcopic lesion is, the greater the chance that there is early invasion. Small-surfaced lesions are almost always preinvasive (see p. 50).

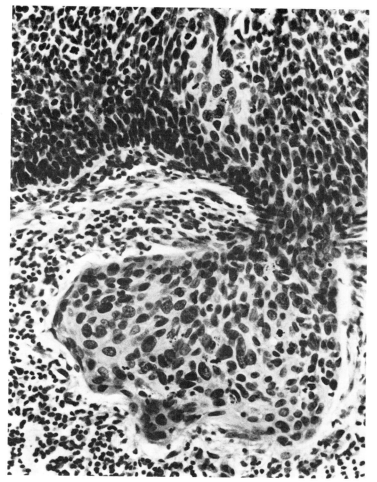

Fig. 4.**38** **Typical early stromal invasion.** The cells of the invasive focus show cytoplasmic clearing; the surrounding stroma is loose and infiltrated by round cells

Microcarcinoma (Stage Ia2)

According to the definition given above (p.19), microcarcinoma forms a small, measurable tumor that may be several millimeters in size and that can be seen with the naked eye on histologic slides (Fig. 4.40). The location of microcarcinoma has already been described (p.44).

Irrespective of its origin in the ectocervix or the endocervical canal, microcarcinoma forms a circumscribed tumor mass, usually just under the intact surface (Fig. 4.41). Less commonly, the surface is ulcerated (Figs. 4.42 and 4.44). Typical stromal changes are always present, and are confined to the immediate vicinity of the tumor (Figs. 4.42–4.44; see also Fig. 3.17). The changes include edema and a variable round-cell infiltrate, and resemble those seen with early stromal invasion. The blood vessels are more numerous and of larger caliber (Figs. 4.42 and 4.44).

Should invasion arise from a gland, the tumor lies deep in the stroma; the distance from the base of the surface epithelium may be several millimeters (Figs. 4.40, 20.4). Such a carcinoma may completely escape colposcopic detection.

If this is borne in mind, criteria for the colposcopic diagnosis of microcarcinoma depend on its location and its relationship to the surface. If it is situated high in the endocervical canal, it is well out of range of the colposcope.

Fig. 4.**39** **Early stromal invasion** arising from the base of carcinoma in situ (CIN 3) on the surface. Note the cytoplasmic clearing of the invasive bud and the inflammatory reaction around it

Fig. 4.**41** **This segment from a conization specimen** contains a small carcinoma arising from atypical epithelium on the surface. It invades to a depth of 4 mm. Its horizontal extent is 8 mm, exceeding the current definition of Stage Ia2. There is a distinct inflammatory response

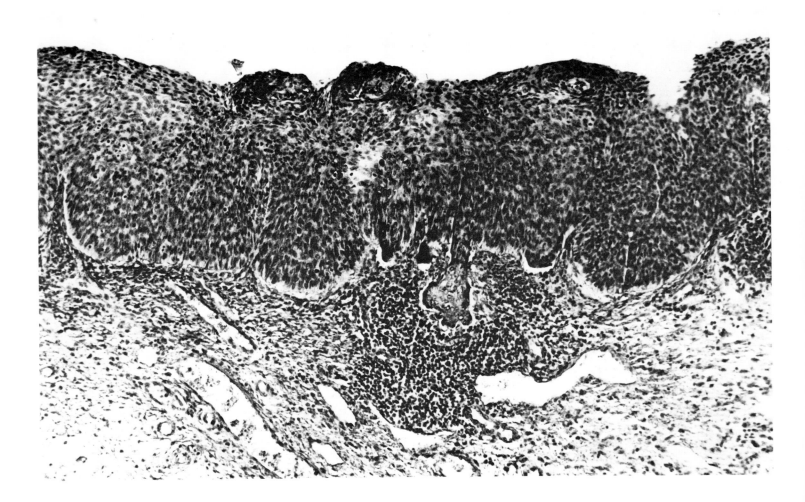

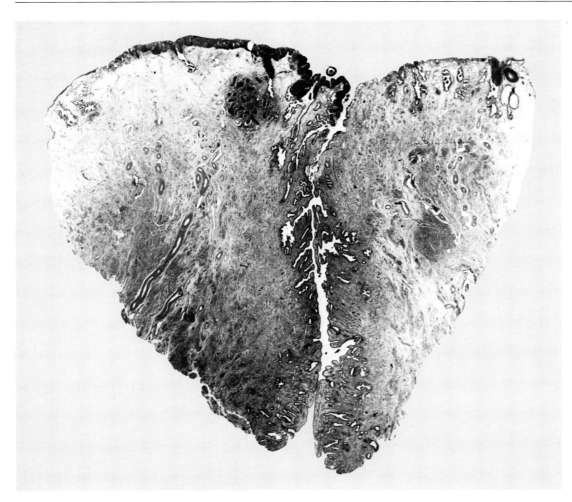

Fig. 4.**40 Conization specimen.** The left lip contains a microcarcinoma, which shows no connection with the surface epithelium. It measures approximately 3 mm in diameter, and reaches 6 mm in depth. This lesion can be seen with the naked eye in histologic sections. The surface and some crypts show carcinoma in situ (CIN 3), extending beyond the external os on the left

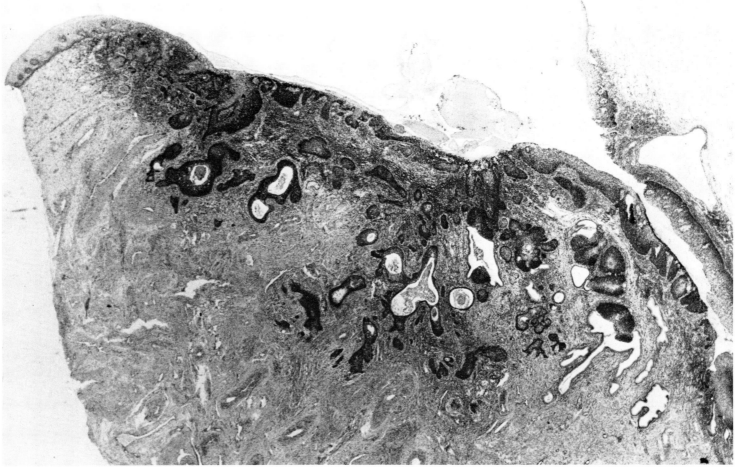

4.**41**

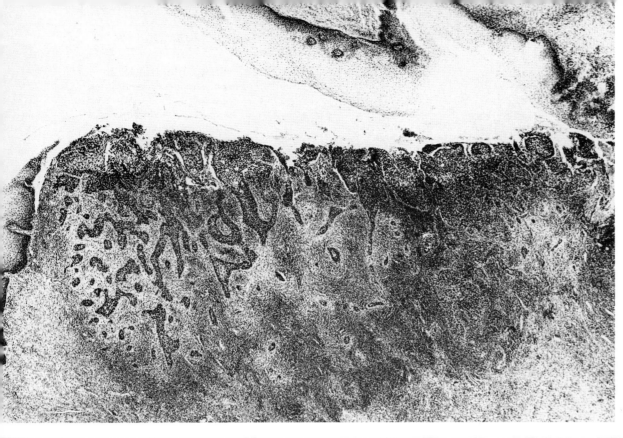

Fig. 4.**42** **Microcarcinoma on the external cervix.** The surface is ulcerated and there is, marked stromal reaction limited to the tumor. Superficial spread, 5 mm; maximum depth, 2 mm

Fig. 4.**43** This microcarcinoma invades to a depth of 2 mm. Its surface is focally ulcerated. The stromal reaction is marked

Fig. 4.**44** This microcarcinoma invades on a broad front. Its surface is ulcerated. There is increased vascularity, with many dilated and thin-walled capillaries

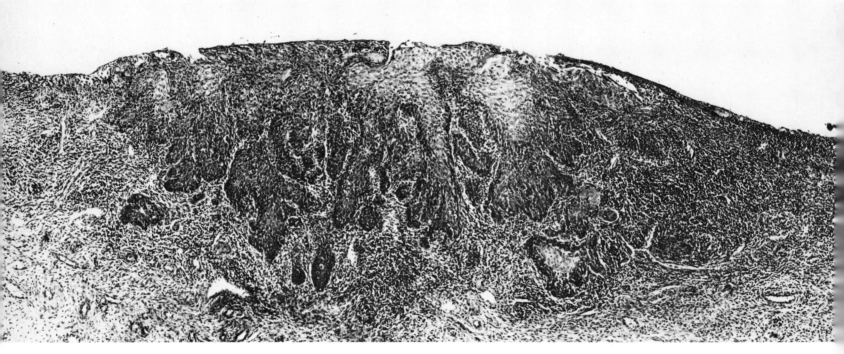

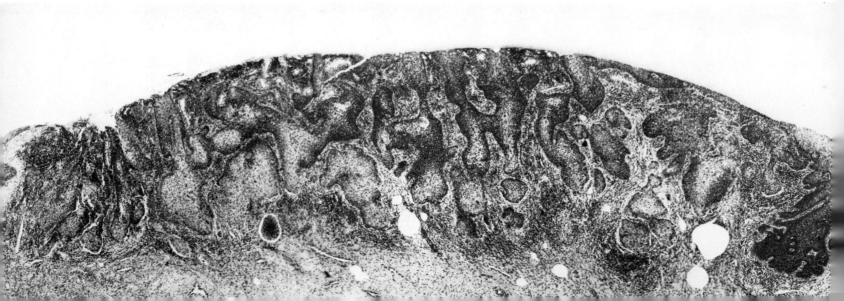

Clinically Invasive Carcinoma

It is not possible to distinguish colposcopically between squamous carcinoma and the less common adenocarcinoma. In spite of the various growth patterns invasive tumors may display (see p. 20), the colposcopic appearance is quite uniform. The surfaces of both the exophytic and endophytic types are irregular, fissured, and papillary.

Of particular importance is endophytic carcinoma, which causes little distortion of the shape of the cervix, the surface being merely ulcerated (Fig. 4.45; see also Fig. 3.19). Such a carcinoma may be overlooked. For this reason, flat ulcers should always be probed by a sound (see p. 111), as the cancerous tissue is easy to penetrate, whereas normal tissue and papillomas offer an elastic resistance. This does not apply to the rare scirrhous carcinomas, that are difficult to diagnose and may be discovered only by conization (Fig. 4.46).

It is often impossible to diagnose purely endocervical tumors by colposcopy. Deep-seated carcinomas may be visualized if the canal is capacious, or by opening the canal with an endocervical speculum. Unless the volume of a tumor is large, it may elude detection (Fig. 4.47), in which case one speaks of an *occult carcinoma*. This term has been used synonymously for microcarcinoma (11), but should be reserved for the designation of larger cancers that nevertheless cannot be diagnosed clinically and colposcopically. Classically, such tumors are detected by conization, carried out for the evaluation of atypical epithelium seen on the surface or in the canal.

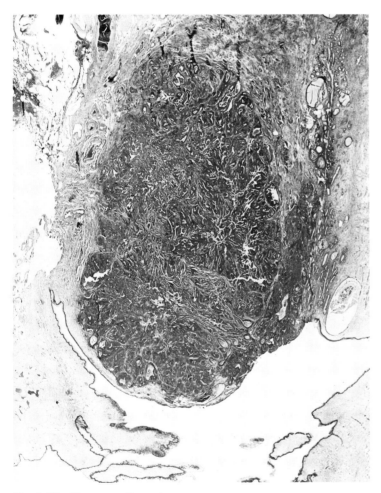

Fig. 4.45   Macrosection obtained at radical hysterectomy, with attached vaginal cuff, containing a predominantly endophytic squamous cell carcinoma with a flat, ulcerated surface

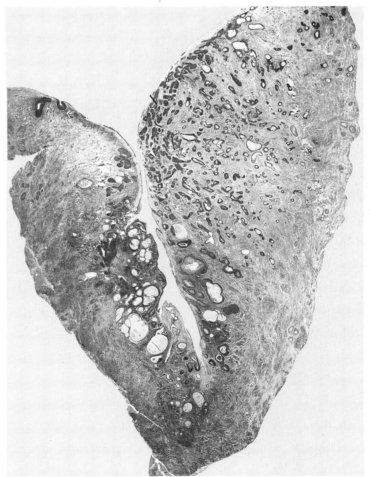

Fig. 4.46   Conization specimen showing extensive involvement of the crypts by carcinoma in situ (CIN 3) on the left. The lip on the right contains nests of invasive carcinoma. Note the absence of any stromal reaction

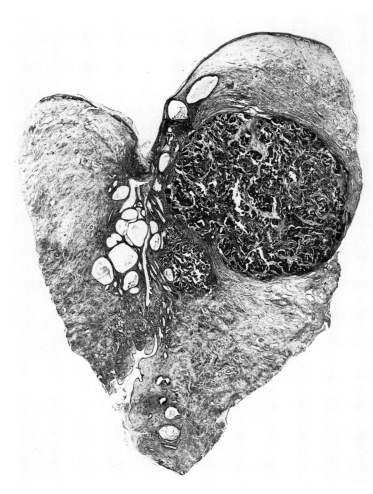

Fig. 4.**47   Conization specimen** containing two clearly circumscribed tumors lying under the surface epithelium. Note that the contour of the cervix is not distorted

Condylomatous Lesions

The colposcopic appearance of condylomatous lesions depends on their surface configuration. It is easy to see how the typical finger-like processes of papillary growths are determined by the histologic architecture (Fig. 4.48). Similarly, the epithelial excrescences of spiked condylomas account for the more or less tightly packed "spikes" (Figs. 4.49, 3.32). Keratinization (Fig. 3.30) may give the surface a homogenous, pearly finish, which may mask further structural details.

The markedly elongated stromal ridges or papillae are also important determinants of colposcopic configuration. Each contains a blood vessel, or several vessels of varying caliber (Fig. 4.50). Unless obscured by keratosis, these are easily visible.

Flat condylomas may appear colposcopically as punctation (Fig. 4.51) or mosaic, depending on whether the supporting stroma forms papillae or ridges (see p. 80). Because of the thickness of the epithelium and the height of the stromal papillae (Figs. 3.30, 3.32, and 3.33), the surface configuration of these lesions is coarser than that of similar colposcopic lesions due to atypical epithelia (Fig. 14.6).

It may be impossible to distinguish between a flat condyloma and an atypical epithelium (20, 21). Under no circumstances may it be assumed that lesions that occur outside the transformation zone are always condylomatous and not due to CIN.

Although supported by tall stromal papillae, the slightly altered glycogen-containing epithelium (Figs. 4.52, 3.34–3.36) of "condylomatous cervicitis and vaginitis" (see p. 178) is diffuse and poorly circumscribed; the poorly keratinized papillary spikes give rise to a white stippling colposcopically (Figs. 11.86, 11.87).

Fig. 4.**49   Typical "spikes" of an essentially flat condyloma.** The degree of cellular and nuclear atypia places this lesion in the CIN spectrum

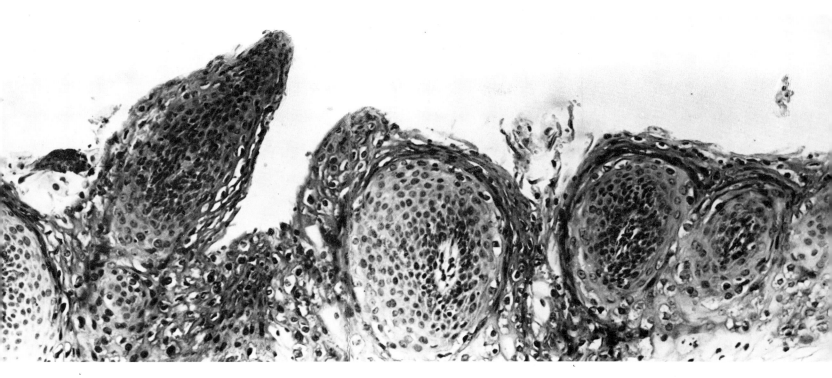

Fig. 4.**48** **Finger-like excrescences** of a papillary cervical condyloma. The cellular and nuclear pleomorphism is suggestive of dysplasia

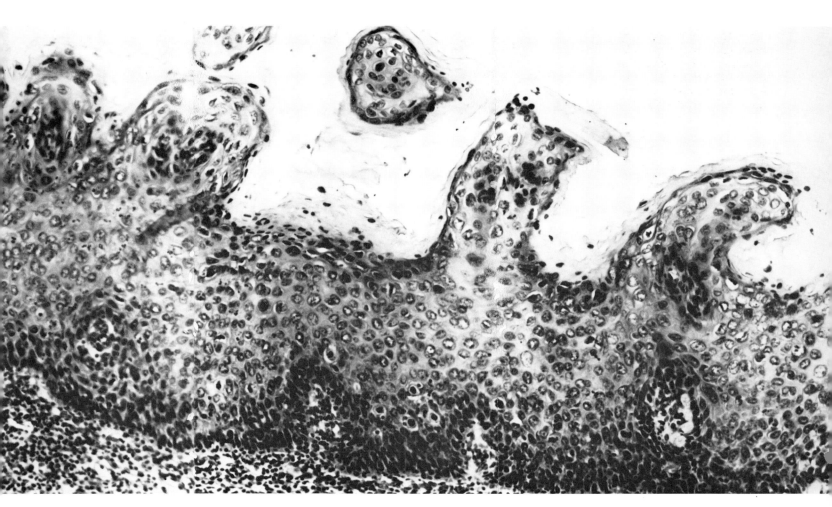

4.**49**

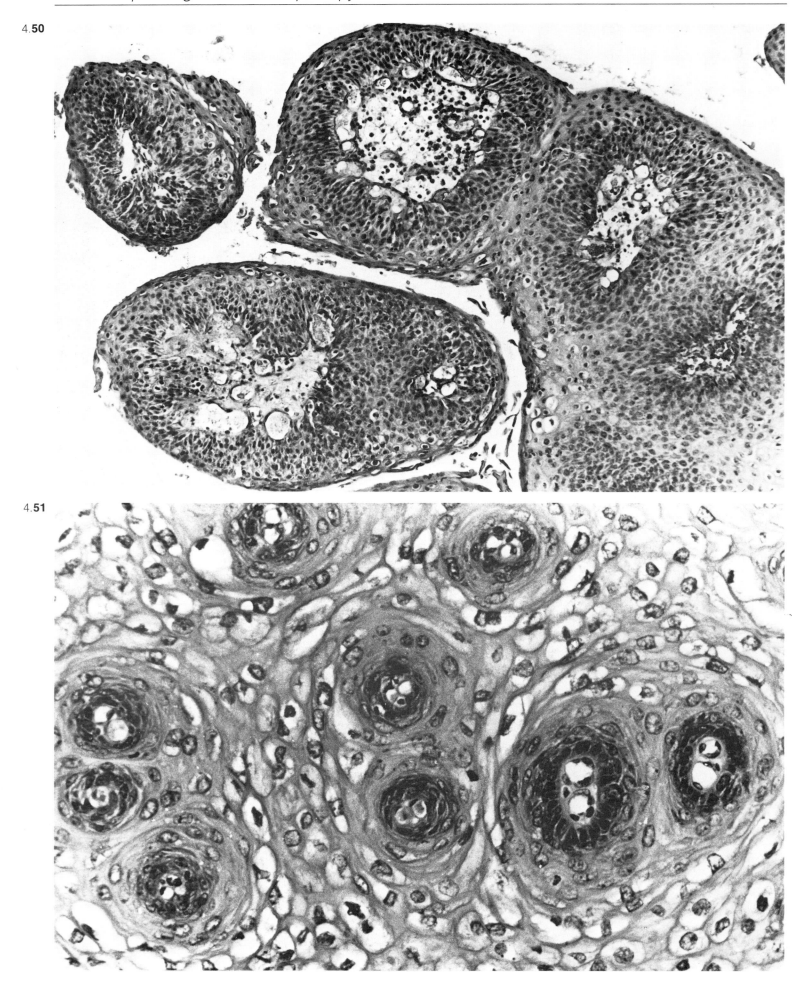

4.50

4.51

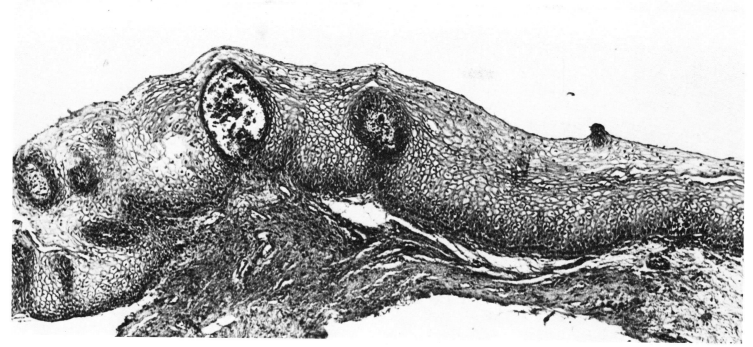

Fig. 4.**52** **Biopsy from a patient with "condylomatous vaginitis"** representing a distorted form of normal squamous epithelium. The broad stromal papillae and gently undulating surface enable it to be recognized

In contrast to acanthotic or atypical epithelium, which may also be characterized by prominent stromal papillae, condylomatous lesions usually contain a certain amount of glycogen (Figs. 4.51, 4.52; see also Figs. 3.31–3.36) and 3.40). In this way, an appearance may be produced that has hardly been mentioned in the colposcopic literature to date: an *iodine-positive mosaic* (see. Figs. 11.83, 11.85). This applies especially to flat condylomas but patchy iodine uptake may also be seen with papillary lesions (see Fig. 11.78).

Fig. 4.**50** **The hefty stromal papillae of this papillary condyloma** contain numerous capillaries, some of which are dilated. There is only mild cellular and nuclear pleomorphism

Fig. 4.**51** **Tangential cut through a flat condyloma.** The stromal papillae that perforate the epithelium account for the colposcopic appearance of punctation

Adenocarcinoma in Situ and Microinvasive Adenocarcinoma

There is as yet no specific colposcopic appearance on which the diagnosis of adenocarcinoma in situ, or indeed early invasive adenocarcinoma, can be made. Since 1961, 48 cases of adenocarcinoma in situ and 11 cases of small or early invasive adenocarcinomas have been diagnosed in conization specimens at our clinic. The detection of the 59 cases was entirely incidental, the tumor being associated with squamous CIN or microinvasive squamous cell carcinoma, the presence of which was the indication for conization. In 11 of the 59 cases, the colposcopic examination showed no atypia, in spite of visible transformation zones.

A previous study (24) showed that more than half of the early invasive adenocarcinomas arose in the endocervical canal in its distal portion. Most cases were detected because of coexistent squamous atypia of the ectocervix.

References

1   De Brux J, Dupré-Froment J. La métaplasie active indifférenciée immature. Ann Anat Pathol 1961;6:347.

2   Burghardt E. Über die atypische Umwandlungszone. Geburtshilfe Frauenheilkd 1959;19:676.

3   Burghardt E. Early histological diagnosis of cervical cancer. Stuttgart: Thieme; Philadelphia: Saunders, 1973.

4   Burghardt E, Holzer E. Die Lokalisation des pathologischen Cervixepithels, 1: Carcinoma in situ, Dysplasien und abnormes Plattenepithel. Arch Gynäkol 1970;209:305.

5   Castano-Almendral A, Beato M. Die Frühstadien des Plattenepithelcarcinoms des Collum uteri, 2: Histometrische Untersuchungen. Arch Gynäkol 1968;205:428.

6   Coppleson M. The new colposcopic terminology. J Reprod Med 1976;16:214.

7   Coppleson M. Report of Committee for Transformation Zone. London, 1981.

8   Coppleson M, Reid B. Preclinical carcinoma of the cervix uteri. Oxford: Pergamon Press, 1967.

9   Coppleson M, Pixley E, Reid B. Colposcopy. Springfield, IL: Thomas, 1978.

10 Dietel H, Focken A, Das Schicksal des atypischen Epithels an der Portio. Geburtshilfe Frauenheilkd 1955;15:593.

11 Fidler HK, Boyd JR. Occult invasive squamous carcinoma of the cervix. Cancer 1960;13:764.

12 FIGO news: changes of the 1985 FIGO report on the result of treatment in gynecological cancer. Int I Gynaecol Obstet 1987;25:87.

13 Glatthaar E. Studien über die Morphogenese des Plattenepithelkarzinoms der Portio vaginalis uteri. Basle: Karger, 1950.

14 Gore H, Hertig AT. Definitions. In: Gray LA, ed. Dysplasia, carcinoma in situ and microinvasive carcinoma of the cervix uteri. Springfield, IL: Thomas, 1964:83.

15 von Haam E, Old JW. Reserve cell hyperplasia, squamous metaplasia and epidermization. In: Gray LA, ed. Dysplasia, carcinoma in situ and microinvasive carcinoma of the cervix uteri. Springfield, IL: Thomas, 1964:41.

16 Hamperl H, Kaufmann C. Ober KG. Histologische Untersuchungen an der Cervix schwangerer Frauen. Arch Gynäkol 1954;184:181.

17 Hamperl H, Kaufmann C. Ober KG, Schneppenheim P. Die "Erosion" der Portio (Die Entstehung der Pseudoerosion, das Ektropion und die Plattenepithelüberhäutung der Cervixdrüsen auf der Portiooberfläche). Virchows Arch [A] 1958;331:51.

18 Hinselmann H. Das klinische Bild der indirekten Metaplasie der ektopischen Zylinderzellenschleimhaut der Portio. Arch Gynäkol 1928;133:64.

19 Howard L Jr, Erickson CC, Stoddard LD. A study of the incidence and histogenesis of endocervical metaplasia and intraepithelial carcinoma. Cancer 1951;4:1210.

20 Meisels A, Fortin R, Roy M. Condylomatous lesions of the cervix, 2: cytologic, colposcopic and histopathologic study. Acta Cytol 1977;21:379.

21 Meisels A, Morin C, Casas-Cordero M, Roy M, Fortier M. Condylomatöse Veränderungen der Cervix, Vagina und Vulva. Gynäkologe 1981;14:254.

22 Meyer R. Die Epithelentwicklung der Cervix und Portio vaginalis uteri und die Pseudoerosio congenita. Arch Gynäkol 1910;91:579.

23 Meyer R. Die Erosion und Pseudoerosion des Erwachsenen. Arch Gynäkol 1910;91:658.

24 Pickel H. Die Lokalisation des Adenocarcinoma in situ. Arch Gynäkol 1978;225:247.

25 Reid B, Coppleson M. Natural history: recent advances. In: Jordan JA, Singer A, eds. The cervix. Philadelphia: Saunders, 1976: 317.

26 Schneppenheim P, Hamperl H, Kaufmann C, Ober KG. Die Beziehungen des Schleimepithels zum Plattenepithel an der Cervix uteri im Lebenslauf der Frau. Arch Gynäkol 1958;190:303.

27 Song J. The human uterus. Springfield, IL: Thomas, 1964.

28 Stafl A. New nomenclature for colposcopy. Obstet Gynecol 1976;4:123.

29 Stafl A, Mattingly RF. Colposcopic diagnosis of cervical neoplasia. Obstet Gynecol 1973;41:168.

30 Stafl A, Mattingly RF. Angiogenesis of cervical neoplasia. Am J Obstet Gynecol 1975;121:845.

31 Stafl A, Linhartová A, Dohnal V. Das kolposkopische Bild der Felderung und seine Pathogenese. Arch Gynäkol 1963;199:223.

32 Treite P. Die Frühdiagnose des Plattenepithel-Karzinoms am Collum uteri. Stuttgart: Enke, 1944.

5

The Colposcope

MEDICAL LIBRARY
ODSTOCK HOSPITAL
SALISBURY SP2 8BJ

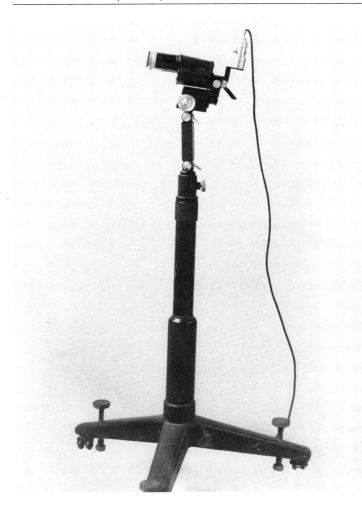

Fig. 5.**1** **First colposcope by Leitz** with a fixed mounting, the type used by *Hinselmann* (from the collection of the Graz Frauenklinik)

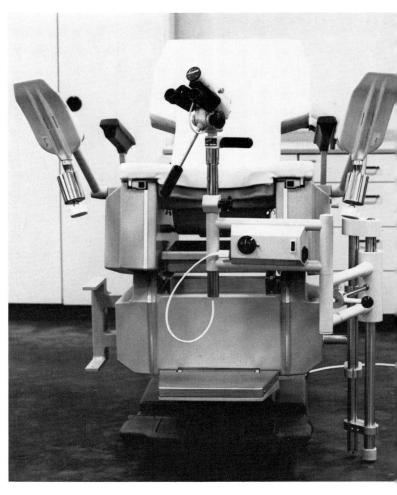

Fig. 5.**2** **Leisegang** (Berlin) **colposcope** (model I), which is mounted on the examination table

Hinselmann used Leitz lenses mounted on a pile of books for his first colposcopic examination (1). An ordinary lamp normally used for gynecologic examination was the light source; when placed above the operator's head, it allowed illumination of the cervix. The first colposcope was a fixed binocular instrument mounted on a tripod and equipped with a light source and a mirror to center the light on the field to be examined (Fig. 5.1).

The modern colposcope is based on this prototype, but differs from the original in that the magnification varies between 6 and 40 times, as opposed to the initial 7.5 times. A 10 times enlargement is most suitable for routine use. Higher magnification enables recognition of minor features, but is not necessary for accurate diagnosis. The colposcope should be equipped with a *green filter* that can be easily swung into position: it filters out red and thereby enhances the vascular appearance by making the vessels dark.

The colposcope may be mounted in different ways. For routine use, a swivel arm attached to the examiner's chair is most suitable (Fig. 5.2). This can be easily adjusted by hand in both vertical and horizontal directions. The mobile but mounted colposcope is independent of the examination couch, and may be moved from place to place (Fig. 5.3a). It may also

be fitted with a swivel arm and, when the wheels are locked, may be used in the same way as the examination-table mounted model. Recently, colposcopes mounted on the wall have become available that are easy to handle on account of their mobility, (Fig. 5.4). The head of the instrument may be tilted up, down, and sideways. There is usually no need for the fine adjustment, as a sharp focus can be achieved just as easily by positioning the instrument at the right working distance, the latter being between 20 and 24 cm, depending on the model.

The most important accessories are the photographic equipment and the teaching arm (Fig. 5.3b). Colpophotography is described in more detail elsewhere (see pp. 240–242, Documentation of Colposcopic Findings). The teaching arm is an invaluable aid. Although only monocular, it offers the beginner under instruction by an experienced colposcopist a visual display that no atlas can replace. The eyepiece can of course be adjusted to individual requirements. The observation tube is designed to be long enough for the presence of the second person not to disturb the patient (see Fig. 6.1).

Simple low-power instruments without any accessories are also available (Fig. 5.4), as well as more sophisticated ones with an electrically operated zoom lens and fine adjustment and camera (Fig. 5.3). The prices vary accordingly. For routine

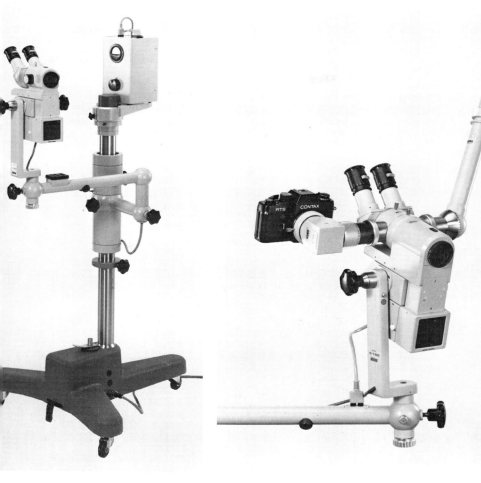

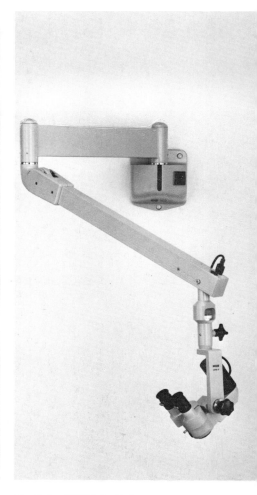

Fig. 5.**3 a** **OPMI 1 H—Zeiss colposcope,** Oberkochen. Basic equipment with quintuple magnification changer and fine power

Fig. 5.**3 b** **OPMI 6 SH—Zeiss colposcope,** Oberkochen. Basic equipment with zoom magnification changer and power fine focus

Fig. 5.**4** **OPMI 9—Zeiss colposcope,** Oberkochen, wall mounted with swivel arm

use, the simple colposcope is quite adequate, but for teaching both a camera and an observation tube are mandatory.

Reference

1 Hinselmann H. Die Ätiologie, Symptomatologie und Diagnostik des Uteruscarcinoms. In: Veit J, Stöckel W, eds. Handbuch der Gynäkologie, vol. 6:1. Munich: Bergmann, 1930:854.

6
Colposcopic Training

As with the learning of any endoscopic method, the pupil must become familiar with the instruments and the technique of the examination. Furthermore, he or she must learn to recognize and evaluate the colposcopic findings in the vagina and the cervix.

Mastery of the Instruments and Technique of Examination

The colposcope is a relatively simple instrument (see Chapter 5), the handling of which should pose no difficulty even for the beginner. As with ordinary binoculars, the eyepieces can be individually adjusted. The instrument is focused by moving the swivel arm to the required working distance, which varies from instrument to instrument. It is usually unnecessary to use the fine focus. The built-in light source provides optimal illumination.

It is helpful for the beginner to examine various objects as if with a magnifying glass: these may include one's own hand, small print, or a coin. The various color filters and enlargements may be tried out at the same time.

The beginner commonly makes the mistake of choosing too high a magnification. For routine use, magnification of 10 times is quite adequate. Higher magnification is needed only for the delineation of certain details. Lesser enlargements may be used for panoramic photographs, provided the camera is able to cope with the various magnifications.

Colpophotography is simple and produces high-quality pictures as long as the cervix is well exposed (see Chapter 16) and the camera correctly focused.

Understanding the Colposcopic Findings

Basic knowledge of colposcopic theory is a prerequisite to its practical application. Appreciation of cervical pathology is essential (see Chapter 3). Only by correlating colposcopic and histologic changes can the colposcopic findings be correctly interpreted (see Chapters 4 and 15). Finally, a connecting thread must be woven between the various colposcopic appearances to formulate a concept of physiologic and pathologic processes that take place on the cervix.

It is best to obtain a biopsy of a colposcopically suspicious area as soon as it is detected, rather than to wait for the result of cytology. If one wishes to reduce the number of biopsies, one can wait for the result of cytology and obtain another smear if the findings of the initial one are normal. Under no circumstances should a colposcopically suspicous but cytologically negative lesion be ignored.

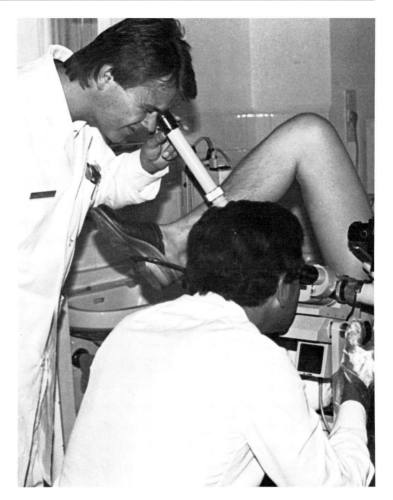

Fig. 6.**1** **The teaching arm** is an ideal method for demonstrating the colposcopic appearances

Practical Application
of the Equipment

Needless to say, one must be familiar with the colposcopic appearance before one can put the instrument to use. To this end one needs a well-illustrated textbook, or a set of teaching slides, or both. Once this knowledge is acquired, it is particularly helpful for the beginner to work with an experienced colposcopist who can demonstrate and explain each individual appearance step by step. This is best done with a teaching arm (Fig. 6.1), which, however, is unfortunately not fitted to every colposcope. Even so, the taking of the target biopsy should be demonstrated and eventually practiced by the pupil. In the training of the specialist, this is the method of choice.

The already practicing physician, for whom this type of training is impractical, is advised to study carefully the theoretical aspects. It is hoped that he or she will be able to find a suitable institution in which even a short time can be spent learning the practical application. Nowadays colposcopy courses are available both for beginners and the more advanced; individual problems can be discussed with the faculty.

Further knowledge and perfection of the method can be acquired only by practice. The time it takes and the degree of excellence reached depend on the way the colposcope is used. Ideally, colposcopy should be an integral part of every gynecologic examination. This is a convenient way to gain experience; it will also convince the practitioner that the method is not as costly and time-consuming as often stated. With repeated use of the method, a colposcopically unaided speculum examination will become unthinkable.

This method will above all expedite recognition of benign appearances, which are of fundamental importance. It will also pave the way for understanding the dynamics of the cervical events, which, if taking the wrong turn, will lead to the development of atypia. The beginner is advised to start with the study of ectopy and to continue with observation of the protean manifestations of the transformation zone. Only by familiarizing oneself with the above appearances can one recognize those that are no longer benign.

There are of course colposcopic appearances that are easy to categorize as benign or highly suspicious, even for the beginner. In between, however, is a whole spectrum of appearances, the evaluation of which is difficult (see Chapter 14). The same applies to cytology. The degree of uncertainty depends on the experience of the examiner. Only by obtaining a biopsy of every doubtful lesion can the beginner who is already in practice accelerate the learning process and avoid serious mistakes. By correlating the colposcopic with the histologic appearance in this way, the practitioner will gain confidence, and the number of unnecessary biopsies will decrease.

The chance of missing a significant finding is considerably reduced by the simultaneous use of cytology. Cytology, however, cannot be relied upon as the sole screening method, but should always be complemented by colposcopy; only in this way can the colposcope be put to best use.

7

Colposcopic Instrumentation

7.1

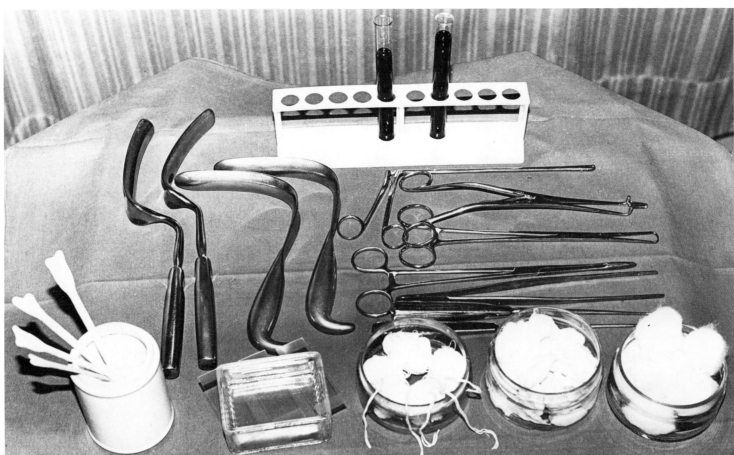

7.2

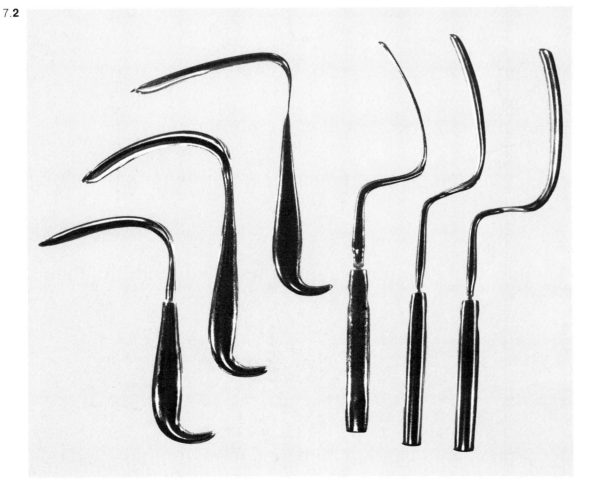

Fig. 7.1 **Instruments for colposcopic examination:** specula, anatomic forceps, tenacula, endocervical speculum, and biopsy instruments: *above*, iodine solution in test tubes; *below*, cotton-wool swabs, tampons, and utensils needed for obtaining and fixing cytology smears

Fig. 7.2 **Vaginal retractors of various sizes,** with the back blades on the left and front blades on the right

The colposcopic armamentarium is not expensive. In addition to the colposcope, one needs specula, biopsy instruments, an endocervical speculum, anatomic forceps, tenacula, and containers for cotton-wool swabs (Fig. 7.1).

Specula

Vaginal retractors (Fig. 7.2) or duckbill specula (Fig. 7.3) may be used. The retractors are useful for providing a clear view of the vagina. A disadvantage is that the front blade is best held by an assistant; however, the assistant can, in turn, expedite the examination by passing instruments and solutions (see Fig. 9.1). The self-retaining duckbill speculum has the advantage that it can be manipulated by the colposcopist alone (see Fig. 9.2). Because of the varying capacity of the vagina, specula of various types and sizes may have to be used.

Forceps

Anatomic forceps (Fig. 7.4, left) should have a minimum length of 20 cm, and are needed to hold dry and moist cotton-wool swabs. They are more practical than tenacula.

Endocervical Speculum

The endocervical speculum (Fig. 7.4), right), or similar instruments, allow inspection of the endocervical canal and are employed to best advantage in the multigravida. Ideally, the distal dilating jaws should be able to be displaced laterally from the remaining shaft of the instrument, so that visibility is not obscured when the instrument is introduced into the canal.

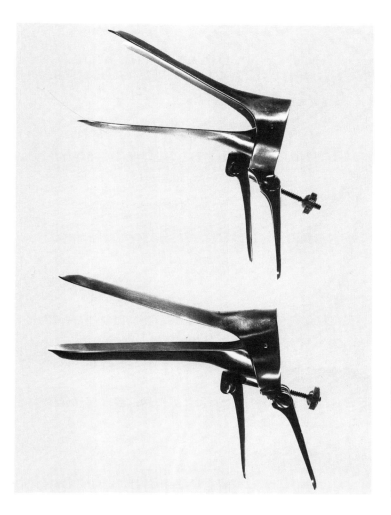

Fig. 7.**3** **Duckbill specula** of various calibers

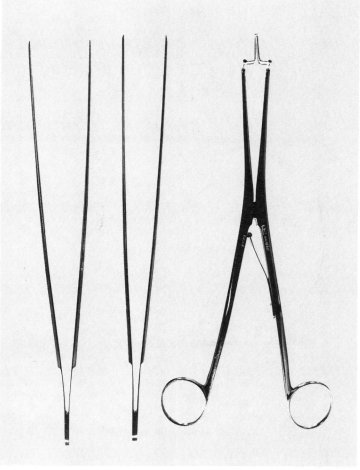

Fig. 7.**4** **Anatomic forceps (left) and endocervical speculum (right)**; the latter allows better exposure of the endocervical canal

Containers

The walnut-sized cotton-wool swabs are stored in sterilized metal cylinders. For the examination, they are placed in a bowl from which they can be easily removed with forceps. For the acetic acid test (see p. 114) they are soaked in 3% acetic acid and handled by forceps. Lugol's solution (see p. 117) is put into test tubes, which are placed in a rack. Tampons, which can be removed by the patient (Fig. 7.5), may be kept in a sterilizable metal container.

Biopsy Instruments

There are several types of biopsy instruments (Fig. 7.6). They are usually pistol-shaped, and have a scissors-like action, with shafts measuring between 20 and 25 cm.

Sharp curettes of various sizes are needed for scraping the endocervical canal, as well as for biopsy of clinically invasive cancers. For curettage of a narrow endocervical canal, instruments with fine, sharp grooves are more practical than spoon-shaped ones.

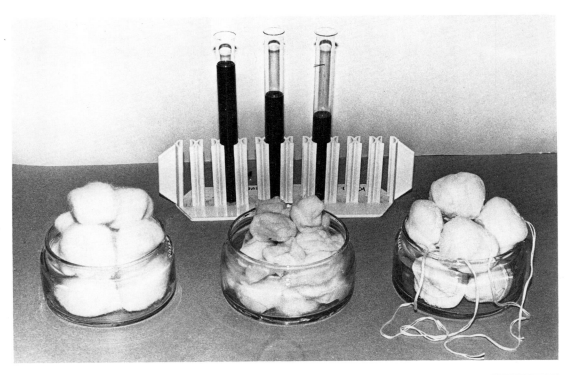

Fig. 7.5 **Iodine solution in test tubes:** far left, dry cotton-wool swabs; middle, cotton-wool swabs saturated with acetic acid; right, tampons with strings used to arrest bleeding following biopsy

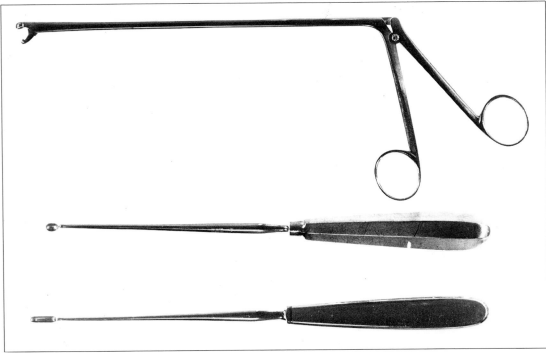

Fig. 7.6 *From top to bottom:* punch biopsy forceps, sharp spoon-shaped and grooved biopsy instruments used for endocervical curettage

Tenacula

To prevent slipping of the biopsy punch, and to obtain a true target biopsy, fixation of the cervix is sometimes necessary. With the tenaculum (Fig. 7.7, below) it is easy to grip and position the cervix without causing any pain. Cervical polyps can be avulsed easily with polyp forceps (Fig. 7.7, above).

Chrobak's Sound

Chrobak's sound (Fig. 7.8) is useful to distinguish between invasive carcinomas, on the one hand, and papillomas or flat ectocervical ulcers on the other (see p. 164–165). It is a thin sound with a bulbous head. In contact with normal tissue or benign tumors, it encounters an elastic resistance; however, it sinks into soft malignant tissue as if it were butter.

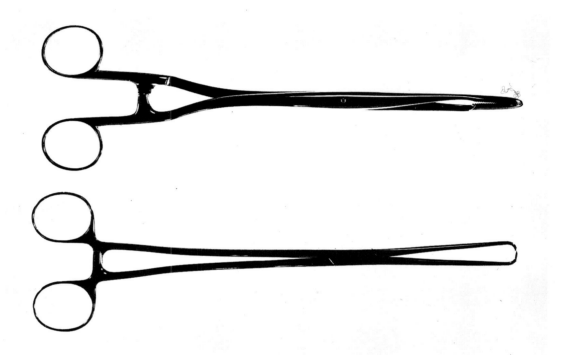

Fig. 7.**7** *Above:* polyp forceps for avulsing cervical polyps; *below:* tenaculum for gripping and fixing the cervix

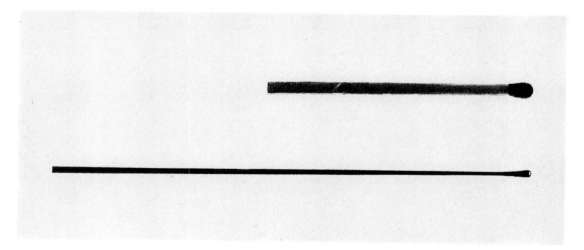

Fig. 7.**8** **Chrobak's sound**

8

Special Colposcopic Techniques

The application of the acetic acid test and the Schiller test, as well as the use of the green filter, can all be traced back to Hinselmann. They form an integral part of every colposcopic examination, even today. A host of other techniques have been suggested, however, that have no place in routine diagnostic practice, but are of use for delineation of certain problem areas only.

Acetic Acid Test

Initially, Hinselmann used a 3% solution of acetic acid mainly to get rid of mucus (3, 4). After removal of the vaginal secretions with dry cotton-wool swabs (see Chapter 9) the cervical epithelium is still masked to some extent by a film of mucus. This is especially so in cases of ectopy. Cleansing the cervix (see p. 127) with acetic acid enhances the colposcopic features. This applies especially to the demonstration of the grape-like structure of columnar epithelium in ectopy. However, all epithelial lesions become more distinct: the color changes are accentuated, and the various structures become more easily distinguishable from each other (Fig. 8.1 a, b).

Ectopy shows a distinct color change after application of acetic acid. The intense dark red ectopic columnar epithelium becomes paler and displays shades of pink to white. At the same time, the grape-like structures become more pronounced because of swelling and enlargement of the villi. The acetic acid therefore not only affects the mucus, but also interacts with certain epithelia, making them swell and change their color (Fig. 8.2 a, b).

Similar changes may be effected on altered epithelia, as first described by Burghardt in 1959 (1) in connection with the definition of the *atypical transformation zone*. He found that the epithelial swelling caused by acetic acid turns atypical epi-

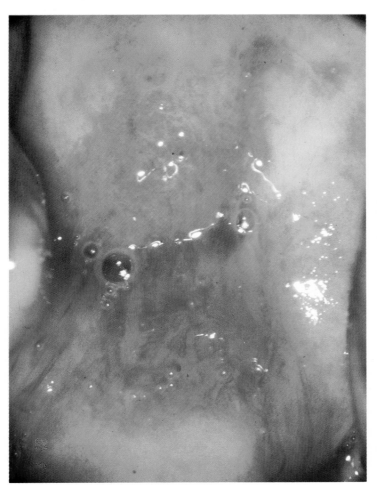

Fig. 8.**1 a** **Typical transformation zone** before the application of acetic acid. The fine details are clouded by mucus

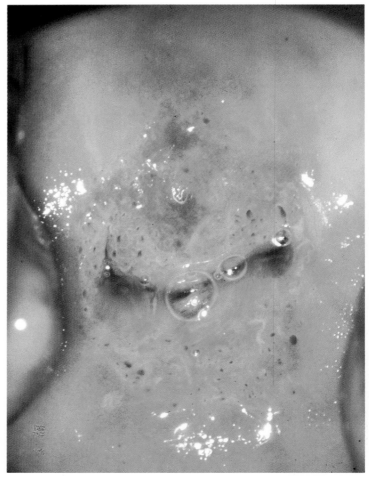

Fig. 8.**1 b** **Removal of the mucus after acetic acid** allows the emergence of the transformation zone with its gland openings

thelium white and accentuates its surface contour (Fig. 8.3 a, b). The mosaic and punctation patterns also became more distinct, and the red partitions or the fine petechiae stood out against the white epithelium (Fig. 8.4 a, b).

Since the effect on pathologic epithelium is not as rapid as on ectopic columnar epithelium, one must always wait for its appearance. The white epithelium that appears after application of acetic acid should not be confused with leukoplakia.

Occasionally, however, poorly keratinized surface lesions will become visible only after the cleansing action of acetic acid, when they immediately change from pale white to gray, do not undergo swelling, and do not change with time.

Acetic acid therefore plays a decisive role in colposcopic diagnosis (see Chapter 9), and no colposcopic examination is complete without it.

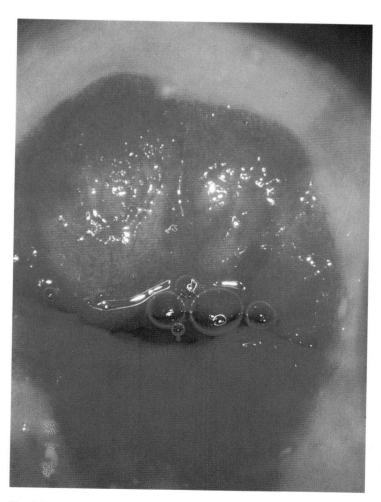

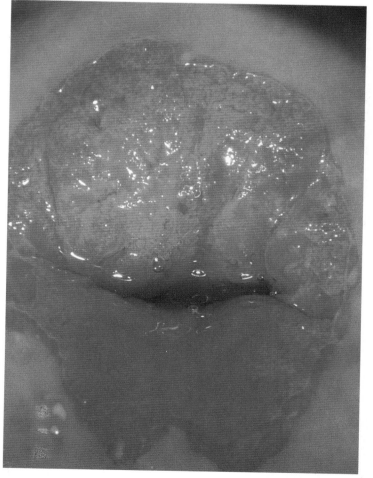

Fig. 8.**2 a** **Large, intensely red area around the external os.** The border with the normal squamous epithelium seems abrupt. The apparent alteration extends into the cervical canal

Fig. 8.**2 b** **Application of acetic acid evokes the grape-like structure of the mucosa covered by columnar epithelium.** Note the blanching of the previously intensely red area caused by the swelling of the columnar epithelium. In the adjacent squamous epithelium on the posterior lip of the cervix, individual gland openings indicate that transformation has occurred

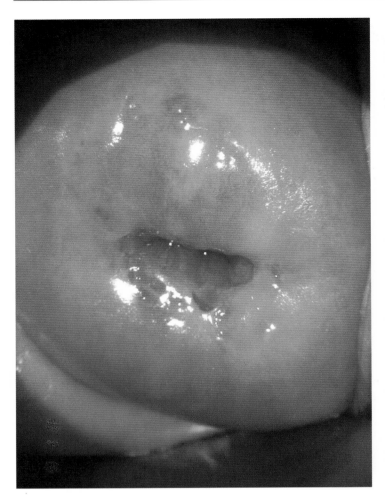

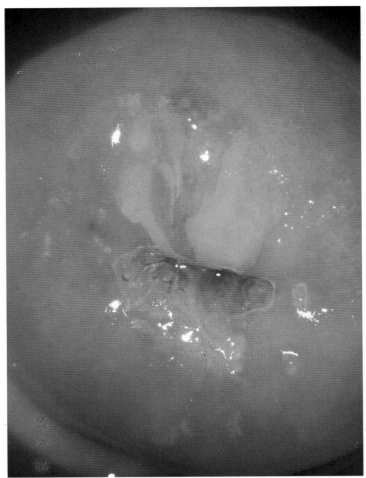

Fig. 8.3 a   An indistinct red area on the anterior lip of the external os. On the posterior lip there is a small, intensely red area

Fig. 8.3 b   Application of acetic acid reveals a number of sharply demarcated white areas on the anterior lip. There are some cuffed gland openings near the white areas. Histology showed moderate dysplasia (CIN 2). The area on the posterior lip is columnar epithelium with a narrow transformation zone on the edge of it

Fig. 8.4 a   Prior to the application of acetic acid, the transformation zone is inconspicuous. Only the experienced colposcopist will detect an early lesion at the 12-o'clock position, outside the transformation zone

Fig. 8.4 b   The white color and mosaic pattern of histologically severely dysplastic epithelium (CIN 3) are due to cellular edema caused by acetic acid

8.**4a**

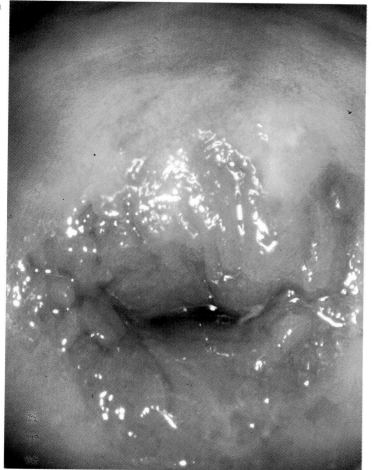

8.**4b**

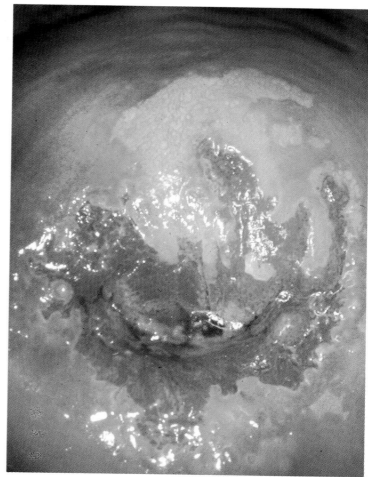

Schiller Test

Lugol's iodine solution was first used in clinical diagnosis by Schiller in 1929 (6), and it has been employed advantageously ever since (5, 7–14). Hinselmann applied it in his so-called expanded colposcopy (4). Unfortunately, its value is being debated at the present time. Some eminent colposcopists do not use it or do not refer to it, which is also unfortunate because the *Schiller* test may yield important additional information for the evaluation of colposcopic morphology. The 1% iodine solution consists of

> iodine, 2 g;
> potassium iodide, 4 g;
> distilled water, 200 g.

The *Schiller* test depends on the interaction between iodine and glycogen. The glycogen-containing vaginal epithelium of women of childbearing age takes up iodine to produce an intense mahogany brown. Glycogen-free epithelium does not stain (Fig. 8.5) with iodine. Such an area is referred to as *Schiller positive* or *iodine negative*. This, however, is a simplification, as these designations do not indicate the full spectrum of reactions obtained with iodine.

1. Iodine solution stains *normal glycogen-containing squamous* epithelium uniformly deep brown. Such epithelium is found during the reproductive period, when under the influence of estrogens (Fig. 8.5).

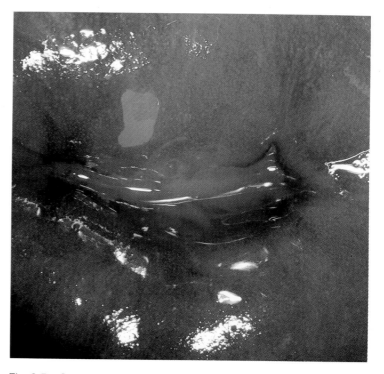

Fig. 8.**5 Original squamous epithelium** displays uniform mahogany staining with iodine. Note a sharply demarcated iodine-negative area at the 11-o'clock position, referred to as Schiller-positive

2. Columnar epithelium does not take up iodine (Fig. 8.6) nor does thin regenerating epithelium, seen during the early stages of squamous metaplasia or ascending healing (Fig. 8.7). Failure to stain with iodine is useful for the assessment of inflammatory lesions, which, because of their increased vascularity and dilatation of the capillaries, may mimic punctation, but their margins are indistinct and do not react significantly with iodine (Fig. 8.8 a, b).

3. Developing atypical epithelium, on the other hand, reacts with iodine as described below (5) even while still thin. This is an important difference between the normal and the unusual transformation zone.

4. A colposcopic lesion, as well as the whole length of the vagina, may display all shades between tan and the chestnut brown of normal squamous epithelium (Fig. 8.9). The vagina may also have a stippled brown appearance, especially during menopause, when the effect of estrogen is waning. The postmenopausal cervix and vagina stain light brown to yellow (Figs. 8.10 and 11.3).

The various shades of brown of the *normal transformation zone* depend on the *maturity*, that is, the glycogen content, of the squamous epithelium (Fig. 8.11). The squamous epithelium in the fully developed transformation zone stains mahogany brown. The transformation zone in such cases can be recognized only by the gland openings and the retention cysts (Fig. 8.12a, b). The deep-brown color distinguishes it from the unusual transformation zone, as atypical and acanthotic epithelia are glycogen-free.

8.6

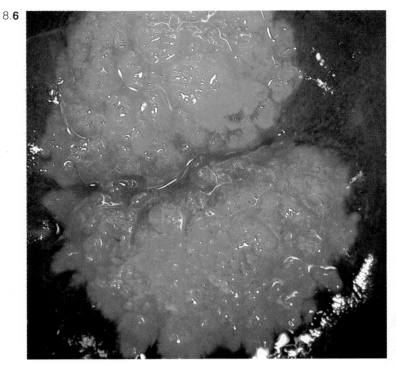

8.7

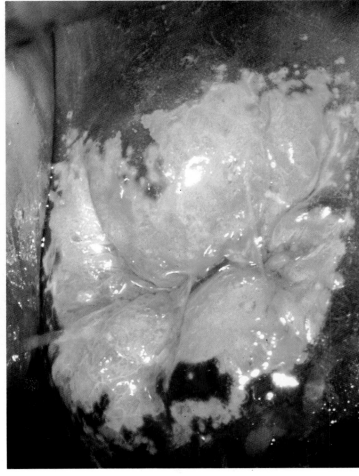

Fig. 8.**6** **The columnar epithelium of an ectopy does not stain with iodine,** and merely shows a slight discoloration due to the thin film of solution veiling it. The original epithelium stains characteristically deep brown

Fig. 8.**7** **The typical transformation zone does not stain with iodine.** Note the contrast with the mahogany color of original squamous epithelium

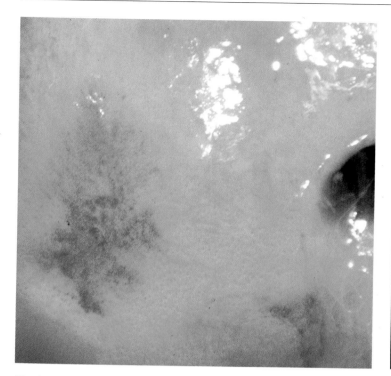

Fig. 8.8 a   Red, inflamed area lateral to the external os

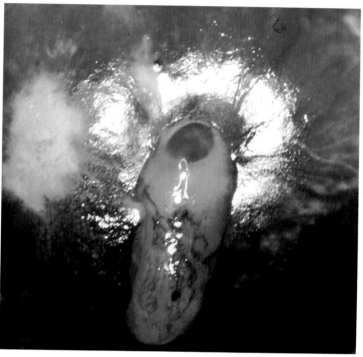

Fig. 8.8 b   This area does not stain with iodine, and is poorly demarcated from the adjacent deep-brown original epithelium

8.9

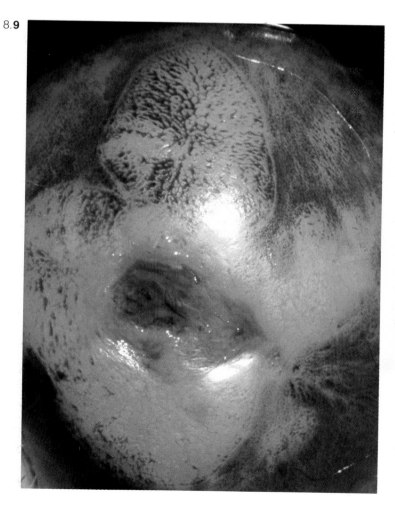

8.10

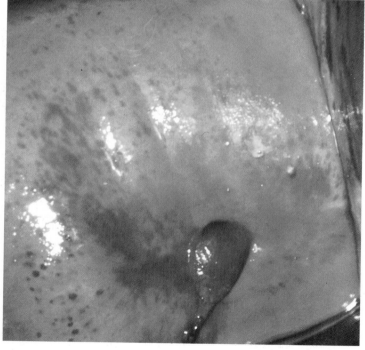

Fig. 8.9   This transformation zone has a stippled appearance with iodine, due to the various stages of development of the metaplastic epithelium

Fig. 8.10   Yellowish light-brown of atrophic epithelium after iodine staining. At least some of the dark spots are due to subepithelial hemorrhages

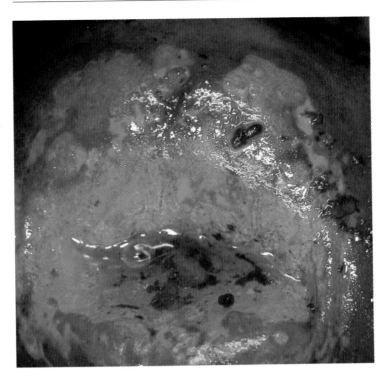

Fig. 8.**11** **When transformation is more advanced, various shades of brown may appear,** according to the maturity of the metaplastic epithelium

Fig. 8.**12 a** **Very different appearance of the transformation zones of the two lips.** On the anterior lip, the squamous epithelium is attenuated over retention cysts, and blood vessels course over their surfaces. The posterior lip displays aceto-white epithelium and gland openings

Fig. 8.**12 b** **Surprising reaction with iodine.** The epithelium covering the retention cyst is fully mature and contains glycogen. The area on the posterior lip, which stains partly yellow or not at all with iodine, was carcinoma in situ (CIN 3) histologically

8.**12 a**

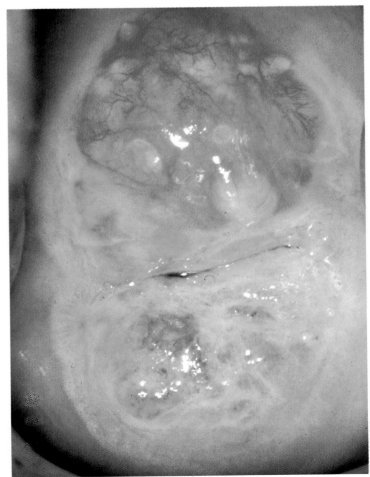

8.**12 b**

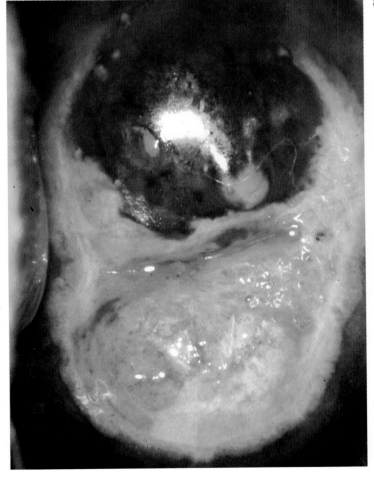

8.**13**

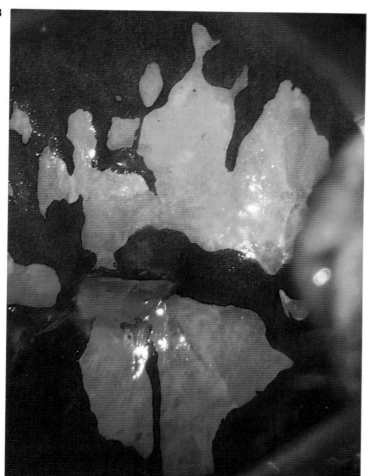

5. Iodine solution reacts with colposcopic lesions to produce a characteristic canary yellow shade, especially when due to *acanthotic or atypical epithelia* (Figs. 8.13–8.16) that are glycogen-free. Large transformation zones may become distinctly yellow, in which case the designation *unusual transformation zone* may be used. In some cases, only portions of the transformation zone stain yellow (Fig. 8.16). Such areas should be regarded with suspicion, should be carefully searched for, and should always be biopsied.

8.**14**

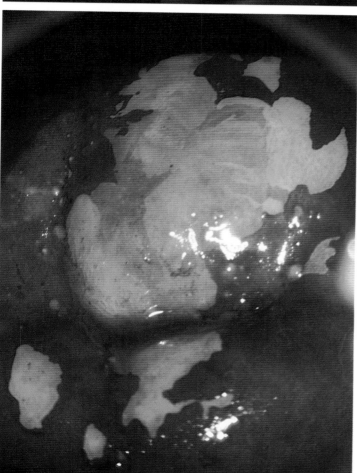

Fig. 8.**13** **Bizarre shape of inconspicuous iodine-yellow areas,** the contours of which remained unchanged over 5 years. Histology showed acanthotic epithelium

Fig. 8.**14** **Inconspicuous iodine-yellow area with different color tones,** from yellow to brown, corresponding to sharply demarcated epithelial fields. Histology showed acanthotic epithelium

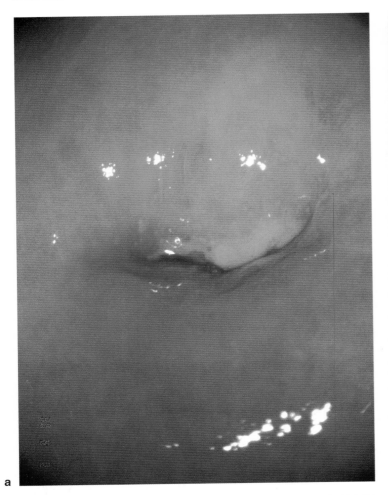

a

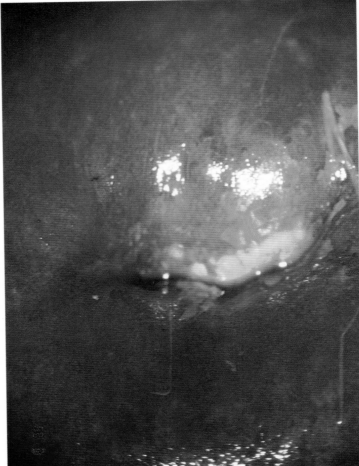

b

Fig. 8.**15a   Only after the application of acetic acid does** a small, easily missed white area appear on the anterior external os

Fig. 8.**15b**   After application of iodine, the area on the external os appears bright yellow. Histology showed moderate dysplasia (CIN 2) in the cervical canal

Fig. 8.**16   Patchy uptake of iodine by a partially unusual transformation zone.** Histology showed carcinoma in situ (CIN 3). On the left, within the transformation zone, there is a small condylomatous area with iodine-positive punctation. At 12 o'clock there is an isolated inconspicuous iodine-yellow area

6. The colposcopist who uses the Schiller test routinely will often see well-demarcated areas with a characteristic canary yellow color that otherwise escape colposcopic detection. Such an area, which is otherwise inconspicuous, is referred to as an *inconspicuous iodine-yellow area,* and is usually due to *acanthotic epithelium* (Fig. 8.5).

If the exact location of the inconspicuous iodine-yellow area has been noted, subsequent colposcopic examination after the effect of iodine has subsided can detect a fine color difference between this area and normal squamous epithelium (Fig. 11.51).

7. Not only the nuances of color, but also the borders between normal and altered epithelia may be viewed to advantage with the help of iodine. The epithelial borders within colposcopic lesions also become distinct (Fig. 8.4; see also Figs. 14.19b and 15.2). There is no better way to demonstrate the sharpness and clarity of epithelial borders. This is of great diagnostic import, as poorly circumscribed colposcopic areas are hardly ever significant (Figs. 8.6–8.9, 8.11).

The following is a summary of the various iodine reactions which are of diagnostic value.

Normal and benign reactions

1. Iodine positive = deep brown = normal glycogen-containing epithelium
2. Iodine negative = no reaction with iodine solution = columnar epithelium, immature transformation zone, inflammatory lesions
3. Weak reaction with iodine = various lighter shades of brown = waning estrogen effect, normal transformation zone in its various stages of development

Abnormal and suspicious reactions

4. Iodine-yellow area = characteristic canary yellow discoloration = mosaic, punctation, unusual transformation zone
5. Colposcopically inconspicuous iodine yellow area
6. Sharp demarcation in cases of (4) and (5)

The rapid action of iodine, together with its special significance, makes it an important diagnostic aid for the assessment of colposcopic findings (see Chapter 14).

References

1 Burghardt E. Über die atypische Umwandlungszone. Geburtshilfe Frauenheilkd 1959;19:676.
2 Friedell GH, Hertig AT, Younge PA. The problem of early stromal invasion in carcinoma in situ of the uterine cervix. Arch Pathol 1958;66:494.
3 Hinselmann H. Die Essigsäureprobe: Ein Bestandteil der erweiterten Kolposkopie. Dtsch Med Wochenschr 1938; 64:40.
4 Hinselmann H. Die Kolposkopie. Wuppertal: Girardet, 1954.
5 Kern G. Carcinoma in situ. Berlin: Springer, 1964.
6 Schiller W Jodpinselung und Abschabung des Portioepithels. Zentralbl Gynäkol 1929;53:1056.
7 Schiller W. Early diagnosis of carcinoma of the cervix. Surg Gynecol Obstet 1933;56:210.
8 Schiller W. Early diagnosis of carcinoma of the portio uteri. Am J Surg 1934;26:269.
9 Schiller W. Zur Frühdiagnose des Karzinoms der Portio uteri. Monatsschr Krebsbekämpfung 1934;2:7.
10 Schiller W. Pathology of the cervix. Am J Obstet Gynecol 1937;34:430.
11 Schiller W. Leukoplakia, leukokeratosis, and carcinoma of the cervix. Am J Obstet Gynecol 1938;35:17.
12 Younge PA. A gynecologist's evaluation of methods of early cancer diagnosis. In: Homburger F, Fishman WH, eds. The laboratory diagnosis of cancer of the cervix. New York: Karger, 1956.
13 Younge PA. Cancer of the uterine cervix: a preventable disease. Obstet Gynecol 1957;10:469.
14 Younge PA, Kevorkian AY. Carcinoma in situ of the cervix: the problems of detection and evaluation in regard to the therapy. London: Churchill, 1959. (Ciba foundation study group 3:83–103.)

9

The Colposcopic Examination

Positioning the Patient

The patient is examined in the lithotomy position. We prefer stirrups, which support only the feet and heels and allow bending of the knees and good separation of the thighs (Fig. 9.1). The examination stool should be adjustable to the required height. Provision should be made for proper positioning of the pelvis.

Exposure of the Cervix

The self-retaining duckbill speculum (see Fig. 7.3) may be used to expose the cervix. When inserted and opened, the speculum may be correctly positioned and held by the examiner's free hand (Fig. 9.2). The speculum should be as large as can be tolerated by the patient without discomfort. The tips of the blades should be in the fornices, which should be widely separated. This procedure provides a good view of the cervix and surrounding vaginal fornices, and also everts the lips of the multiparous cervix, allowing the lower portion of the endocervical canal to come into view; in this way, a pseudoectopy may be produced. The examination is useless and even dangerous if the vagina and cervix are poorly exposed, as important lesions may be missed and wrong diagnoses made.

We prefer vaginal retractors with a flat anterior and a grooved posterior blade, available in different lengths and widths (see Fig. 7.2). Placing the tips of these in the fornices should result in good exposure of the vagina and at times eversion of the lower canal. It is a great advantage to have a wide field of view at the vaginal opening (Fig. 9.3). The fact that the anterior retractor must be held in place by an assistant is a drawback (Fig. 9.1), but the assitant's free hand can expedite the examination. Even the patient herself may hold the anterior retractor once it is in the right position. The colposcopist guides the posterior blade and conducts the examination at the same time (Fig. 9.4).

The retractors are particularly useful if the cervix is difficult to expose because of anatomic deformity, such as stenosis or atrophy. In such circumstances, a second anterior speculum may be inserted on one or the other side (Fig. 9.5).

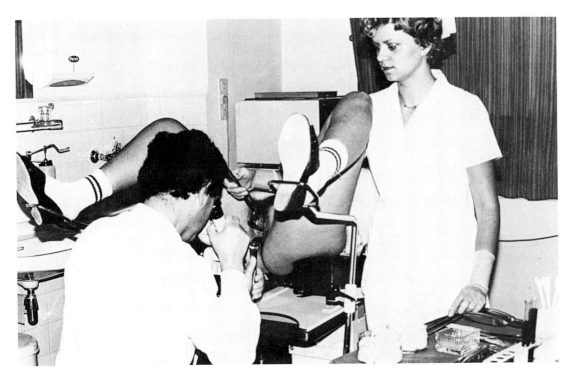

Fig. 9.**1 Colposcopic examination using vaginal retractors.** The anterior retractor is held by an assistant, who can also perform other tasks. Accessories are displayed on the tray

Initial Inspection

After exposing the cervix, one should assess the nature of the cervicovaginal secretions and note any obvious lesion in the fornices or on the cervix.

Removal of Mucus and Discharge

Vaginal secretions, which obscure the view, may be removed gently with cotton-wool swabs (see Fig. 7.5) held by forceps (see Fig. 7.4). Loss of epithelium and bleeding due to traumatic manipulation must be avoided.

First Colposcopic Examination

The cervix and exposed portions of the vagina can now be observed colposcopically. Differences in color, surface contour, and margins between lesions and normal tissues should be carefully noted.

Special attention should be paid to the blood vessels, which are better displayed at this stage of the examination than after the application of acetic acid (see Fig. 11.30). For this purpose, the green filter is particularly useful, as it shows the terminal angioarchitecture etched out in black, allowing a degree of discrimination not otherwise achieved. Routine use of this filter is recommended.

Acetic Acid Test

The whole cervix, and particularly all the visible lesions, are carefully dabbed with swabs saturated with acetic acid (see Fig. 7.5). The swabs are held with forceps, which also squeezes out the fluid. The lesions should be swabbed, not wiped, to avoid injury to the epithelium. Excess acetic acid may be soaked up by dry swabs.

Second Colposcopic Examination

The most important part of the colposcopic examination follows the application of acetic acid. The well-displayed changes can now be subjected to detailed scrutiny, which allows their definition and assessment. It is particularly important to observe any color change and swelling of the epithelium caused by the acetic acid. These are two important criteria by which colposcopic findings can be classified (see Chapter 14). It is important to realize that it may take a minute or so for maximal changes to develop.

Schiller Test

Approximately 3 ml of Lugol's iodine is poured into the posterior fornix (Fig. 9.6) from a test tube (see Fig. 7.5), and by manipulating the anterior retractor, the cervix is immersed in the fluid pool. Alternatively, one can apply the iodine in the same way as the acetic acid, by using swabs. Again, any excess is removed with dry swabs.

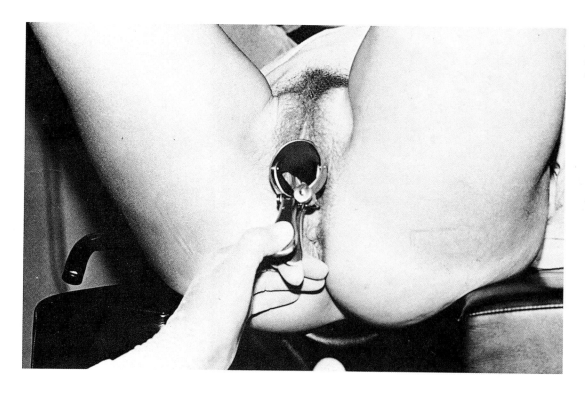

Fig. 9.**2 Examination with the duckbill speculum,** which can be easily manipulated by one hand

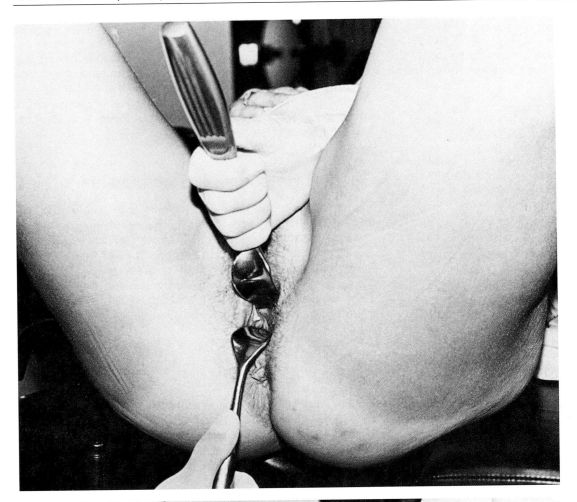

Fig. 9.3 **If the right size is chosen, retractors allow optimal exposure.** The anterior retractor is held by an assistant

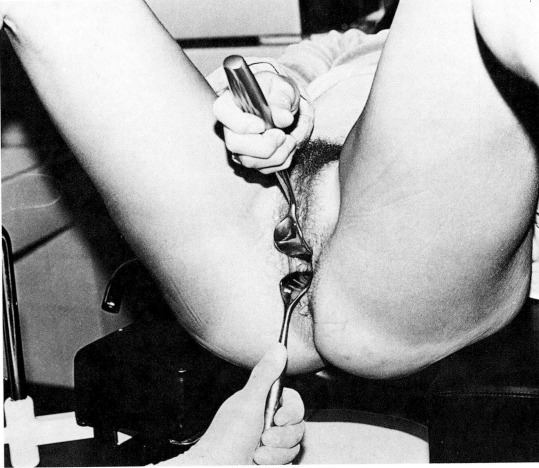

Fig. 9.4 **If an assistant is not available, the anterior retractor may be held by the patient** once it has been properly positioned by the examiner

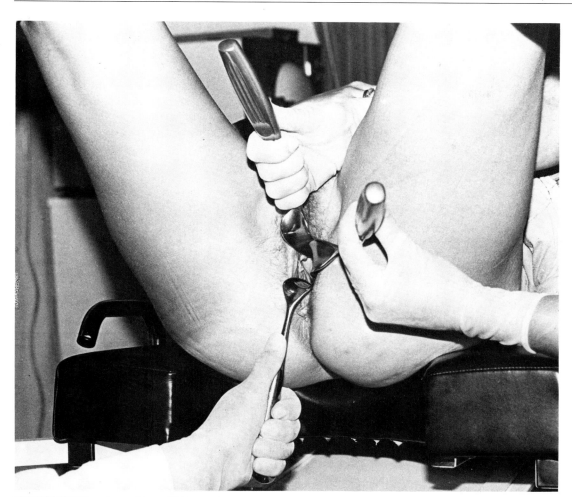

Fig. 9.**5** Exposure may be aided by inserting a third retractor

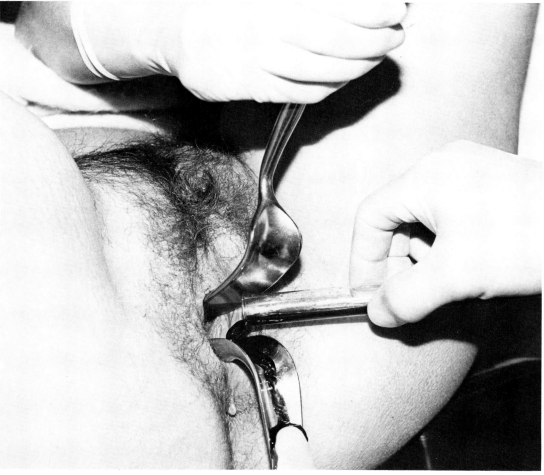

Fig. 9.**6** **The Schiller test** is performed by pouring several milliliters of Lugol's iodine from a test tube into the posterior fornix. The cervix is then immersed in the pool by manipulating the anterior retractor. Excess fluid is removed with dry swabs. This method produces more uniform staining than using wet swabs

Final Colposcopic Inspection

The final step in the examination, which follows the application of iodine, was introduced by Hinselmann very soon after the publication of Schiller's test, but is nowadays omitted by many colposcopists. The experienced colposcopist, however, would not do without it. Its value is inestimable (see Chapters 8 and 14). First, iodine may reveal typically yellow, sharply demarcated lesions previously unsuspected. Second, the exact color tone a lesion assumes may be of diagnostic value (see p. 117). Finally, there is no better way of demonstrating the sharp borders between normal and newly formed epithelia than with Lugol's iodine. Evaluation of a seemingly typical transformation zone is not complete without the Schiller test.

Following the examination of the cervix, the retractors are withdrawn slowly, so that any changes in the vagina may be observed.

Documentation of the Colposcopic Findings

This is carried out with photographs or sketches. To avoid taking too many pictures, it is best to photograph the cervix after the application of acetic acid. For further details, see Chapter 16.

Obtaining Smears

The time at which the smear is obtained depends on the method used. If one uses a cotton-tipped applicator or a platinum loop or aspirates the posterior fornix pool or the endocervical canal, it is best to take the smear immediately after the initial exposure of the cervix and prior to the mopping up of the secretions. Directed cytology smears can be taken from visible lesions on the ectocervix or from the endocervical canal during the initial colposcopic inspection.

If one elects to scrape the surface with an Ayre's spatula (see Fig. 7.1) the sequence of the colposcopic examination may have to be changed. The smear may be obtained at the same time, as described above, or it may be directed by taking it after removal of the vaginal secretions. Without exerting too much pressure, the loosely adherent or already exfoliating surface layers of some lesions may be easily detached by the spatula. This procedure, however, may cause bleeding, making the colposcopic examination more difficult. A delicate touch, however, should prevent bleeding.

If one still wishes to use Ayre's spatula, but without risk of bleeding interfering with the colposcopic examination, the taking of the smear may be delayed until after the acetic acid test has been completed. It is not true that the cell sample one wishes to obtain has already been removed. Scraping at this stage should be more vigorous, as bleeding is unlikely to interfere with the Schiller test.

We prefer Ayre's spatula in our clinic. The timing of obtaining the smear has been changed several times during the last 30 years. We have not found that the diagnostic accuracy of cytology is improved by any particular timing. In our experience, however, the numerical ratio of atypical to normal cells in abnormal smears is heavily weighted in favor of the former if the smear is taken after the application of acetic acid rather than prior to removal of the mucus.

For obtaining smears from the cervical canal, the Ayre's spatula may be used if one end is formed to a spine which can enter the canal deeply enough. A cytobrush is used for the same purpose.

Target Biopsy

Biopsies should be taken only after the colposcopic examination has been completed. Depending on the site of the suspicious lesion, either a punch biopsy or endocervical curettage should be carried out. Occasionally, both procedures are necessary.

Punch Biopsy

The instrument for punch biopsy is pistol-shaped, with a long shaft (see Fig. 7.6). Under colposcopic control, the instrument may be positioned on the area where the biopsy specimen is to be obtained. Although the cervix tends to slip away on pressure, it is usually easy to grasp and remove the desired tissue with the biopsy forceps. The procedure is virtually painless. The specimen is approximately 5 mm in size, and is covered on one side by epithelium (see Fig. 18.1). Several specimens may be taken from larger lesions. Bleeding is usually mild, but may occasionally be excessive. The patient should be given some type of sanitary pad. We prefer a sterilized, self-removable tampon (see Fig. 7.5), which is shown to the patient prior to insertion and which she is instructed to remove on the same day. The bleeding always stops within a few hours.

If the cervix gives way under pressure or slips away from the instrument, it must be "fixed." This is best done with a tenaculum (see Fig. 7.7). The point at which the cervix is grasped must be away from any lesions. This manipulation is not painful.

The tissue remains in the concavity of the instrument's jaw. The instrument is then immersed in fixative in a specimen jar, and the specimen is shaken free.

Loop Diathermy Excision

A variety of wire loops have been used in Europe for decades for diathermy excision or cervical biopsies. Cartier (1977) has revived and perfected the technique. The procedure can be performed under local anesthesia by injecting a solution of ornipressin (see p. 271). It is appropriate for lesions of different sizes that can be removed with a margin of healthy tissue. The excision is performed with a very small amount of pressure on the loop. After removal of the tissue, the wound, which hardly bleeds after infiltration, is coagulated with a ball electrode.

Endocervical Curettage

First, the patient must be warned that this procedure may be painful, as it is done without a general anesthetic. Fixing the cervix, as described for punch biopsy, is rarely necessary.

The procedure is performed with sharp, spoon-shaped or grooved curettes (see Fig. 7.6); the latter are particularly useful for insertion through a narrow os. The canal is scraped in a circumferential manner. Tissue that remains in the cavity of the jaws of the instrument may be rinsed in the fixative. Residual tissue fragments on the surface of the cervix or around the os may be removed with forceps and then placed in fixative.

During the curettage, the consistency of the cervical wall should be noted. If it is firm and regular, it is unlikely to harbor a deeply invasive carcinoma; such tissue is friable and would disintegrate during curettage. Bleeding is not usually excessive. Nevertheless, the patient should be given a sanitary pad, or a sterilizable, self-removable tampon should be inserted.

Chrobak's Sound

The uterine sound test devised by the Viennese gynecologist Chrobak (1840–1910) is not widely known. It is a simple way of distinguishing between benign and malignant tissue. It is particularly useful in assessing purely endophytic or only slightly ulcerating carcinomas and to distinguish between benign papillomas and exophytic carcinomas. The sound (see Fig. 7.8) easily penetrates cancerous tissue on light pressure, as if going into butter. According to the depth of penetration, even the volume of the tumor can be roughly estimated. Conversely, the sound encounters elastic resistance when in contact with normal tissues or benign tumors. The sound may traumatize atypical epithelium but not normal epithelium.

Duration of Colposcopic Examination

The experienced colposcopist needs less time for the examination described above than would be expected. Careful performance of all steps should not take longer than 3 minutes. Another 2 to 3 minutes may be added if a biopsy is to be taken. It must be stressed again and again that the best result is achieved by the routine use of colposcopy. Once the colposcopist has learned how to handle the instruments and how to interpret cervical changes, 3 minutes' time should be ample.

Reference

Cartier R. Practical colposcopy. Basel: S. Karger, 1977.

10
Colposcopic Terminology

Nomenclature of Hinselmann

At first, Hinselmann (5) recognized only a few colposcopic findings, which he divided into *normal* and *pathologic*:

1. *Normal findings*
   Original mucosa
   Ectopy
   Transformation zone

2. *Pathologic findings*
   Portio leukoplakia
       Ground of leukoplakia (punctation)
       "*Felderung*" (mosaic)

The evolution of this nomenclature is described in Chapter 2. When Hinselmann removed the keratin layer from the surfaces of leukoplakia he detected on their "ground" a punctation. He also found "*Felderung*" to be associated with leukoplakia.

Hinselmann (3, 4) referred to the pathologic findings, which he believed were always due to epithelial precursors of cervical carcinoma, collectively as:

   matrix area.

Only later (6) did he acknowledge the existence of an atypical transformation zone as originally described by Treite (8), which, however, he called:

   abnormal transformation zone.

Quite apart from the above appearances, Hinselmann recognized the significance of *true erosion* (5), which he distinguished from what was previously known simply as *erosion* and is now referred to, in contrast to leukoplakia, as *erythroplakia*. He also suggested that erosions appeared in areas previously occupied by atypical epithelium, which he found to be fragile and of low cohesiveness. The quite flat ulcer caused by endophytic carcinoma was also included in this schema.

Nomenclature of Wespi

Wespi (9) divided the colposcopic findings into four groups: normal appearance of the portio, established portio carcinoma, atypical portio epithelium, and findings of uncertain significance:

1. *Normal appearance of the portio*
   Original portio mucosa
   Ectopy
   Transformation zone

2. *Established portio carcinoma*
3. *Atypical portio epithelium*
   Leukoplakia
   "Ground" (punctation)
   "*Felderung*" (mosaic)
   Colposcopically inconspicuous iodine-negative area

4. *Findings of uncertain significance*

This nomenclature distinguished for the first time between ground (punctation) and *Felderung* (mosaic), on the one hand, and leukoplakia on the other; the concept of a colposcopically inconspicuous iodine-negative area was also new. Prominent among the findings of uncertain significance was a *red area* mainly corresponding to *true erosion.*

The So-Called International Terminology

During the second Congress of Cervical Pathology and Colposcopy in Graz in 1975, a terminology committee met to formulate a new colposcopic nomenclature (1), the aim of which was to reconcile the differing interpretations of various colposcopic appearances and to produce an internationally acceptable terminology. Particular attention was paid to adopting terms that could be translated into all the major languages without ambiguity. Accordingly, "ground" was replaced by "punctation" and "leukoplakia" by "keratosis." A change in emphasis resulted in "erosion" no longer being regarded as suspicious. The term "colposcopically inconspicuous iodine-negative area" was dropped altogether, as the Schiller test was not thought to be a necessary part of colposcopic examination.

Complete agreement, of course, was not achieved. Publication of a version of this terminology as the official international nomenclature was premature (7). Most of the controversies centered around the concept of the "atypical transformation zone" (see p. 85). While in English-speaking countries it was primarily a collective term for *mosaic, punctation, white epithelium, keratosis,* and *atypical vessels,* in Europe the atypical or unusual transformation zone was merely additional to the other terms and of similar significance.

The "international" (as opposed to the European) version of this nomenclature is as follows:

I　*Normal colposcopic findings*
　　A　Original squamous epithelium
　　B　Columnar epithelium (ectopy)
　　C　Transformation zone

II　*Abnormal colposcopic findings*
　　A　Atypical transformation zone
　　　　1　Mosaic
　　　　2　Punctation
　　　　3　(Aceto-)white epithelium
　　　　4　Keratosis
　　　　5　Atypical vessels
　　B　Suspect frank invasive carcinoma

III　*Unsatisfactory colposcopic findings*
　　(squamocolumnar junction not visible)

IV　*Miscellaneous colposcopic findings*
　　A　Inflammatory changes
　　B　Atrophic changes
　　C　Erosion
　　D　Condyloma
　　E　Papilloma
　　F　Others

The weakness of the provisional international nomenclature was the compromise concerning the concept of the atypical transformation zone (see page 85). Because the latter was adopted as an overriding umbrella term, it became necessary to regard even mere diagnostic details characterizing specific findings as diagnostic criteria in their own right. Aceto-white epithelium, for example, can also be found, besides mosaic and punctation, in a transformation zone which is termed "unusual" purely on account of this reaction. Similarly, atypical vessels can never constitute a finding per se but are seen only in association with other lesions, e.g., frankly invasive carcinoma. Finally, the so-called atypical transformation zone only rarely corresponds to histologic atypia.

"Columnar epithelium" should not replace "ectopy," as the latter indicates the location of the columnar epithelium, while the former does not. In addition, the Schiller test should form an integral part of the colposcopic examination (see p. 117). If this test is not employed, the opportunity to observe the sharply circumscribed yellow areas which are so characteristic colposcopically is lost. The place of the Schiller test in colposcopic terminology is more important than the "miscellaneous" category, which can never be complete. Finally, the nontraumatic erosion known to classical colposcopy should be included under the suspicious findings, as preinvasive and even invasive lesions may give rise to erosions.

A Proposal for a New Terminology

Considering these facts, it is clear that the debate on a definitive colposcopic terminology is not yet over. In addition, a predictive categorization of colposcopic findings is more and more becoming the goal in designing a system of terminology. From such a schema it should be possible to assess which histologic change is responsible for which colposcopic appearance. The schema should, of course, concern itself not only with terminology, but also with the various colposcopic appearances as they evolve during the colposcopic examination, including the responses to acetic acid and iodine.

Table 10.**1**　**A European proposal for colposcopic classification** (Burghardt E. et al., Cervix 1989;7:251—4)

Colposcopic conclusions		Colposcopic terms	
Normal findings		a Original squamous epithelium b Columnar epithelium (ectopy) c Normal transformation	
Abnormal findings	Nonsuspicious zone	Unusual transformation	Grade 0
	Doubtful zones	a Unusual transformation b Fine mosaic c Fine punctation d Fine leukoplakia e Erosion	Grade I
	Suspicious zones	a Unusual transformation b Coarse mosaic c Coarse punctation d Thick leukoplakia e Irregular vascularization f Ulcer	Grade II
Frank invasive cancer			
Condylomatous aspects			
Miscellaneous			
Inconclusive findings			

Table 10.2   Terminology of colposcopy (Rome 1990)

I   **Normal colposcopic findings**
  A   Original squamous epithelium
  B   Columnar epithelium
  C   Normal transformation zone

II   **Abnormal colposcopic findings**
  A   Within the transformation zone
    1   Aceto-white epithelium*
      a   Flat
      b   Micropapillary or microconvoluted
    2   Punctation*
    3   Mosaic*
    4   Leukoplakia*
    5   Iodine-negative area
    6   Atypical vessels
  B   Outside the transformation zone, e.g., ectocervix, vagina
    1   Aceto-white epithelium*
      a   Flat
      b   Micropapillary or microconvoluted
    2   Punctation*
    3   Mosaic*
    4   Leukoplakia*
    5   Iodine-negative area
    6   Atypical vessels

III   **Colposcopically suspect invasive carcinoma**

IV   **Unsatisfactory colposcopy**
  A   Squamocolumnar junction not visible
  B   Severe inflammation or severe atrophy
  C   Cervix not visible

V   **Miscellaneous findings**
  A   Non aceto-white micropapillary surface
  B   Exophytic condyloma
  C   Inflammation
  D   Atrophy
  E   Ulcer
  F   Other

* Indicates minor or major change

   Minor changes
     Aceto-white epithelium
     Fine mosaic
     Fine punctation
     Thin leukoplakia

   Major changes
     Dense aceto-white epithelium
     Coarse mosaic
     Coarse punctation
     Thick leukoplakia
     Atypical vessels
     Erosion

At the Sixth World Congress for Colposcopy and Cervical Pathology in São Paulo in 1987, it was decided to prepare a new colposcopic terminology, to be presented at the Congress in Rome in 1990. After intensive discussions, a European group proposed a terminology which included a qualitative assessment of individual colposcopic images. Abnormal findings were to be subclassified into Group 0 (nonsuspicious), Group 1 (doubtful), and Group 2 (suspicious) (Table 10.1). This proposal, published in 1989 (2), was turned down by the Terminology Committee in Rome in 1990. By a majority vote, the Committee accepted the terminology given in Table 10.2.

This terminology is an improvement, insofar as it takes into account the fact that identical colposcopic lesions can be found both within and outside the transformation zone. This nullifies the assertion that all colposcopic lesions develop within an atypical transformation zone, and the concept of the atypical transformation zone no longer appears in the new terminology. Also, the sudivision of mosaic lesions and leukoplakia into minor changes and major changes (albeit in footnotes) implies a certain qualitative assessment.

On the other hand, the new terminology still contains terms—such as aceto-white epithelium and atypical vessels—that were criticized in the previous terminology. This again ignores the fact that there are colposcopic images which show all the attributes of a transformation zone, but whose native color and reaction with acetic acid or iodine show them to be abnormal. Such findings are called "unusual transformation zone" in this book (Figs. 11.39–46, 14.1).

The terminology used in this book is shown in Table 10.3. It generally corresponds to the international terminology, but clarifies its weaknesses.

Table 10.3   Terminology used in the present work

I   Normal colposcopic findings
  A   Original squamous epithelium
  B   Ectopy (columnar epithelium)
  C   Transformation zone

II   Doubtful colposcopic findings
  A   Thin leukoplakia
  B   Fine punctation
  C   Fine mosaic
  D   Unusual transformation zone
  E   Colposcopically inconspicuous iodine-yellow area

III   Suspicious colposcopic findings
  A   Coarse leukoplakia
  B   Coarse punctation
  C   Coarse mosaic
  D   Unusual transformation zone
  E   Erosion (ulcer)
  F   Suspicious invasive carcinoma

IV   Invasive carcinoma

V   Miscellaneous findings
  A   Condylomas
  B   Polyps
  C   Inflammatory changes
  D   Atrophic changes
  E   Others

References

1   Almendral AC, Seidl S. Colposcopical terminology. Chairmen's report. In: Burghardt E, Holzer E, Jordan JA, eds. Cervical pathology and colposcopy. Stuttgart: Thieme, 1978:134—135.

2   Burghardt E, Coupez F, Dexeus S, et al. A European proposal for a classification of colposcopic findings. Cervix 1989;7:251—4.

2a Cartier R. Practical Colposcopy. Basel: Karger, 1977.

3   Hinselmann H. Ausgewählte Gesichtspunkte zur Beurteilung des Zusammenhanges der "Matrixbezirke" und des Karzinoms der sichtbaren Abschnitte des weiblichen Genitaltraktes. Z Geburtshilfe 1933;104:228.

4   Hinselmann H. Die klinische und mikroskopische Frühdiagnose des Portiokarzinoms. Arch Gynäkol 1934; 156:239.

5   Hinselmann H. Die Kolposkopie. Wuppertal: Girardet, 1954.

6   Hinselmann H. Kolposkopische Studien, vol 1. Leipzig: VEB Thieme, 1954.

7   Stafl A. New nomenclature for colposcopy. Obstet Gynecol 1976;48:123.

8   Treite P. Die Frühdiagnose des Plattenepithel-Karzinoms am Collum uteri. Stuttgart: Enke, 1944.

9   Wespi H. Early carcinoma of the uterine cervix: pathogenesis and detection. New York: Grune and Stratton, 1949.

MEDICAL LIBRARY
ODSTOCK HOSPITAL
SALISBURY SP2 8BJ

11

Colposcopic Morphology

Introduction

The best way to describe and depict colposcopic findings is using numerous colpophotographs. The illustrations here have been chosen to portray as faithfully as possible all the important changes, to be compared with appearances as they are encountered from day to day. Colposcopy can be understood only if it is appreciated that the same colposcopic appearance can be produced by a number of biologically different processes. This apparent diagnostic paradox can be resolved only by a knowledge of the histologic basis for it. The colposcopic literature neglects the fact that a lesion is often a composite of a number of quite different epithelial types of differing significance, though sharing a common developmental origin. This is attested to by the constant location of the various epithelia and their clear demarcation from each other, features that provide not only the key for the understanding of colposcopic diagnosis, but also parameters without which no concept of the morphogenesis of cervical carcinoma can be formulated. The fundamental reciprocal relationship between cervical pathology and colposcopic diagnosis is obvious from the above considerations.

Normal Colposcopic Appearances

Original Squamous Epithelium

Like any normal surface squamous epithelium, the native, original squamous epithelium is smooth and uninterrupted by gland openings (Fig. 11.1). This sets it apart from normal squamous epithelium that has arisen through metaplasia and at first sight resembles it. More detailed observation of a surface covered by the latter type of epithelium will reveal the presence of gland openings and retention cysts, which indicate that the area was originally occupied by columnar epithelium (see Fig. 11.8). The original squamous epithelium during the reproductive period displays a reddish color that may vary from pale to intense pink during the various phases of the menstrual cycle. The deep-brown stain with iodine reflects its glycogen content (see Fig. 8.8 b).

Fig. 11.**1** **Original squamous epithelium** of the reproductive period. The surface is completely smooth and displays a fresh reddish color

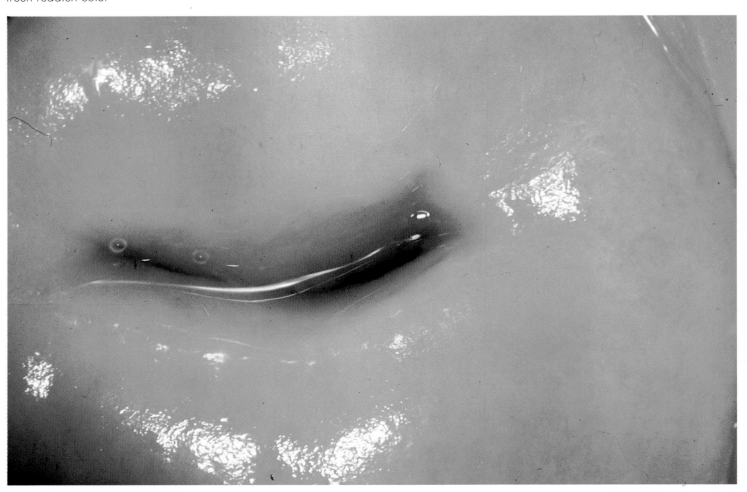

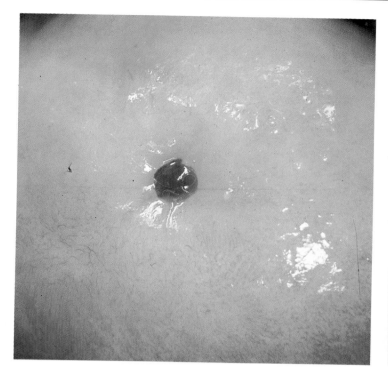

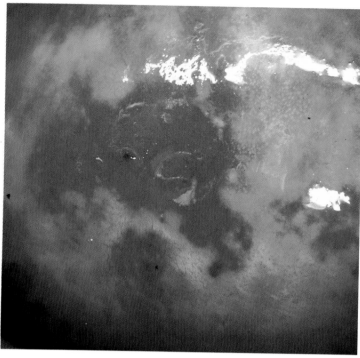

Fig. 11.**2a** **Atrophic post-menopausal squamous epithelium.** Fine blood vessels shine through the attenuated epithelium, which appears pale pink to yellowish

Fig. 11.**2b** The same case after application of iodine. The characteristic stippled appearance is due to focal glycogen retention

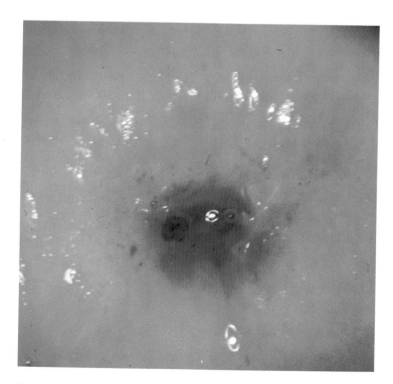

Fig. 11.**3** The loss of glycogen is uniform from the senile epithelium, resulting in homogeneous yellow staining with iodine

Atrophic Squamous Epithelium

After the menopause, the squamous epithelium becomes thin and devoid of glycogen; in addition, the stromal blood supply diminishes. These changes result in a pale epithelium that may display a fine network of capillaries (Fig. 11.2 a).

The epithelial thinning and loss of glycogen are patchy, and result in a stippled appearance with iodine because of its irregular uptake (Fig. 11.2 b). In the aged, the epithelium assumes a uniform light brown to yellow discoloration as a result of complete loss of glycogen (Fig. 11.3).

The thin epithelial covering is fragile and makes the terminal vessels vulnerable to minor trauma, which may result in erosions and subepithelial hemorrhages (Fig. 11.4).

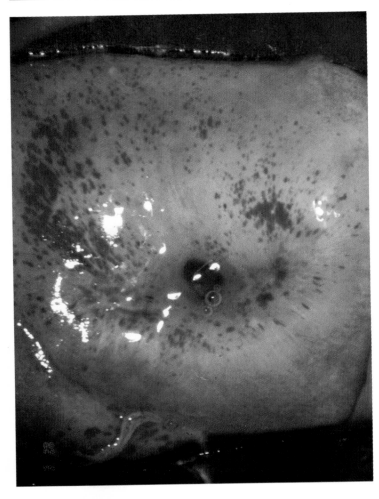

Fig. 11.**4** With advancing age, the squamous epithelium becomes fragile. Subepithelial hemorrhages may appear during vaginal examination. Note the fine vessels that stream toward the os

Ectopy (Columnar Epithelium)

In ideal circumstances, the original squamocolumnar junction is situated at the external os. According to the size, shape, and mouth of the external os, varying portions of the canal may be visible. In cases of a gaping ("shark-mouth") os, the architecture of endocervical mucosa can be clearly seen (Fig. 11.5).

In some circumstances (see p. 70), the columnar epithelium is situated on the ectocervix at some distance from the external os, in which case we speak of ectopic mucosa. As this is a frequent and basic colposcopic finding of fundamental importance for the understanding of cervical carcinogenesis, we are justified in resurrecting the term *ectopy*. The alternative term *columnar epithelium* is quite acceptable, but it cannot indicate its ectopic location. In cases of marked eversion of the endocervical mucosa, its rugose architecture becomes evident (Fig. 11.6). In such cases, it may be more nearly correct to speak of an *ectropion* rather than ectopy.

Ectopy is more often apparent than real. The separated blades of the speculum spread out the fornices and evert the endocervical canal, so that it appears as part of the covering of the ectocervix (Fig. 11.7).

The fresh and intact ectopy appears classically as a "red patch" (Fig. 11.8 a). Macroscopically it may look highly suspicious to the inexperienced. More detailed colposcopic examination reveals its unique papillary architecture, which identifies its real nature. It is always iodine-negative (Fig. 11.8 b).

Ectopy is usually hidden by mucus secreted by the columnar epithelium. Acetic acid helps to remove the mucus (see p. 114), revealing a distinctive papillary structure. At the same time, it causes the tissue to swell, throwing the mucosal architecture into sharp relief, and giving the papillae a grape-like appearance. The intense red of the red patch changes to pink or whitish (Fig. 11.9).

The squamocolumnar junction is usually sharp and step-like (Figs. 11.5, 11.9 and 11.10). Careful observation of the margin, however, often reveals a slender seam, the white color and gland openings of which indicate the initiation of transformation (Fig. 11.7). It is therefore important to pay close attention to the margins in ectopy in order not to overlook significant colposcopic lesions.

Ectopic columnar epithelium is less resilient and more vulnerable to trauma than squamous epithelium. It is subject to contact bleeding even during hasty speculum examination. Any contact bleeding, however, should raise the possibility of a papillary carcinoma. Although neoplastic papillary fronds tend to be coarse and irregular, they may be mistaken for benign changes.

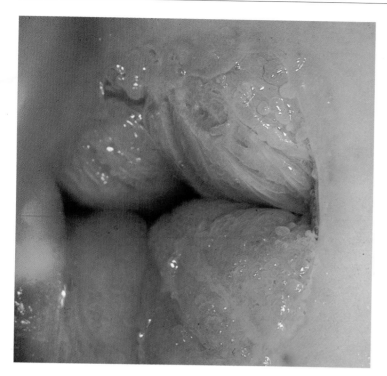

Fig. 11.5 The original squamocolumnar junction of this gaping cervix is most distinct. The anterior lip displays a thin rim of transformation zone. The rugose structure of the endocervical mucosa is clearly seen

Fig. 11.6 **Eversion of the endocervical mucosa,** with its rugose architecture thrown into sharp relief. This may be referred to as *ectropion*

Fig. 11.7 **Apparent eversion (ectopy) of a cervix with a patulous os,** due to wide separation of the speculum. A thin rim of transformation zone is visible near the junction with the original squamous epithelium

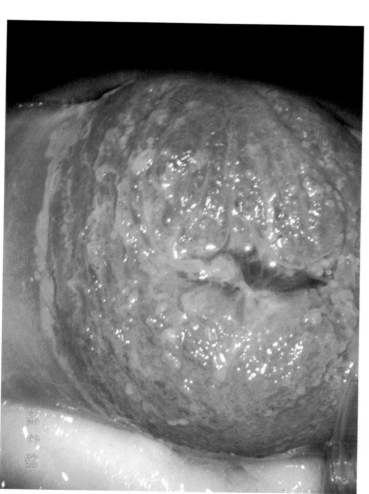

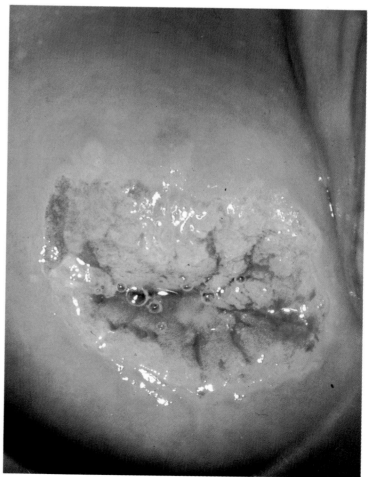

11.6

11.7

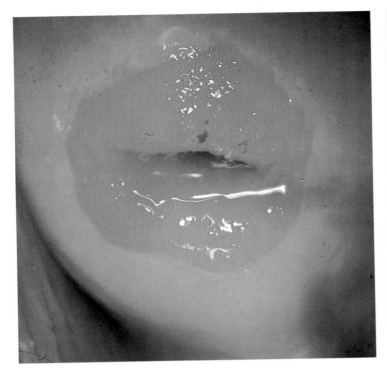

Fig. 11.8 a   Ectopy prior to application of acetic acid. The gland openings at the 10-o'clock position indicate preceding transformation

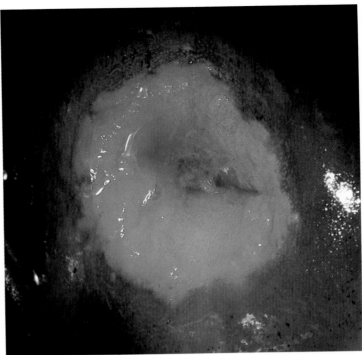

Fig. 11.8 b   An ectopy does not take up iodine; it is merely discolored by the thin film covering it. The demarcation from the deep-brown original squamous epithelium is indistinct

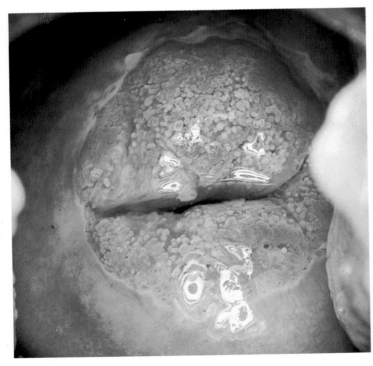

Fig. 11.9   Classical appearance of ectopy following acetic acid application. The grape-like structure is unmistakable. Note the whitish rim of transformation zone at the periphery

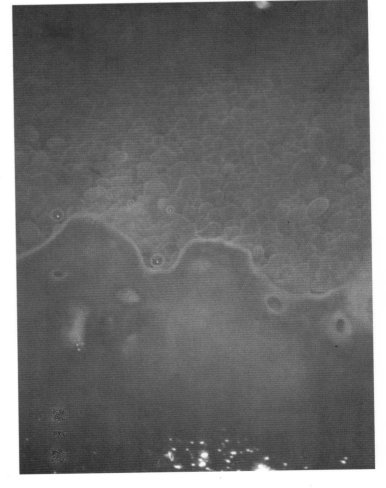

Fig. 11.10   Step-like border between the grape-like structure of the ectopy and the squamous epithelium. Note the gland openings at the periphery of the squamous epithelium, indicating completed transformation at the edge of the previously larger ectopic area

Transformation Zone

The transformation zone can appear as a nonspecific red area. Sometimes there is a fine vascular pattern (Fig. 11.11 a). Application of acetic acid turns the previously red epithelium grayish-white. Within the transformation zone, there are openings of cervical glands and small islands of residual columnar epithelium. The demarcation from the original squamous epithelium is unclear (Fig. 11.11 b).

The process of transformation begins characteristically at the squamocolumnar junction. The flat epithelial seam around the periphery of an ectopy can be distinguished from the original squamous as well as columnar epithelium by its variable color and by the presence of gland openings (Figs. 8.2, 11.10, 11.12). It is impossible to tell colposcopically whether the transformation process at this site is due to ascending healing (see p. 75) or squamous metaplasia (see p. 74).

Pari passu with peripheral transformation of an ectopy, the surface contour of its central portion undergoes changes. The papillae become coarse and fused, resulting in only slight fissuring of the surface. These changes signify the initiation of squamous metaplasia. Fields of metaplastic epithelium within a transformation zone may vary widely in their maturation,

easily verifiable by the Schiller test, which is a particularly sensitive indicator of epithelial maturity (Fig. 11.12 b).

The topographic progress of the transformation may be haphazard, and its stage of evolution can vary significantly from one part of the periphery to another. Islands of squamous epithelium may appear in a sea of columnar epithelium; these must have arisen by metaplasia (Fig. 11.13; see also Fig. 12.8). The metaplastic epithelium may form tongues or finger-like processes that interdigitate with intact columnar epithelium (Fig. 11.14). Even when most of an ectopy is fully transformed, small islands of columnar epithelium may remain; this appearance is referred to as transformation zone with ectopic rests (Fig. 11.15). The study of the same transformation zone over many years is particularly informative (see Chapter 12).

The transformation of an ectopy may not always proceed to completion. The newly formed squamous epithelium may fully mature, whereas other parts of an ectopy may remain intact for long periods (Fig. 11.16). A fully transformed ectopy (fully developed transformation zone) may closely resemble the "ideal" cervix. The new squamocolumnar junction is situated again at the external os. The squamous epithelium of such a transformation zone can be distinguished from original squamous epithelium only by the presence of gland openings, more prominent vessels (Fig. 11.17), or retention cysts (Fig. 11.18). Undulations due to numerous retention cysts (nabothian follicles), with long vessels coursing over their surface, are also characteristic (Fig. 11.19). The vasculature in such cases is so typical that the presence of deep-seated and otherwise invisible cysts can be easily deduced (see Fig. 14.10).

Fig. 11.**11 a** **Typical transformation zone** before the application of acetic acid. There are small, unremarkable vessels at the edge of the reddish area on the posterior lip of the cervix

Fig. 11.**11 b** After application of acetic acid, the previously reddish epithelium is grayish-white. Gland openings and small islands of residual columnar epithelium are signs of the transformation zone

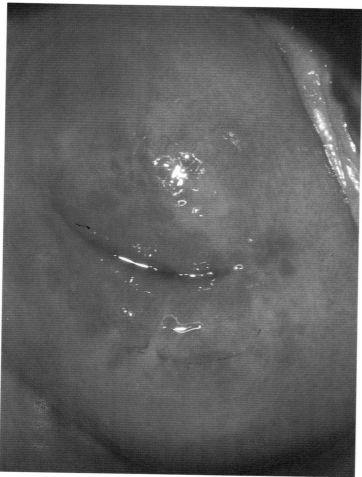

11.**11 a**

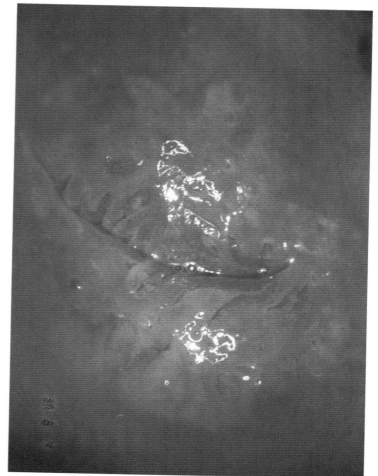

11.**11 b**

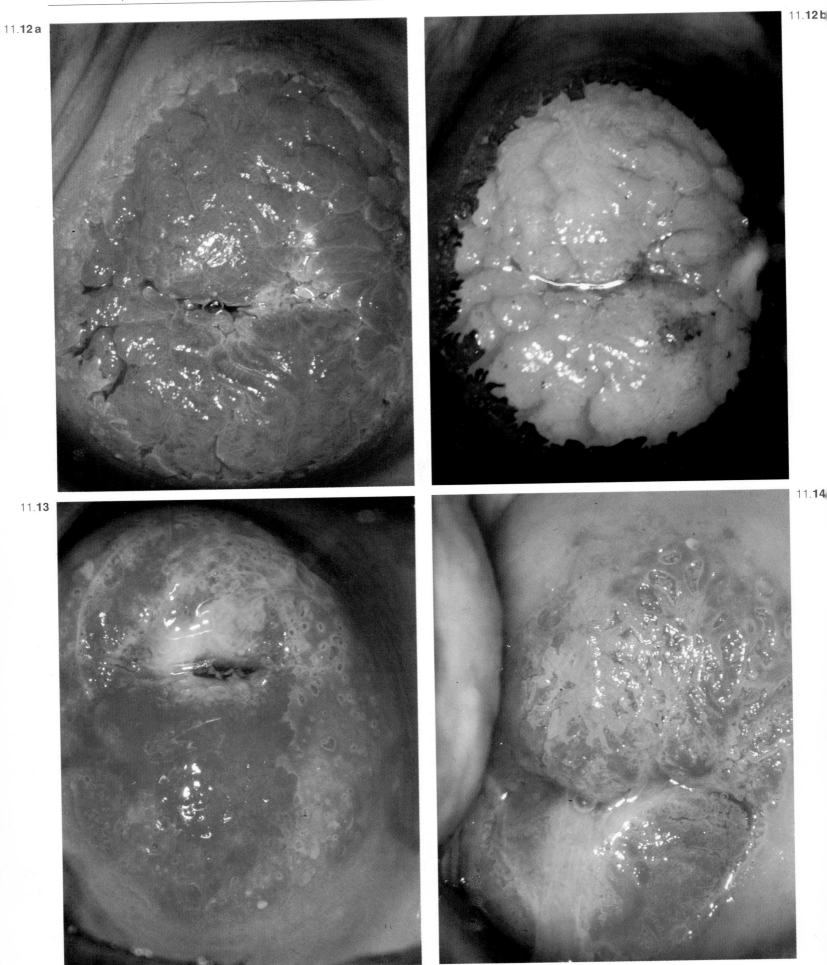

11.**15**

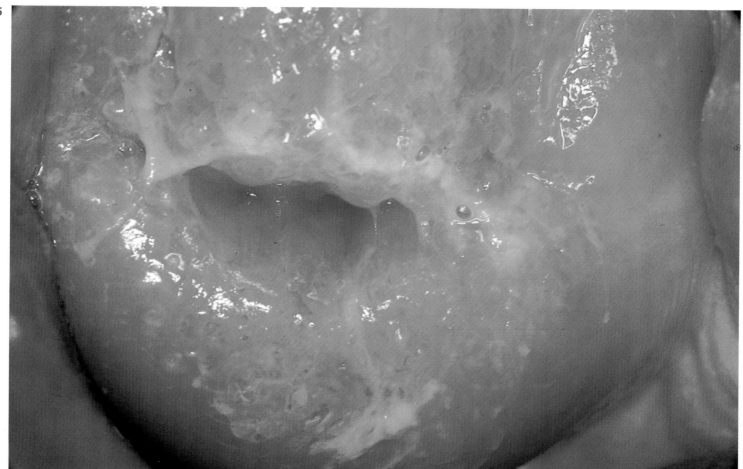

◁ Fig. 11.**12a Transformation zone** Centrally, within this ectopic area, the villi become plumper and fuse to form a flat surface eventually

◁ Fig. 11.**12b** The same case following application of iodine. The transformed epithelium is already mature and contains glycogen. Gland openings are well displayed. The central part does not take up iodine, which merely covers it like a veil

◁ Fig. 11.**13 Advanced transformation zone.** Here too, the process begins peripherally and spreads toward the center in an irregular manner. Note the smooth surface in spite of the incomplete transformation. There are numerous gland openings

◁ Fig. 11.**14 Finger-like processes of metaplastic epithelium** extend centrally from the periphery and interdigitate with islands of columnar epithelium. The transformation involves only the anterior lip

Fig. 11.**15 Transformation zone** with residual islands of grape-like columnar epithelium on the anterior lip

Fig. 11.**16 Partial transformation.** The transformation zone on the anterior lip takes up only a small portion of the ectopy, which is largely unchanged, apart from enlargement and fusion of its papillae

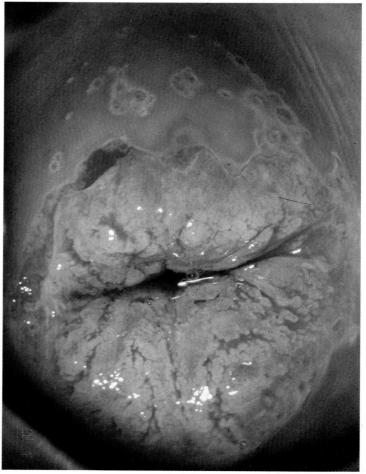

11.**16**

11.**17**

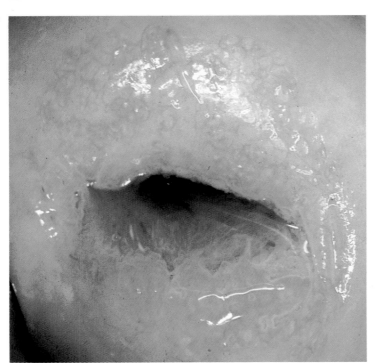

Fig. 11.**17** **Well-established transformation zone.** Although the color of the new squamous epithelium is hardly distinguishable from that of the original, the border of the transformation is marked by fine blood vessels. The new squamocolumnar junction is abrupt

Fig. 11.**20** Coarse plaque of keratosis with a partly fissured surface: histologically carcinoma in situ (CIN 3) ▷

Fig. 11.**18** **Several nabothian follicles covered by smooth squamous epithelium.** They are the only indicators of preceding transformation. Blood vessels character- istically course over the sur- face of the retention cyst on the right

Fig. 11.**19** **Numerous na- bothian follicles in an estab- lished transformation zone.** The long regularly branching blood vessels that shine through the attenuated epithe- lium are typical

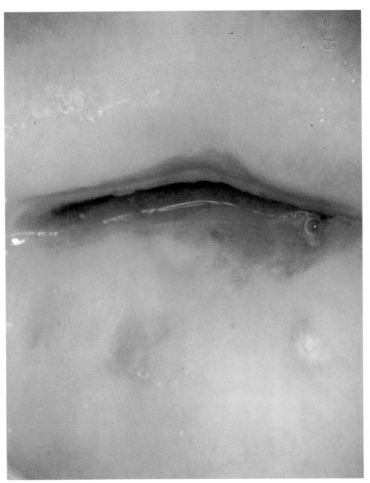

11.**18**

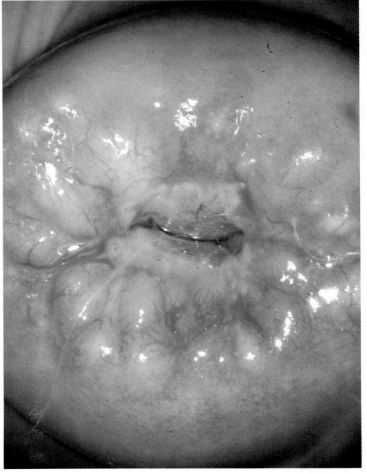

11.**19**

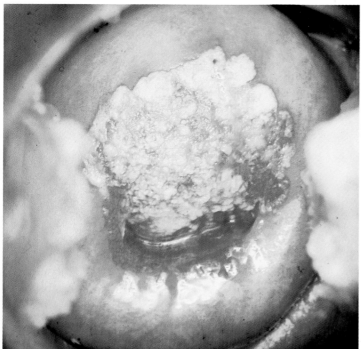

Fig. 11.**21 Sharply demarcated but only slightly keratotic area** on the posterior lip; histologically, acanthotic epithelium with parakeratosis. Note the thin seam of transformation zone on the anterior lip

Abnormal Colposcopic Findings

Leukoplakia

In many cases leukoplakia can be seen with the naked eye (Fig. 11.20), but sometimes only with the colposcope (Fig. 11.21). Histologically one sees parakeratosis or true keratinization (see p. 76), which cannot be distinguished colposcopically. A colposcopically delicate white patch, however, usually corresponds to parakeratosis, while hyperkeratosis usually produces a thick, rough-surfaced plaque. Fine leukoplakias are well circumscribed (Fig. 11.21), their surface being either flat or finely pitted. When keratinization is marked, the margins become obscured by the overlapping horny layer. The surface may be smooth, but is more commonly pitted, and may even have a mosaic appearance. Partial shedding or removal of the keratin may result in a plaque-like appearance, referred to as *plaquelike leukoplakia.*

If the keratin layer is completely removed, the underlying epithelium may display a certain pattern, which is often punctation (Fig. 11.22) and which Hinselmann designated as *ground* (base) of leukoplakia (12, 13). Leukoplakia may be found within or outside the transformation zone, in the latter

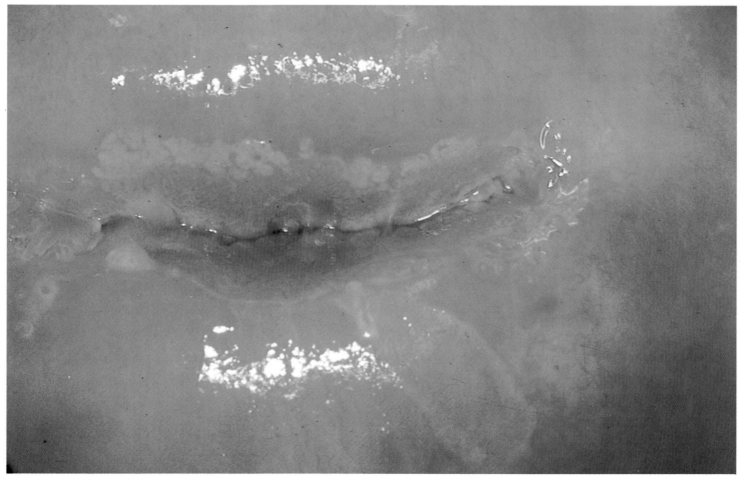

11.**21**

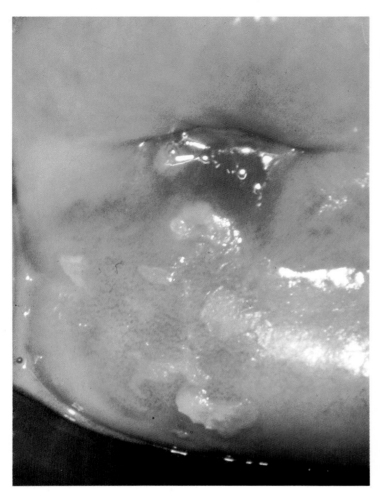

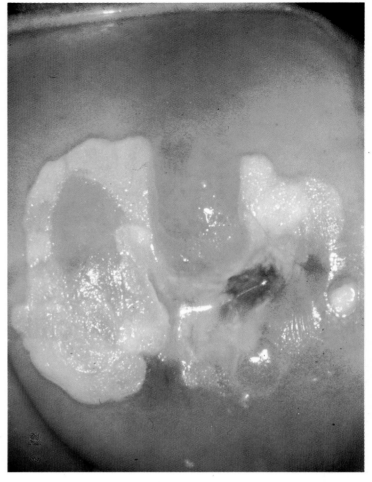

Fig. 11.**22**   **Ground of leuko-plakia.** Where the keratin layer has been peeled off, punctation appears. Histologically, keratinizing acanthotic epithelium

Fig. 11.**23a**   **Pronounced leu-koplakia** displayed by most of a well-circumscribed lesion. Note the sharp border close to the external os at the 11-o'clock position. Conization specimen showed carcinoma in situ (CIN 3) with early stromal invasion

case arising from original squamous epithelium. It is important to appreciate that the type of epithelium underlying leukoplakia cannot be predicted colposcopically. The epithelium may be acanthotic, especially when the leukoplakia is fine. When cornification is more pronounced, the underlying epithelium may show the features of carcinoma in situ, early stromal inva-sion, and even deeper invasion, or only acanthosis (Figs. 11.23 and 11.24). Even the Schiller test cannot provide further diagnostic clues (Fig. 11.23 b). Moderate-sized leukoplakias typically stain canary yellow with iodine, which also enhances their sharp demarcation.

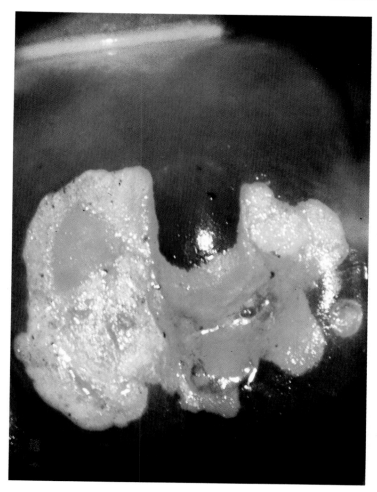

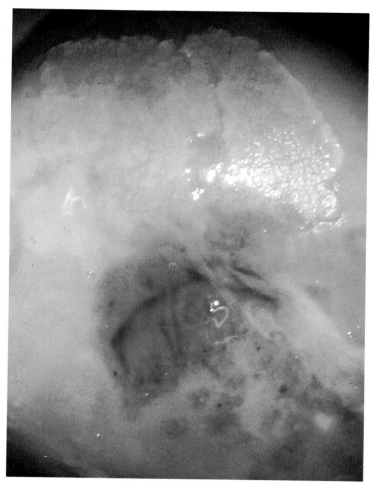

Fig. 11.**23 b**   After application of iodine, the border seen in Fig. 11.**23 a** is accentuated. The leukoplakia is outside the transformation zone. A plaque-like arrangement of the keratin is suggested. Histologically, keratinizing acanthotic epithelium

Fig. 11.**24 Leukoplakia outside the transformation zone,** on the anterior lip. Histologically, acanthotic epithelium

Punctation

As already mentioned, one may find punctation under the keratin layer of a leukoplakia. Usually the punctation is imprinted on a uniform surface which is not disturbed either by gland openings or nabothian follicles, or by any other signs of a transformation zone. The degree to which punctation is expressed depends on the type of underlying epithelial abnormality. The type of punctation, as well as of mosaic, is of decisive value in colposcopic evaluation. As was stated above, the colposcopist must be aware that similar colposcopic appearances may be due to either benign acanthotic epithelium or atypical epithelium, which differ only in arrangement and degree of expression. In practice there are two types of punctation of diagnostic importance:

a) *fine punctation* and
b) *coarse punctation.*

There are good diagnostic criteria to distinguish between the two types. A gray zone nevertheless exists between the two, and it is not always possible to categorize a given case as one or the other. Such appearances should always be regarded with suspicion: biopsy should be carried out, or cytology should be repeated. *Fine punctation* characteristically imparts delicate stippling to an otherwise circumscribed grayish-white to reddish area (Fig. 11.25). When the epithelium is keratinized, the dots may appear white, but they are usually red and remain in the same plane as the surface epithelium even after the application of acetic acid. The "dots" in fine punctation are close together (Fig. 11.22). Fine punctation is often combined with equally fine mosaic (Fig. 11.25). Fine focal punctation may be due to inflammation, in which case the margins of the inflamed area appear indistinct after application of iodine (see Figs. 11.89 and 11.90 b).

In *coarse punctation*, the petechiae are more pronounced. Not only are they bigger, but they are more widely separated (Figs. 11.26 – 11.28). In extreme cases, punctation appears in the form of papillae; the term *papillary punctation* is then used (Fig. 11.29). With higher magnification, corkscrew capillaries can be seen in the papillae. After application of acetic acid, coarse punctation stands out from the plane of the surrounding surface epithelium (Fig. 11.27 a, b). Coarse punctation may be combined with coarse mosaic. The two patterns may overlap, with intermingling of dots and fissures (Fig. 11.28).

Fig. 11.**27 a** **Atypical yellow-ish-reddish area** showing focal punctation

Fig. 11.**27 b** After acetic acid application the area of punctation swells, stands out from the surface, and becomes white. Histologically, carcinoma in situ (CIN 3). An island of fully mature squamous epithelium is seen in the transformation zone of the anterior lip

Fig. 11.**28** **Combination of quite coarse punctation and coarse mosaic.** Histologically, carcinoma in situ (CIN 3)

Fig. 11.**29** **Pronounced papillary punctation.** Histologically, carcinoma in situ (CIN 3) with early stromal invasion

Fig. 11.**25** **Sharply circumscribed area of fine punctation merges with fine mosaic outside the transformation zone.** Histologically, acanthotic epithelium

Fig. 11.**26** **Slightly prominent punctation,** coarser than in Fig. 11.**25**. The entire, sharply demarcated area apparently lies within unaltered squamous epithelium. Histology showed carcinoma in situ (CIN 3)

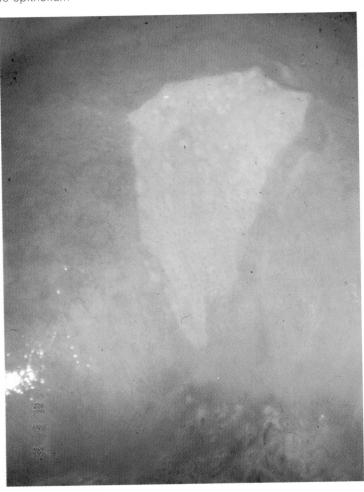

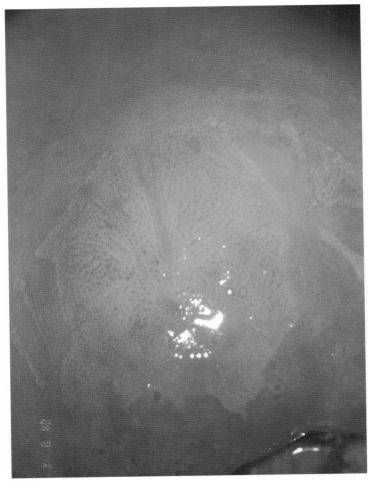

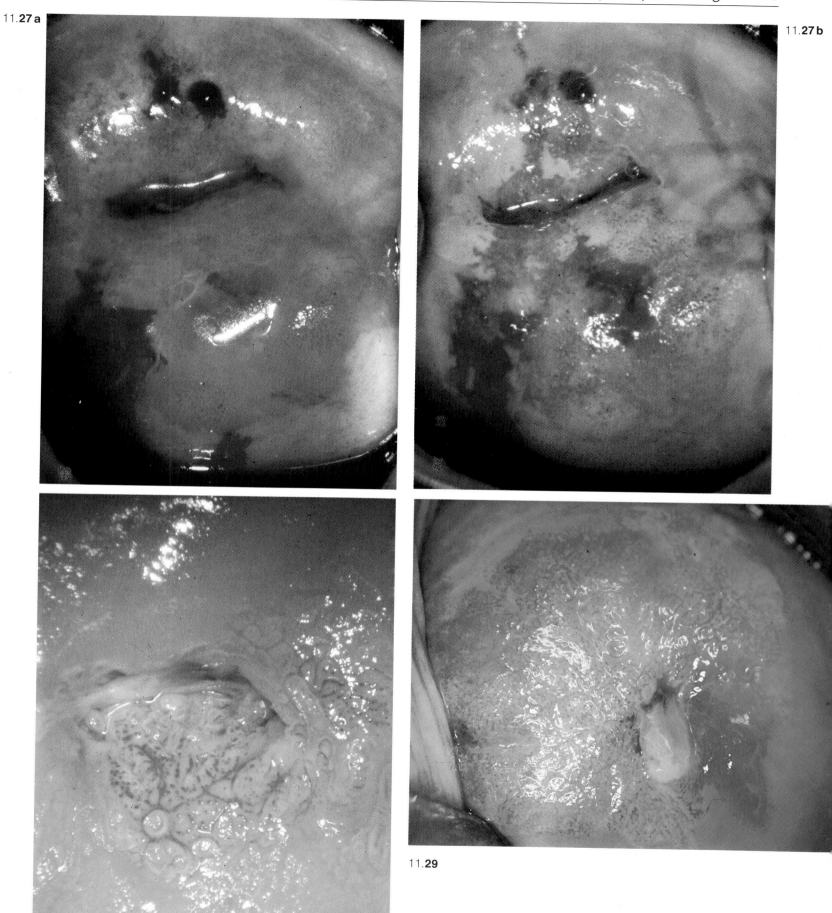

11.27 a

11.27 b

11.28

11.29

Mosaic

The above remarks about punctation also apply to mosaic. As with punctation, the morphologic manifestations of mosaic are also determined by epithelial changes, which allow distinction between

a) *fine mosaic* and
b) *coarse mosaic.*

Fine mosaic, like fine punctation, occurs in sharply demarcated areas in the plane of the surface epithelium. The appearance of such an area prior to application of acetic acid may be quite nonspecific and may remind one of a relatively vascular transformation zone, which, however, is usually devoid of gland openings or cysts (Figs. 11.30–11.34, 11.37). A distinct color change to gray-white occurs with acetic acid application, and the margins become sharp. The blood vessels become less conspicuous (Fig. 11.30 b). The whole area remains in the same plane as before. The mosaic pattern is delineated by the fine network of pale red lines. Such an area may not display the mosaic pattern throughout its entirety; in places, the surface may be uniform and flat because the epithelium is not supported by elongated stromal papillae.

It is often difficult to classify mosaic as fine or coarse (Fig. 11.35). Such intermediate forms are mostly caused by lower grade dysplasias (CIN 1–2), which may also produce various forms of punctation, depending on the degree of atypia and epithelial architecture.

Coarse mosaic is characterized by greater irregularity of the mosaic pattern. The network of fissures is more pronounced and intensely red. The furrows are more widely spaced, and the epithelial cobbles between them are bigger and more variable in shape than in the fine form (Figs. 11.33–11.37).

The swelling due to acetic acid makes the structures stand out (Fig. 11.37); the maximal effect may take a minute to develop. The metamorphosis can be observed before one's very eyes as the coarse structure of the mosaic and punctation gradually appears. In contrast, the effect of acetic acid on fine mosaic is immediate and is not intensified with time.

Hinselmann thought mosaic (which he termed "*Felderung*") was due to glandular involvement by squamous epithelium (4). Certainly in such cases one can see small white spots that stand out clearly against the reddish background. If the glands (filled with squamous epithelium) are closely packed together, the appearance may simulate a coarse mosaic (Fig. 11.38). Since in such cases the nature of the epithelial plugs in the glands cannot be determined colposcopically, biopsy is recommended.

As mentioned previously, gland openings and nabothian follicles are not usually found within areas of punctation or mosaic. Like leukoplakia, mosaic and punctation may also be found outside the transformation zone, in original squamous epithelium (Figs. 11.24–11.26, 11.35; see also Fig. 11.51). This fact is fundamental to the understanding of the morphogenesis of punctation and mosaic (see p. 80) as well as to the understanding of epithelial atypia. Punctation and mosaic may occur in isolated fields (Figs. 11.24 to 11.26, and 11.35) and may coexist with other lesions (see Figs. 15.1 and 15.3). In the latter case the more peripherally located lesions usually represent lower-grade (more mature) lesions, such as dysplasia or merely acanthotic epithelium.

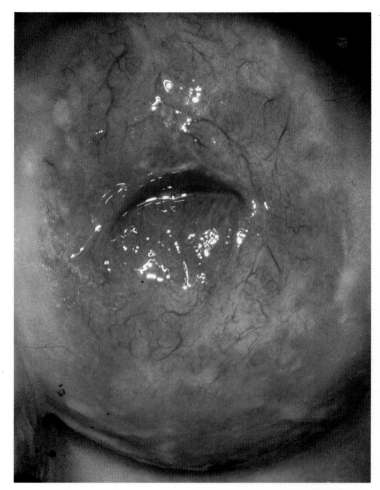
11.3

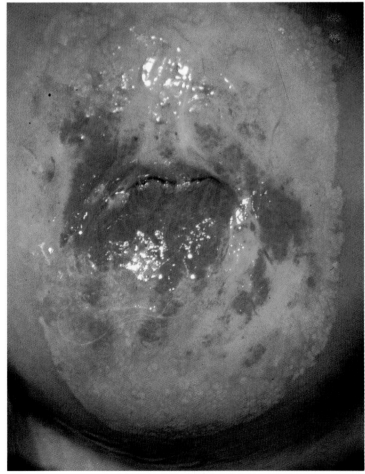
11.3

11.31

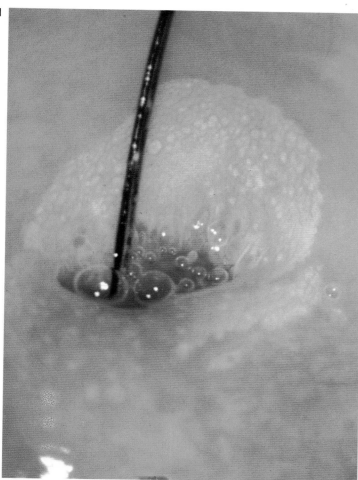

11.32a

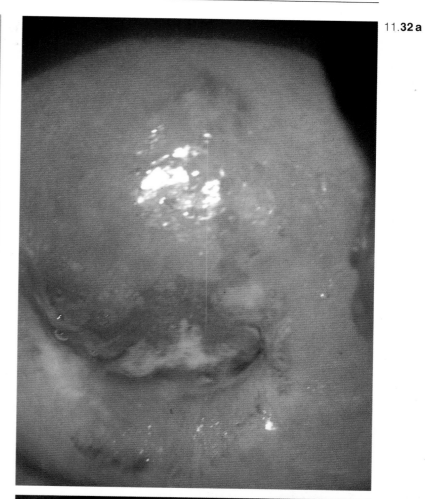

11.32b

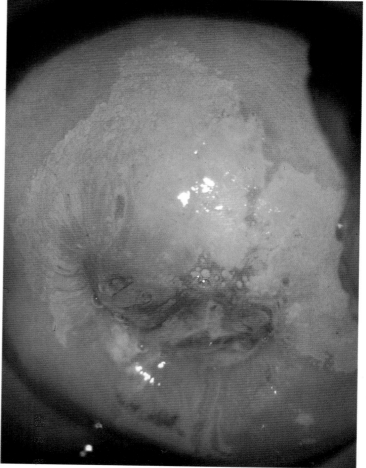

Fig. 11.**31** **Fine mosaic,** mainly on the anterior lip of the external os, after application of acetic acid. Histology showed acanthotic epithelium. The string of an IUD is visible

Fig. 11.**32a** **Indistinct lesion** outside an intensely red area around the external os. There is increased vasculary on the posterior lip at the edge of the area on close examination

Fig. 11.**32b** **Unexpectedly large, fine mosaic** appears mainly on the anterior lip after the application of acetic acid. The whitish points in the narrow transformation zone are glands filled by squamous epithelium. Histology showed acanthotic epithelium

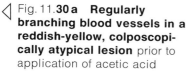 Fig. 11.**30a** **Regularly branching blood vessels in a reddish-yellow, colposcopically atypical lesion** prior to application of acetic acid

Fig. 11.**30b** **Acetic acid suppresses the vascular pattern,** but brings out a sharply demarcated fine mosaic with a distinct change in color tone. Histologically, acanthotic epithelium

11.**33 a**

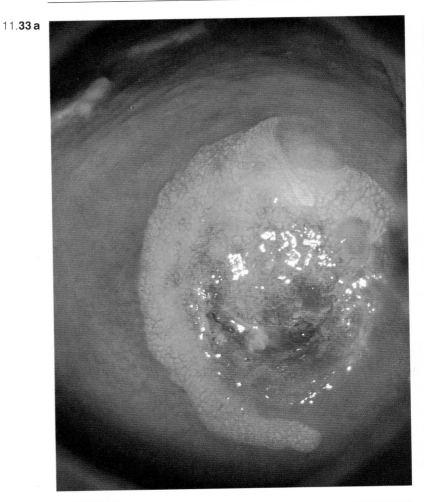

11.**33 b**

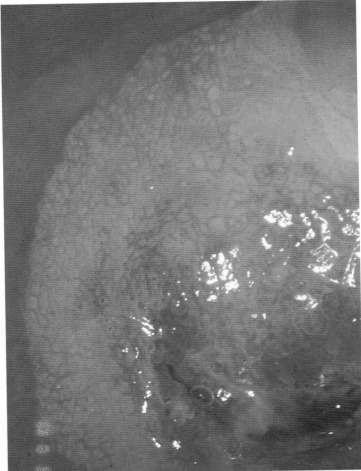

Fig. 11.**33 a**   **Transformation zone** surrounded by a semicircular area that turns whitish after the application of acetic acid, and shows a clear mosaic

Fig. 11.**33 b**   Higher magnification shows that the mosaic is coarser and more irregular than in Figs. 11.**30**—11.**32**. Histology showed mild dysplasia (CIN I)

Fig. 11.**34**   **Coarse, irregular mosaic** at the edge of a transformation zone after the application of acetic acid. Histology showed moderate dysplasia (CIN 2). On the anterior lip there is a regular vascular pattern in a mature transformation zone

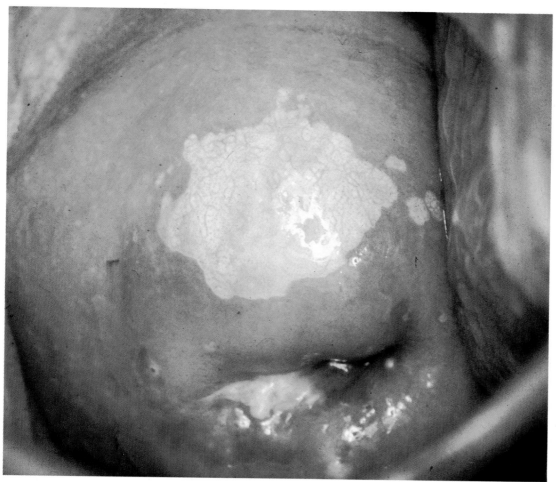

Fig. 11.**35** **Fine to coarse mosaic outside the transformation zone** involving original squamous epithelium: histologically, moderate dysplasia (CIN 2)

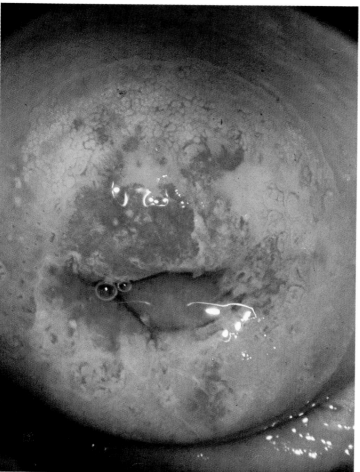

Fig. 11.**36** **Moderately to distinctly coarse mosaic** around the os: histologically, severe dysplasia (CIN 3)

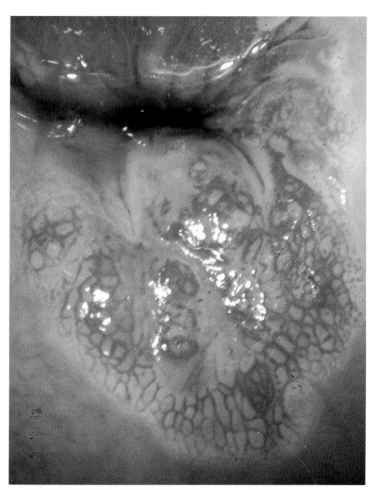

Fig. 11.**37** **Coarse mosaic intermingling with coarse punctation on the posterior lip.** Its border with an unusual transformation zone is sharp. The latter returned carcinoma in situ (CIN 3) and the former severe dysplasia (CIN 3) histologically

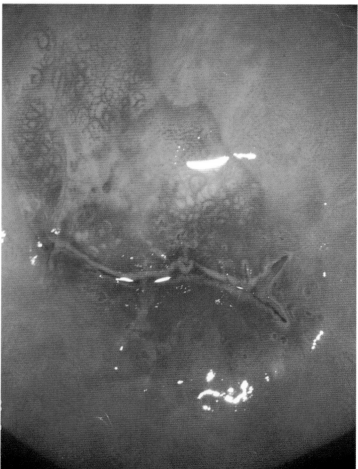

Fig. 11.**38** **Coarse mosaic** at the edge of an unusual transformation zone with cuffed gland openings and solid white points. The points correspond to atypical squamous epithelium in the glands. Histology showed carcinoma in situ (CIN 3)

Unusual (Atypical) Transformation Zone

As already explained (see p. 85), we do not use "atypical transformation zone" as an umbrella designation to encompass practically all the abnormal colposcopic appearances such as leukoplakia punctation, and mosaic, as these also occur outside the transformation zone (Figs. 11.24–11.26, 11.35; see also Figs. 11.51 and 15.3). Naturally, it would be possible to expand the concept of transformation to every type of colposcopic lesions, as all atypical epithelia are the result of transformation, whether of columnar or original squamous epithelium. It appears more reasonable, however, to confine the use of the term "transformation zone" to its original context, that is, the area where columnar epithelium is converted to squamous. This area is characterized by the presence of ectopy. In contrast, areas of potential change within the squamous epithelium cannot be predicted. Thus, the statement that cervical cancer arises in an atypical transformation zone is fundamentally wrong. In order to avoid any misunderstanding, we eschew the term "atypical transformation zone" (4, 8, 28) and use the designation *"unusual transformation zone"* for a specific colposcopic appearance.

The unusual transformation zone does not display the patterns of mosaic, punctation, or leukoplakia, but does usually contain gland openings, and even retention cysts. It corresponds in principle to the normal transformation zone, but differs from it in several important respects. It is characterized, therefore, by the hallmarks of transformation (e.g., gland openings, retention cysts, residual islands of columnar epithelium) yet differs from normal in the following features, either singly or in combination (4):

1. A dull to yellow-red color prior to application of acetic acid.
2. A more pronounced color change from red to white with acetic acid application (white epithelium).
3. Cuffed gland openings.
4. A richer vascularity with occasional atypical vessels.
5. A characteristic yellow tinge after application of iodine, with at least part of its circumference being sharply demarcated.

These criteria do not always signify the development of atypical epithelium. In the course of transformation, an acanthotic epithelium may also develop, showing only slight keratinization and no elongated stromal papillae, and thus will not appear colposcopically as keratosis, punctation, or mosaic. When compared to normal, acanthotic epithelium undergoes a more distinct color change with acetic acid, and its junction with original squamous epithelium is sharply defined (Fig. 11.30). In spite of these differences, it is not always possible to distinguish colposcopically between acanthotic epithelium and CIN in the course of unusual transformation. Even the whitish epithelium of CIN may be only relatively discrete, so that its differentiation from a normal transformation zone may be equally difficult (Fig. 11.40). A variegated appearance, not suspected otherwise, may be produced with the Schiller test (Fig. 11.40).

There may be hints of the presence of an unusual transformation zone prior to application of acetic acid, of which the most difficult to evaluate are the color tones. Any shade of red other than the fresh red of the normal transformation zone should be viewed with suspicion. Grayish red tones, which give the transformation zone an opaque appearance, and yellow shades, which are probably due to marked inflammatory in-filtration of the stroma (Figs. 11.41a and 11.44a), are particularly worrisome. In such cases, acetic acid usually induces a distinct white color change and reveals their sharp borders (Figs. 11.41b and 11.44b). A rich vascular bed is suggestive of unusual transformation but is not pathognomonic of epithelial atypia. Only in the presence of atypical vessels arranged in a haphazard manner is such a possibility highly likely (Fig. 11.42).

Actually, the best criterion is the acetic acid test. The more marked the color change and the greater the swelling, the higher the likelihood of epithelial atypia (Figs. 11.43 and 11.44b). However, the spectrum of color changes is wide (Figs. 11.45 and 11.46a).

11.**39**

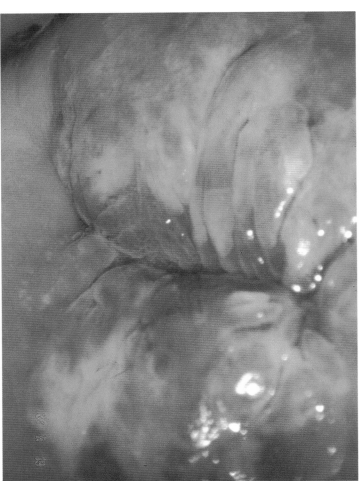

Fig. 11.**39** **Unusual transformation zone** with gleaming whitish epithelium after application of acetic acid. There are only isolated gland openings. Histology showed carcinoma in situ (CIN 3)

Fig. 11.**40 a** **Characteristic appearance of the unusual transformation zone,** distinguished from the typical transformation zone only by the aceto-white epithelium and some cuffed gland openings. There are numerous gland openings. Histologically, mild dysplasia (CIN 1)

Fig. 11.**40 b** The Schiller test reveals a variegated appearance due to admixture of atypical epithelium and fully mature brown squamous epithelium

Fig. 11.**41 a** Prior to application of acetic acid, the unusual transformation zone is an indistinct grayish red to reddish yellow. Several nabothian follicles shine through the reddish surface epithelium

Fig. 11.**41 b** The white change is produced by acetic acid. Some gland openings are cuffed. The lesion between the 11-o'clock and 12-o'clock positions is due to glandular involvement. Histologically, mild dysplasia (CIN 1)

Fig. 11.**42** **Markedly vascular transformation zone on the posterior lip.** Some atypical vessels are seen among the dense vascular network. Histologically, carcinoma in situ (CIN 3)

Fig. 11.**43** **Typical unusual tansformation zone** with numerous-cuffed gland openings. Intense aceto-white epithelium. Histologically, severe dysplasia (CIN 3)

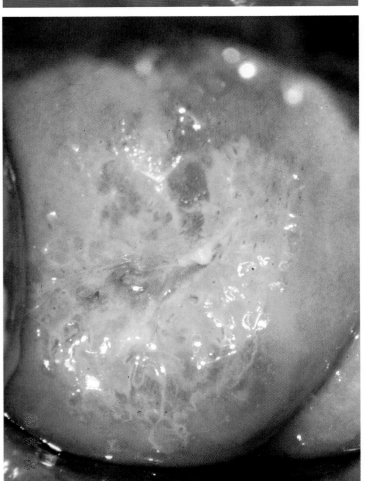

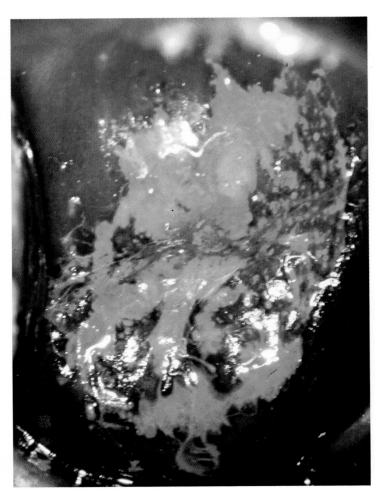

11.4

11.**41 a**

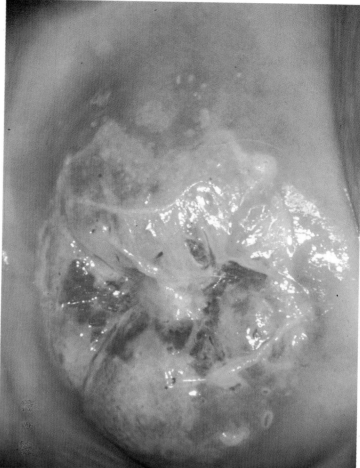

11.**41 b**

11.**42**

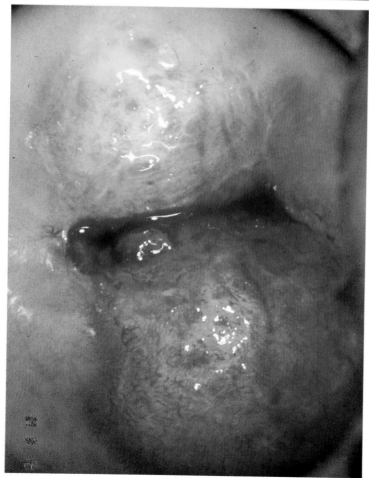

11.**43**

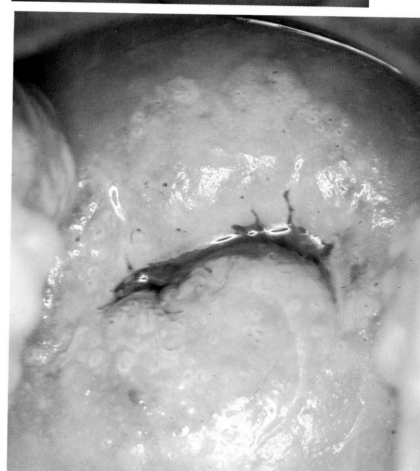

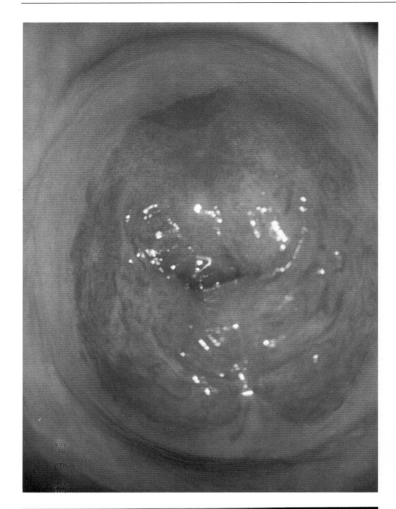

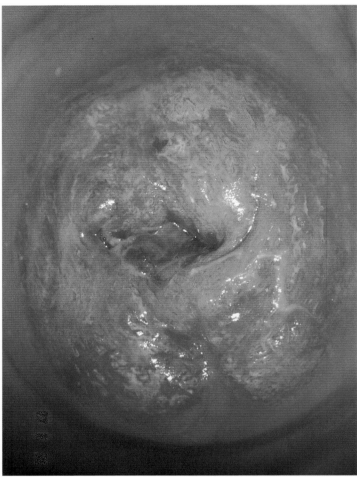

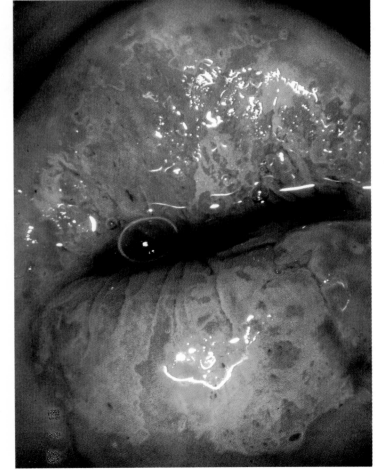

Fig. 11.44a Angry red transformation zone, sharply demarcated from the original squamous epithelium

Fig. 11.44b Patchy appearance after application of acetic acid. Between the coarse and irregular white patches there are reddish areas with cuffed gland openings and solid epithelial pegs in the glands. Histology showed carcinoma in situ (CIN 3)

Fig. 11.45 Unusual transformation zone on the posterior lip and also on the anterior lip between the 12-o'clock and 3-o'clock positions as well as between the 9-o'clock and 10-o'clock positions. The aceto-white epithelium was histologically carcinoma in situ (CIN 3), whereas the pale pink area on anterior lip was thin metaplastic epithelium

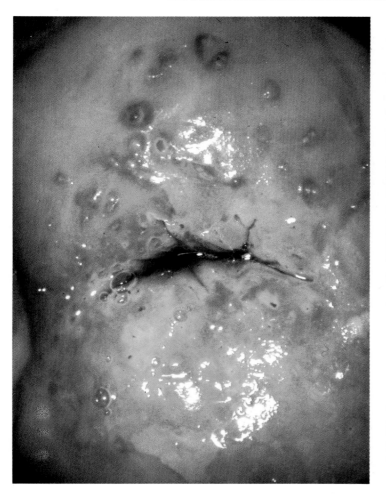

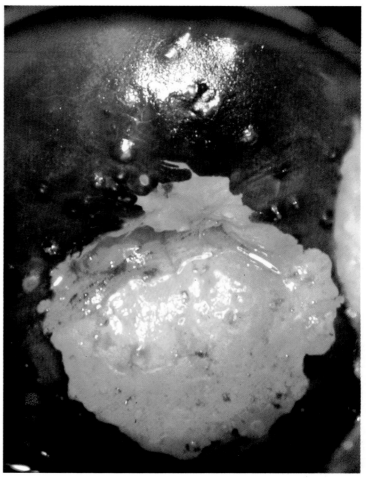

Fig. 11.**46 a** **Unusual transformation zone** involving the entire posterior lip as well as the area of the external os between the 11-o'clock and 1-o'clock positions. Note the whiteness of the epithelium and the gland openings, some of which are cuffed. Histologically, carcinoma in situ (CIN 3)

Fig. 11.**46 b** **After iodine staining,** the pathologic epithelium clearly stands out against the fully mature squamous epithelium in the transformation zone

Erosion (Ulcer)

The old colposcopic literature made use of the term *true erosion* because in those days all macroscopically visible lesions of the cervix were designated as erosions. Currently, the term is restricted to cases of epithelial defects. If these are deep, with exposure of the stroma, one speaks of an *ulcer*.

To regard erosion as an abnormal colposcopic finding is correct insofar as erosions do not occur normally in women of childbearing age. The atrophic epithelium of postmenopausal women, however, is prone to develop erosions even during gynecologic examination. Atypical epithelium is particularly vulnerable as it lacks cohesiveness, being more loosely structured than normal squamous epithelium. It is this feature that accounts for the exfoliation of cells detected in smears as well as the swelling induced by acetic acid. The epithelium is also less firmly attached to the underlying stroma, from which it may detach with ease to produce an erosion.

Such erosions are less easy to see when they occur within a colposcopically evident lesion (Fig. 11.47). They are seen to advantage with iodine because the exposed stroma does not stain (Fig. 11.47 b). An erosion may be recognized by its intense red color, its granular floor, and its punched-out margin (Figs. 11.48, 11.49).

It is even more important not to miss larger erosions that result from detachment of whole epithelial fields (Fig. 11.49). Careful examination of the edges of such defects will reveal residual epithelium, which differs from surrounding normal epithelium by its color and acetic acid reaction. Such residual epithelial rims should always undergo biopsy.

As endophytic carcinomas (Fig. 11.50) may masquerade as erosions or flat ulcers, the latter should be probed with Chrobak's sound (see Fig. 7.8). Stroma infiltrated by tumor offers no resistance, the sound sinking into it as into butter. With normal tissues the sound encounters an elastic resistance.

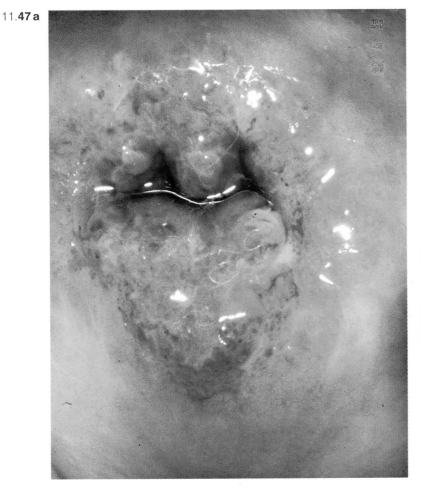

11.47 a

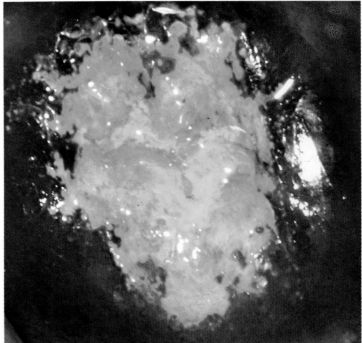

11.47 b

Fig. 11.**47 a**   **True erosion at the outskirts of an unusual transformation zone.** The step-like edge, with pathologic as well as normal squamous epithelium, is well shown in places. Biopsy of the whitish epithelium showed moderate dysplasia (CIN 2)

Fig. 11.**47 b**
After application of iodine, the pathologic epithelium in Fig. 11.**47 a** is typically iodine-yellow, whereas the erosion does not stain at all

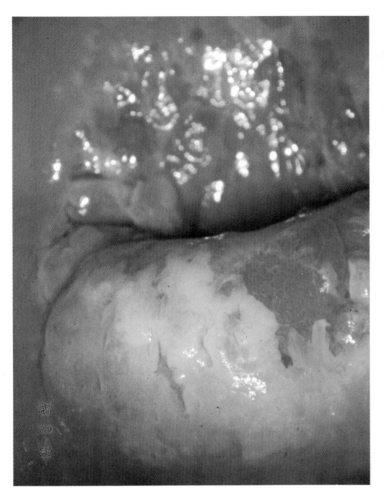

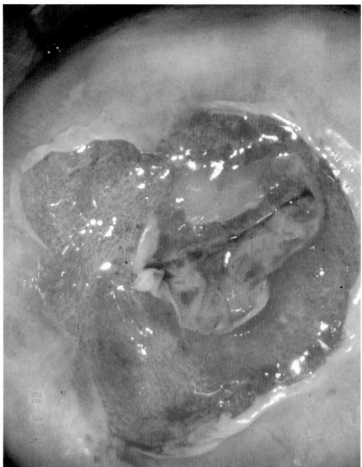

Fig. 11.**48 Typical erosion in an unusual transformation zone.** The epithelial denudation has allowed emergence of the intensely red stroma. The whitish epithelium was severely dysplastic (CIN 3) histologically

Fig. 11.**49 Extensive erosion.** Both centrifugally, and bordering the peripheral normal squamous epithelium, islands of histologically atypical epithelium remain (CIN 3). The texture of the exposed stroma is easily seen

Fig. 11.**50 Flat ulcer to the left of the external os;** its floor is uneven and yellowish to dark red. The diagnosis was invasive squamous cell carcinoma

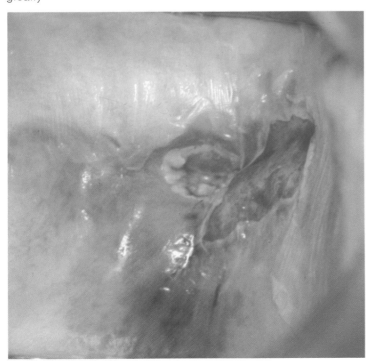

11.51a

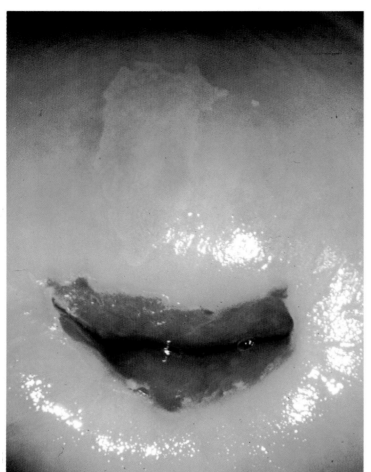

Inconspicuous Iodine-Yellow Area

If one uses the Schiller test routinely as part of every colposcopic examination, time and again one will encounter sharply circumscribed iodine-yellow areas that are otherwise either not visible or overlooked. Such areas are especially striking in cases in which the cervix appears completely normal colposcopically at first sight (Fig. 11.51a and b). If one has the opportunity to examine the patient after the iodine reaction has abated or at some later time, the previously iodine-yellow area will appear grayish and sharply demarcated when consciously searched for.

Besides such unsuspected and isolated foci, iodine-yellow areas are also found in combination with other colposcopic lesions; the latter are therefore really bigger and have different outlines than at first suspected (Fig. 11.52a,b).

Colposcopically inconspicuous iodine-yellow areas are usually caused by benign acanthotic epithelium. Table 14.1, however, shows that this colposcopic appearance carries a low *malignancy index*. This is because the inexperienced colposcopist, who should perform biopsy in the case of every abnormal finding, can miss suspicious lesions that nevertheless declare themselves after iodine staining. This is another reason why the Schiller test is a valuable adjunct to the colposcopic examination.

11.51b

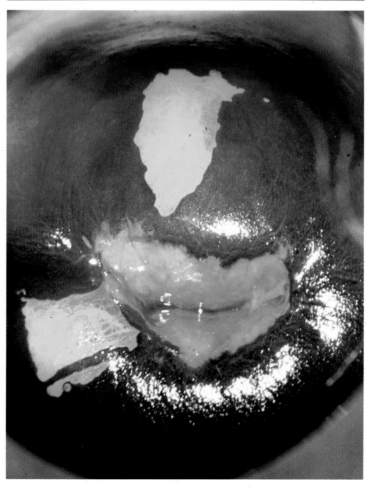

Fig. 11.**51a** Only the nuances in color allow recognition of this lesion arising in original squamous epithelium. Such a lesion can be easily overlooked during routine colposcopy

Fig. 11.**51b** It is remarkable how the above area stands out after application of iodine with its bright yellow color. There is also a second yellow lesion, hardly recognizable in Fig. 11.**51a**. Histologically, acanthotic epithelium

Fig. 11.**52a** **Keratoses** in a vascular transformation zone

Fig. 11.**52b** It is surprising how brown the vascular epithelium becomes with iodine, whereas the presence of the clearly circumscribed iodine-yellow areas could not be suspected before. Histologically, severe dysplasia (CIN 3)

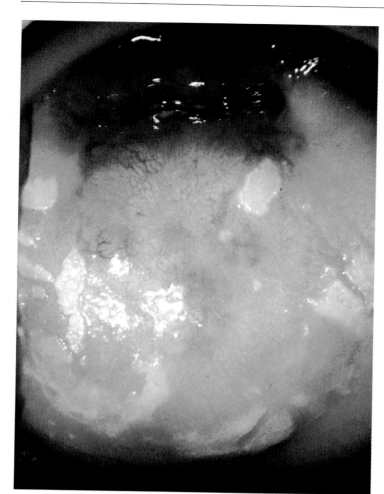

Suspect Invasive Carcinoma

The colposcopic detection of invasive growths depends on their greater size. Foci of *early stromal invasion* that extend to a depth of fractions of a millimeter cannot be seen with the colposcope. Furthermore, such foci arise more often from glands involved by CIN than from atypical surface epithelium (see p. 44). In the latter case, the colposcopic appearances are merely those of the parent surface epithelium, the invasive foci taking root from its base.

Clues to the presence of early invasion are indirect. Our morphometric investigations have shown that the larger the surface extent of a lesion, the higher the likelihood of early stromal invasion (see Fig. 3.66). Table 14.2 shows that in contrast to noninvasive lesions, early stromal invasion is more common when different epithelial types are combined. In some cases, all of the above features are present. Increased vascularity is also suggestive of invasion (Figs. 11.53, 11,56).

Fig. 11.**53   Markedly vascular transformation zone.**
At the periphery, between the 4-o'clock and 6-o'clock positions, there is moderately coarse mosaic as well as clearly delineated mild keratoses (arrows). Biopsy from the transformation zone revealed carcinoma in situ (CIN 3) with early stromal invasion and acanthotic epithelium from the white plaques

.52 b

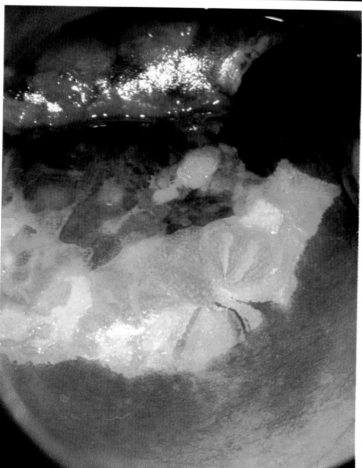

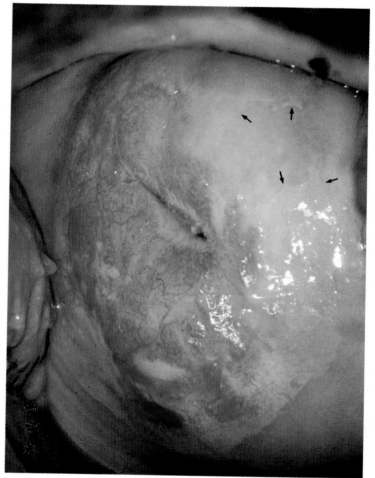

11.**53**

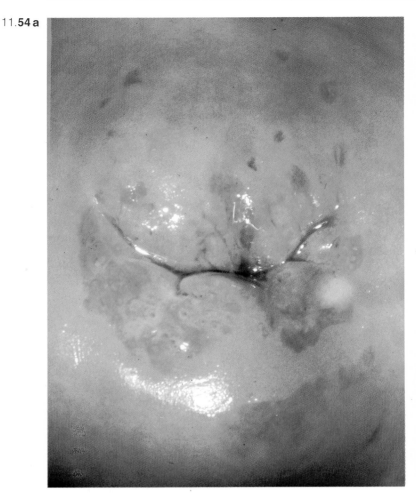

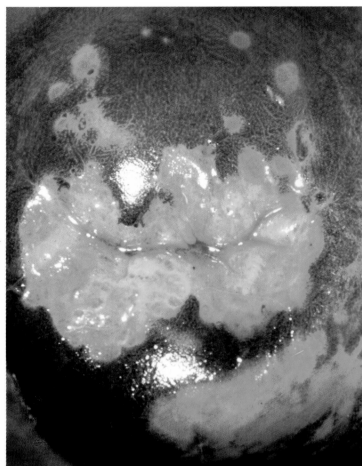

In spite of what has been said about the size of a lesion, quite small lesions can be invasive. The same applies to lesions of low vascularity. Finally, there are cases of early stromal invasion with a surprising paucity of colposcopic changes that hardly raise one's index of suspicion (Figs. 11.54a, b, 11.55).

Colposcopic detection of *microcarcinomas* depends on their size and location. If a microcarcinoma is located entirely within the canal, epithelial abnormalities on the ectocervix will provide no clue to its presence. Ectocervical lesions characterized by focal collections of atypical vessels should be regarded as highly suspicious. Atypical vessels are invariably restricted to the invasive focus (Fig. 11.57). The vessels are often drawn out, have an irregular course, and are prone to bleed.

Somewhat larger tumors produce a slight hump on the surface that gives away their location (Figs. 11.58, 11.59), or appear as a confined polypoid lesion (Fig. 11.61). Diagnosis of an invasive growth arising within an already vascular transformation zone is particularly difficult, if not impossible. Clues to the invasive nature in such cases can be sought only retrospectively by carefully correlating the colposcopic findings with those of histology in conization specimens (Fig. 11.60).

Fig. 11.**54a** **Unusually opaque transformation zone** that merges imperceptibly with the periphery. Note the separate poorly circumscribed reddish area on the posterior lip

Fig. 11.**54b** The iodine-yellow area around the external os was carcinoma in situ (CIN 3) with early stromal invasion. The isolated area on the posterior lip was inflammatory. The speckled brown lesion on the anterior lip is condylomatous colpitis (see p. 181–182)

11.55

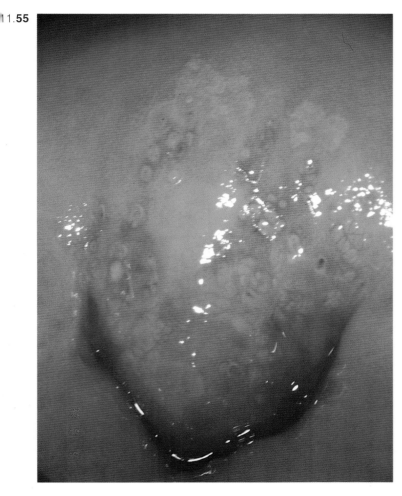

11.56

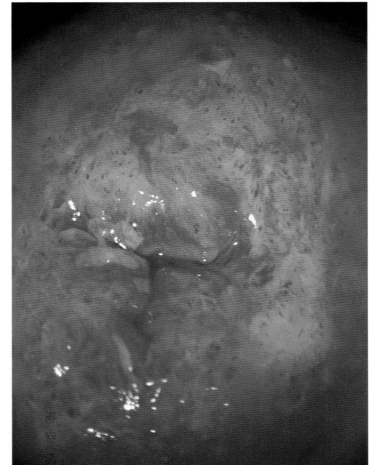

Fig. 11.**55** **Unusual transformation zone** with cuffed gland openings after application of acetic acid. The conization specimen showed severe dysplasia and a carcinoma in situ (CIN 3) with early stromal invasion (stage Ia1)

Fig. 11.**56** **Unusual transformation zone** with a strikingly coarse surface. In the entire area there are irregularly located, comma-shared vessels. The conization specimen showed dysplastic changes (CIN 2), carcinoma in situ (CIN 3), and early stromal invasion (stage Ia1)

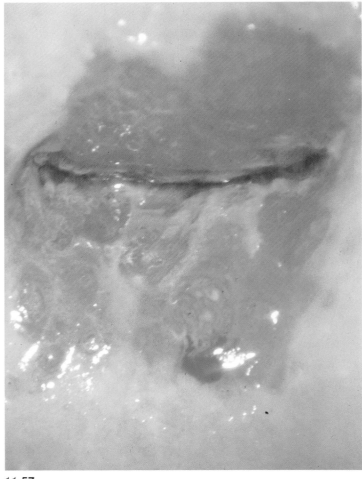

Fig. 11.**57** **Unusual transformation zone**, prior to acetic acid application, harboring a microcarcinoma, just above the bleeding point. Note the irregularly branching vessels. The neighboring reddish areas were carcinoma in situ (CIN 3) histologically. True erosion and regenerating epithelium in the vicinity of the external os on the posterior lip, and regenerating epithelium on the anterior lip

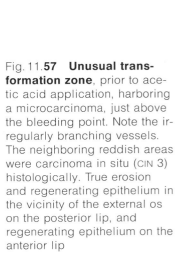

11.**57**

11.**58**

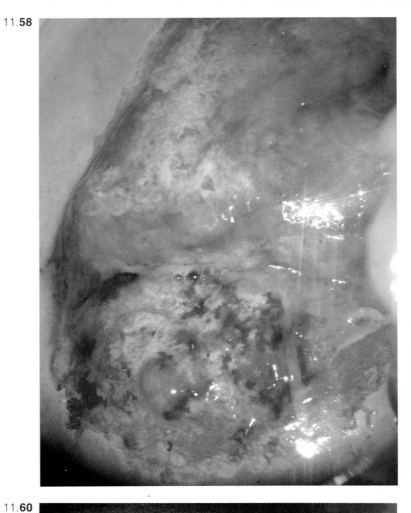

11.**6**

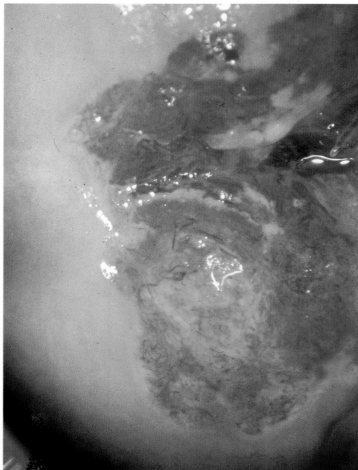

11.**60**

Fig. 11.**58   Large unusual transformation zone** prior to application of acetic acid. The surface of the posterior lip is bulging because of the presence of a small invasive carcinoma, no longer a microcarcinoma. Note the extravasation of blood where the vessels are atypical

Fig. 11.**59   Microcarcinoma** producing a small bulge on the posterior lip. Atypical vessels course over the white surface

Fig. 11.**60   Vascular transformation zone** showing focal hemorrhages. The microcarcinoma occupying the left lateral recess of the external os (arrows) may be easily overlooked

Fig. 11.**61a   Unusual transformation zone** with a coarse surface. The effect of acetic acid is especially marked on the anterior lip: white epithelium with a small polyp in the left corner of the external os

Fig. 11.**61b**   At high magnification the tumor displays numerous atypical vessels. The polyp is a small exophytic carcinoma that has exceeded the limits of a microcarcinoma

11.**61 a**

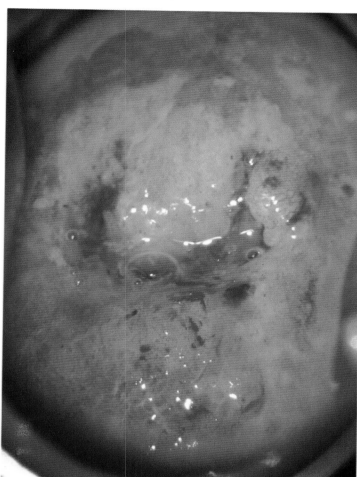

1.**61 b**

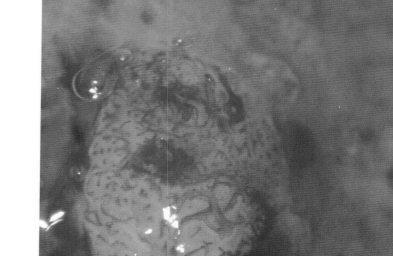

Invasive Carcinoma

Invasive carcinomas are evident with the naked eye. Tumors located entirely within the canal can be seen better with the colposcope, but only if the os is somewhat gaping. In all other cases, colposcopy merely confirms the macroscopic findings.

Distortion of the ectocervical contour depends on the growth pattern of the tumor: exophytic lesions protrude into the vagina as fungating tumors of varying size (Fig. 11.62). Purely endophytic neoplasms, on the other hand, present merely as red or white eroded areas, the true nature of which can be recognized only by their papillary surface and atypical vessels (Fig. 11.59). Flat endophytic carcinomas with ulcerated surfaces may be difficult to diagnose both with the naked eye and with the colposcope (Fig. 11.50). In such cases, palpation and Chrobak's sound (see p. 131) are of value. As invasive carcinomas are most often partly exophytic and partly endophytic, their diagnosis should pose no difficulty. Most carcinomas surround the external os (Fig. 11.64, see also Fig. 11.67). Less often, one or only part of one lip is involved (Fig. 11.62).

The surface of invasive tumors is usually irregularly fissured (Fig. 11.65) and resembles that of a cauliflower. If the papillae are somewhat finer and more regular, their appearance may be confused with that of an ectopy. The degree of ulceration and tissue destruction is greater in more advanced cancers. Occasionally, tumors present as smooth sessile polyps (Fig. 11.66), to be distinguished from benign polyps by their vasculature and by use of Chrobak's sound. An endophytic tumor with a keratotic surface may pose a further diagnostic problem (Fig. 11.67). Mistakes can be avoided by always obtaining a biopsy of a keratotic lesion, the nature of which cannot be determined colposcopically, as the epithelium is masked by keratin.

Invasive cancers afford an excellent opportunity for the study of all kinds of atypical vessels (see p. 223). This should be done after the cervix is cleansed with a dry swab and prior to application of acetic acid, which makes the vessels blanch (Fig. 11.68 a, b). Invasive lesions also become more prominent and whitish with acetic acid (Fig. 11.68). These changes, however, are of no further diagnostic value. Following the acetic acid test, the criteria for the evaluation of atypical epithelia may be applied to the study of preinvasive lesions, which frequently surround an invasive tumor (Fig. 11.69).

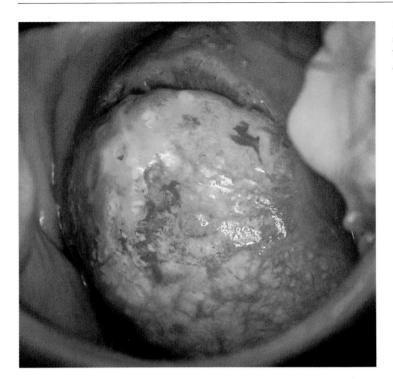

Fig. 11.**62** **Purely exophytic squamous cell carcinoma** on the posterior lip with an ulcerated tip

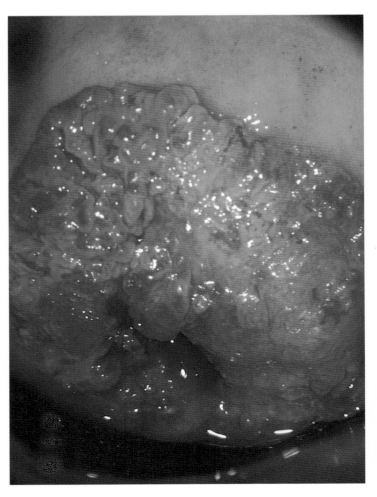

Fig. 11.**63** **Exophytic, papillary verrucous carcinoma** around the external os

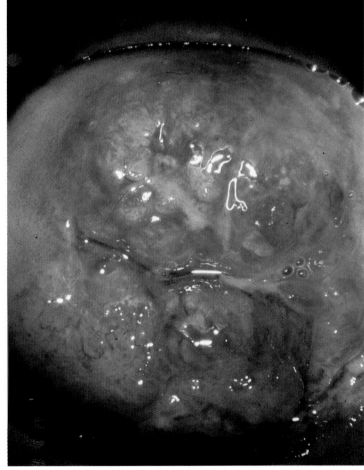

Fig. 11.**64** **This endophytic invasive squamous cell carcinoma** may be mistaken for a merely unusual transformation zone. The markedly atypical blood vessels on the posterior lip are associated as a rule only with invasive carcinomas

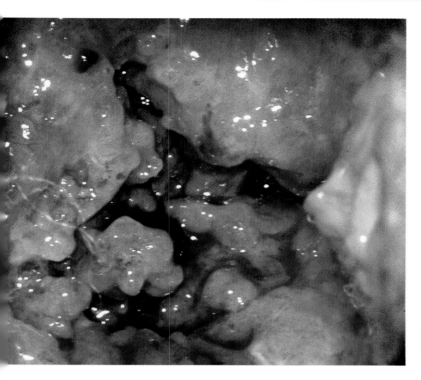

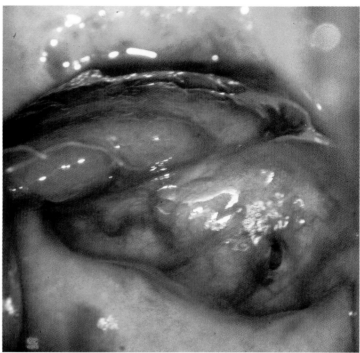

Fig. 11.65 Deeply fissured and coarsely papillary invasive squamous cell carcinoma. The vascular pattern is not pronounced

Fig. 11.66 Polypoid invasive squamous cell carcinoma, which may be mistaken for a large benign cervical polyp.

The color and blood supply of the polyp lower down are reminiscent of those of a nabothian follicle

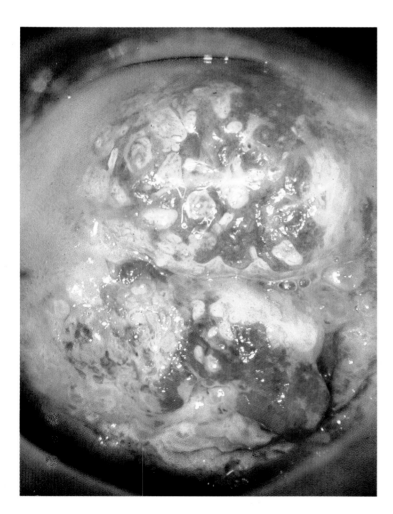

Fig. 11.67 Endophytic invasive squamous cell carcinoma, showing marked hyperkeratosis of its surface

11.**68a**

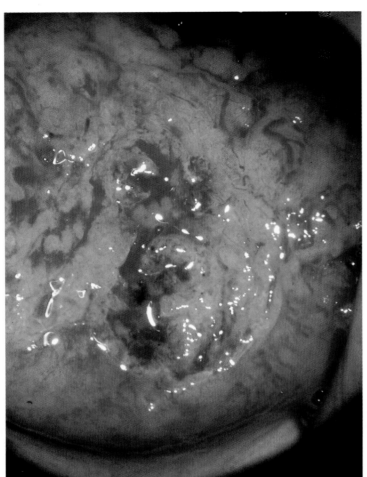

11.**68b**

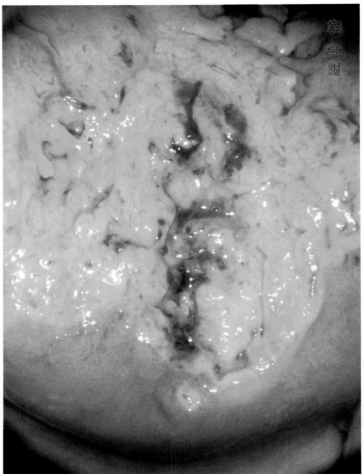

11.**69**

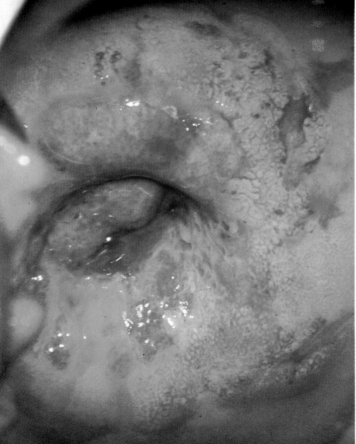

Fig. 11.**68a**   **A somewhat exophytic squamous cell carcinoma,** associated with a variety of atypical blood vessels

Fig. 11.**68b**   The vascular pattern is suppressed by acetic acid, which turns the background white

Fig. 11.**69**   **In situ carcinomatous seam around a squamous cell carcinoma** that is situated predominantly in the canal. Note the flat ulcer on the anterior lip

Adenocarcinoma In Situ and Microinvasive Adenocarcinoma

There are no colposcopic images that suggest the presence of an adenocarcinoma in situ or of a microinvasive adenocarcinoma (19). Since these lesions usually occur with CIN, one finds the colposcopic changes indicative of CIN (Figs. 11.70, 11.71). Furthermore, atypical columnar epithelium is usually located in glands or crypts; when on the surface, it is friable and often eroded (Figs. 11.70 and 11.72). The somewhat larger microinvasive adenocarcinoma (stage 1a2) can occasionally be seen with the colposcope, but cannot be distinguished from squamous cell carcinoma at colposcopic magnification (Fig. 11.72).

Fig. 11.70 In this patient with an unusual transformation zone, the conization specimen showed mild to severe dysplasia (CIN 1−3) as well as an adenocarcinoma in situ on the ectocervix. The latter was present both in glands and in the superficial columnar epithelium

Fig. 11.71 Moderately vascular transformation zone with a few gland openings. Histology showed moderate dysplasia (CIN 2) on the ectocervix. There is an adenocarcinoma in situ in the lower part of the cervical canal

Fig. 11.72 Large, partly eroded transformation zone. The rugae of the ectropionized cervical mucosa are still visible. Histology of the whitish areas showed moderate dysplasia (CIN 2). On the left side of the cervical os there is a 10×3 mm microinvasive adenocarcinoma

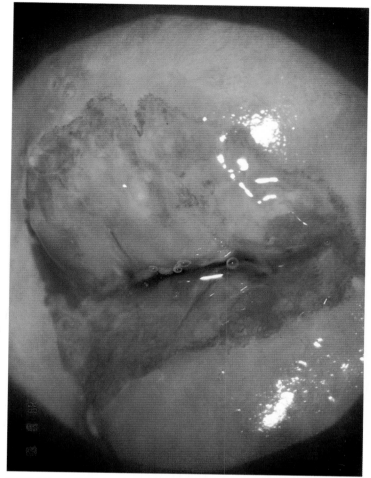

11.70

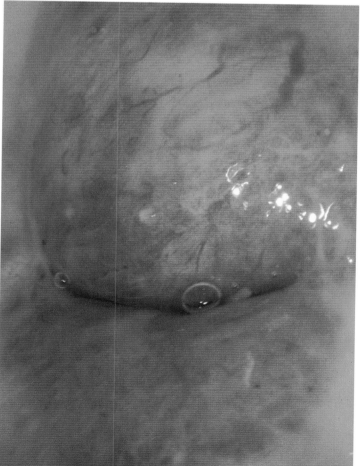

11.71

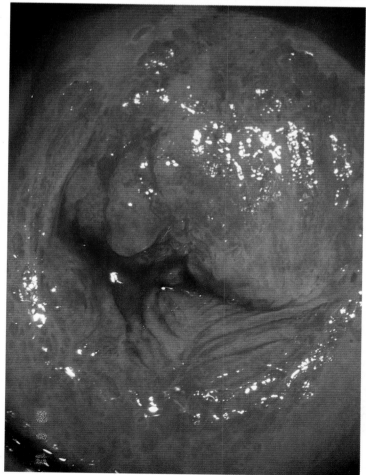

11.72

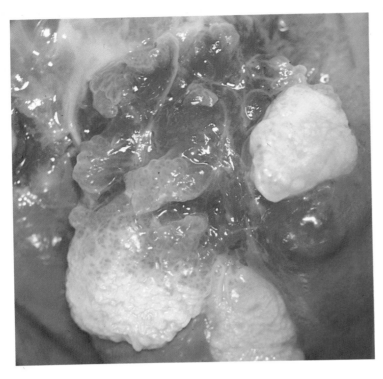

Condylomatous Lesions

The diagnosis of condylomas has attracted a great deal of interest in recent years. The recognition of flat condylomatous lesions on the cervix was crucial for colposcopy, as such changes closely mimic colposcopically suspect findings (16, 17, 18) and yet may be reversible and essentially benign (see p. 94). The delineation of condylomatous colpitis (see p. 181–182) introduced a new dimension to colposcopic diagnosis, as such changes were previously poorly understood.

Condylomata acuminata are usually easy to diagnose colposcopically. An isolated condyloma in the region of the external os, however, may be mistaken for an exophytic carcinoma (Fig. 11.73). Chrobak's sound may be a useful diagnostic aid (see p. 111). The surface of condylomatous lesions is classically papillary (Figs. 11.73–11.75, 11.81, 11.84). The structural details, however, may be concealed by keratin, resulting in a smooth, shiny, mother-of pearl-like surface (Figs. 11.76, 11.80). Not uncommonly, the papillae are fine and finger-like (Fig. 11.77). The color of condylomas varies according to the degree of keratinization and may range from white and grayish red to intense red.

Condylomas are often multiple (Figs. 11.73, 11.79, 13.9) and vary in size, providing a good opportunity to study their

Fig. 11.73 Multiple condylomas around the external os. Only the tips of the large ones show advanced keratinization

Fig. 11.74 Lacerated external os. Note the slightly elevated, fine papillary condyloma in a fold, not easily visible to the naked eye

Fig. 11.75 Fine papillary condyloma as an isolated lesion on the anterior lip of the cervix close to the external os. HPV-16 positive. Histologically, a condyloma without atypia

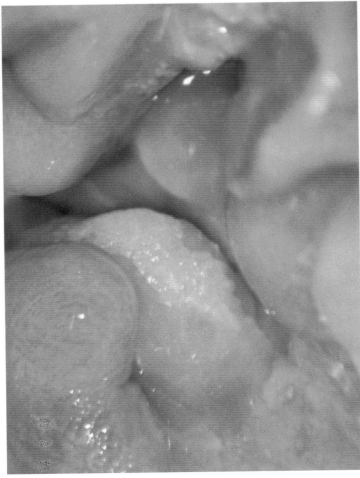

11.74

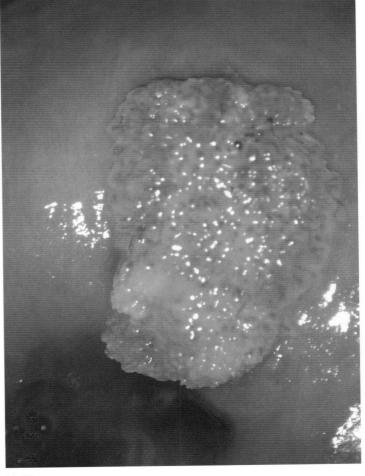

11.75

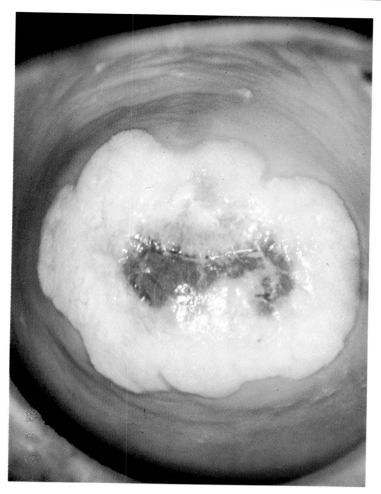

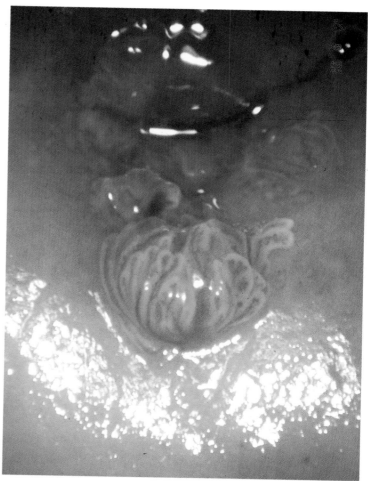

11.**77**

Fig. 11.76 Condyloma with marked keratinization. The keratin layer is so thick that a fissured surface is retained only focally, on the left side

Fig. 11.77 Condyloma characterized by finger-like processes with little in the way of keratinization

Fig. 11.**78** On higher magnification, the vessels within the papillae are comma-shaped and staghorn-like. Their coarseness gives the impression of atypicality

development. Exophytic condylomas may intermingle with flat lesions (Fig. 11.79).

Higher magnification reveals the presence of blood vessels within the papillae of condylomas. They may be comma, corkscrew, or staghorn in shape, and may appear suspicious because of their relatively large caliber (Fig. 11.78). Flat and smooth lesions tend to have a distinctive pearly surface as a result of hyperkeratosis (Figs. 11.79, 11.80). No criteria have been described to distinguish colposcopically between typical and atypical condylomas (18). It is conceivable, however, that the latter may have a coarser structure that may produce coarse punctation or mosaic in analogy with CIN and acanthotic epithelium. The Schiller test shows that condylomatous cells still contain various amounts of glycogen. A stippled, variegated appearance may be produced by focal keratinization (Figs. 11.81b, 11.82). There is also no difference between infection with different HPV types. To distinguish between condylomatous and non-condylomatous lesions of similar appearance, Reid et al. (22) proposed a grading classification which would suggest subclinical HPV infection. However, other authors found this classification unsatisfactory (20).

Occasionally, the degree of glycogen storage by condylomatous epithelium produces the hitherto undescribed, but by

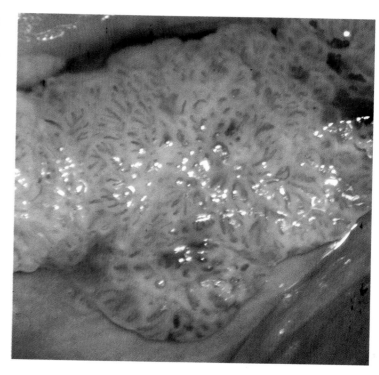

11.**78**

us long-observed, colposcopic appearance of *iodine-positive mosaic or punctation* (Fig. 11.83 a, b). It is problematic whether this picture is typical of and always due to condylomatous lesions. At any rate, such mosaic is caused by glycogen-containing epithelium associated with tall stromal papillae. Histologically, the epithelium in such cases is not merely a variant of normal, but shows features suggestive of flat condylomas (see Fig. 3.35). An iodine-positive mosaic pattern may be produced by colposcopic lesions that, prior to the Schiller test, appear nonspecific apart from their pearly surface. The result of the Schiller test in such cases is all the more surprising (Fig. 11.85 a, b).

Condylomatous lesions frequently coexist with CIN, in which HPV can usually be found (Figs. 11.83 a, b; 11.84).

Every experienced colposcopist will have come across an essentially normal cervix and vagina, the surfaces of which, however, are evenly studded by numerous white dots (Fig. 11.87). These correspond to the tips of elongated stromal papillae that perforate a rather irregular-structured yet glycogen-containing epithelium (see Fig. 4.52). Meisels et al. (18) called this appearance condylomatous cervicitis and vaginitis.

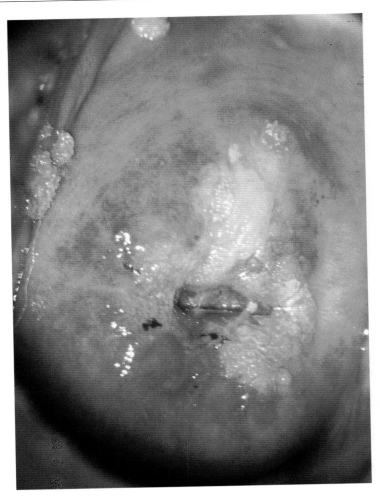

Fig. 11.**79** **Flat condylomas** around the external os. Most of their surface is finely granular, some areas are smooth. HPV-16 and HIV-positive. Small condylomatous lesions dot the cervix and the vagina

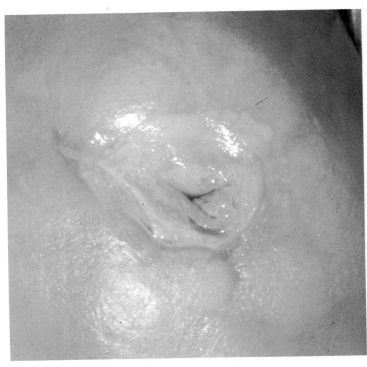

Fig. 11.**80** **Markedly keratinized flat condyloma** surrounding the external os. Note the characteristic pearly, flat surface

11.**80**

1.81a

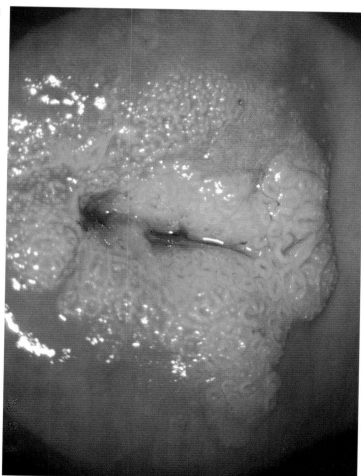

11.81b

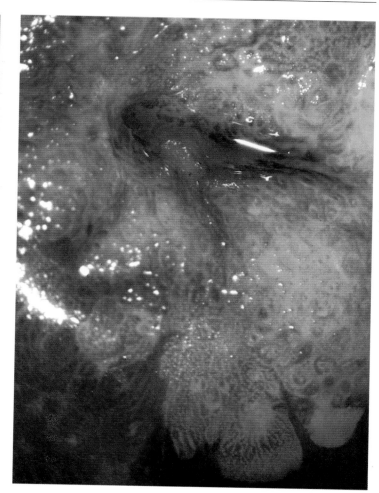

Fig. 11.**81a** **Flat to distinctly elevated condylomas** around the external os and in the lower cervical canal. The same patient as in Fig. 11.**79**, six months later

Fig. 11.**81b** The Schiller test shows the typical patchy brown areas indicating glycogen storage in the condylomas. Histology showed mild dysplasia with koilocytosis (CIN 1)

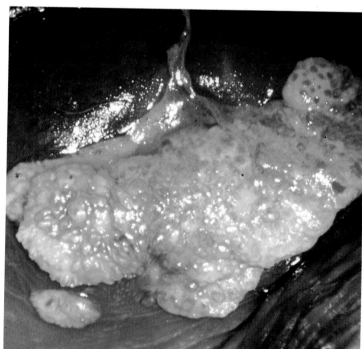

Fig. 11.**82** The brownish color with iodine of glycogen containing patches within the condyloma correlates well with the histologic picture

11.**83 a**

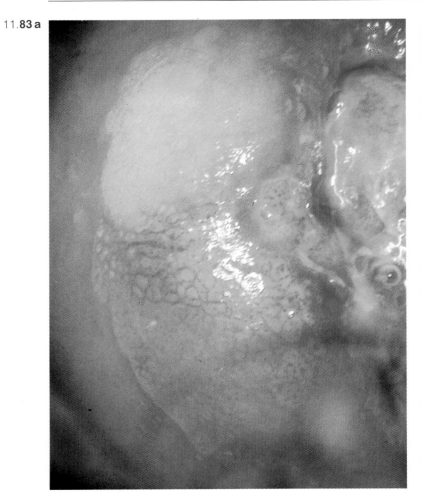

11.**8**

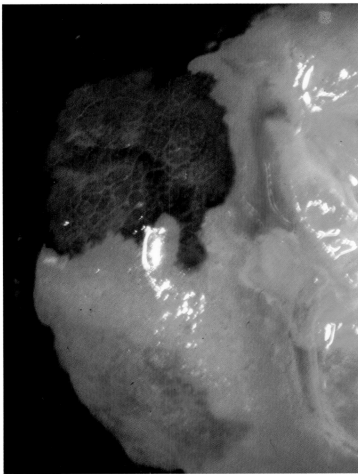

Fig. 11.83 a   A shiny mother-of-pearl surface of a lesion also showing moderately coarse mosaic and punctation: histologically, the white area corresponds to a flat condyloma, the mosaic to mild dysplasia (CIN 1)

Fig. 11.**83 b**   The previously white lesion displays an iodine-positive mosaic pattern after the Schiller test: histologically flat condyloma. The mosaic and punctation, clearly visible before the Schiller test, are stained poorly. Less structured areas are light brown

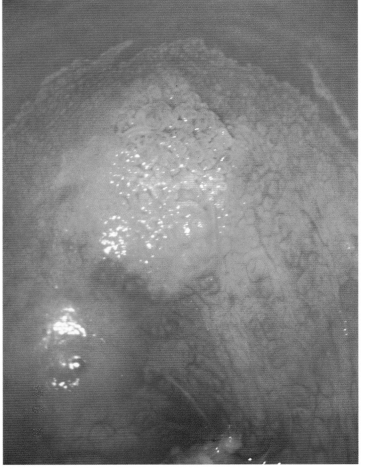

Fig. 11.84   Flat, fine papillary condylamatous excrescences within a mosaic field. The mosaic is HPV-16 positive and histologically shows mild dysplasia (CIN 1)

11.**84**

1.85 a

11.85 b

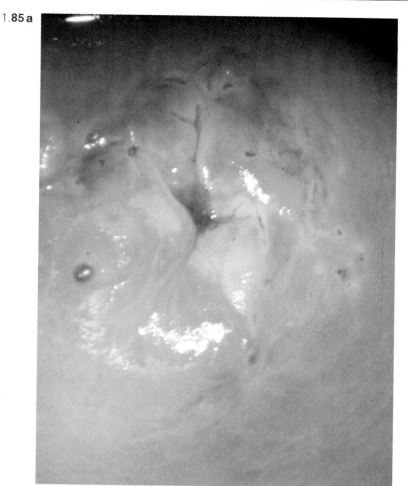

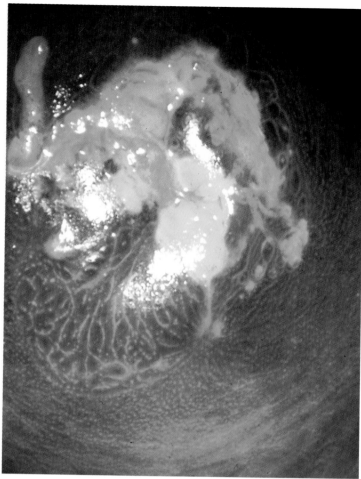

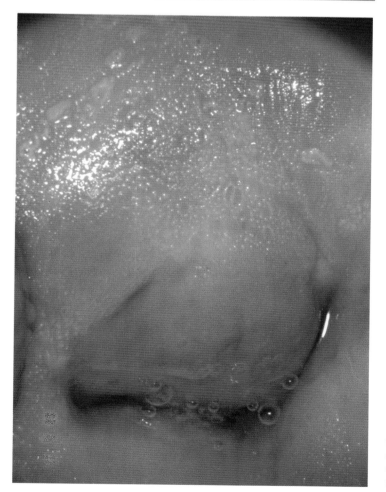

Fig. 11.**85 a** **Lesion around the external os with a shiny pearly appearance.** Note the advanced state of development of the transformation zone clockwise from the 9-o'clock to the 6-o'clock positions. On careful examination, a fine yet clearly delineated lesion is seen between the 6-o'clock and 9-o'clock positions. The white epithelium was an atypical flat condyloma histologically

Fig. 11.**85 b** After the Schiller test, the flat condyloma in Fig. 11.**85 a** has the appearance of iodine-positive mosaic

Fig. 11.**86** **Typical appearance of the cervical mucosa** in a patient with condylomatous vaginitis. There are circumscribed, slightly elevated condylomas whithin the granular area

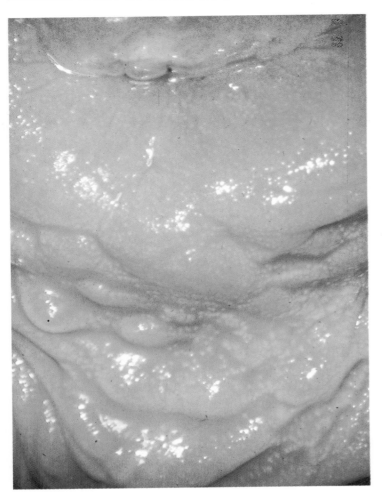

Fig. 11.**87** **The cervix and the vagina are covered by numerous white spots** due to condylomatous colpitis

Miscellaneous Colposcopic Findings

Inflammatory Changes

Diffuse inflammation of the vagina has a nonspecific colposcopic appearance. The appearance of focal lesions is of some significance, due to patchy inflammatory infiltration of the stroma accompanied by dilated capillaries. Diagnostic difficulties arise when such foci become bigger and indiscriminately arranged.

Trichomonal infection produces a typical frothy discharge. Removal of the secretions may reveal numerous red spots covering the cervix (Fig. 11.88 a). The inflammatory foci vary in shape and in distribution. After application of acetic acid, the previously red areas turn whitish, the squamous epithelium being already "loosened up" by the inflammation (Fig. 11.88 b). The damaged epithelium may release its glycogen, with consequent failure to take up iodine. Iodine typically imparts a leopard-skin appearance to inflammatory lesions (Fig. 11.89) and confirms the poor circumscription of larger ones which may otherwise be mistaken for more serious abnormalities.

Colpitis macularis (strawberry cervix) has a unique colposcopic appearance, characterized by uniformly arranged red spots a few millimeters in size; it is usually due to *Trichomonas vaginalis* (Fig. 11.90 a). The inflamed area is always iodine-negative, and its margin is indistinct (Fig. 11.90 b). In severe cases, the vagina is also involved.

.88a

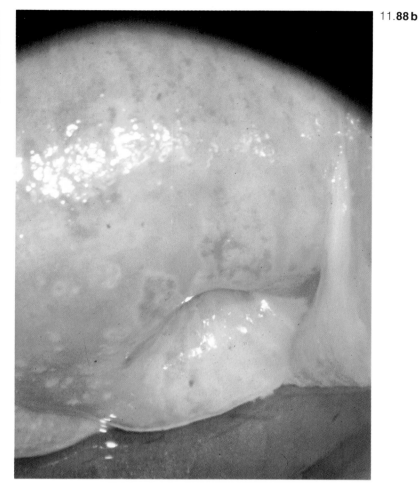

11.88b

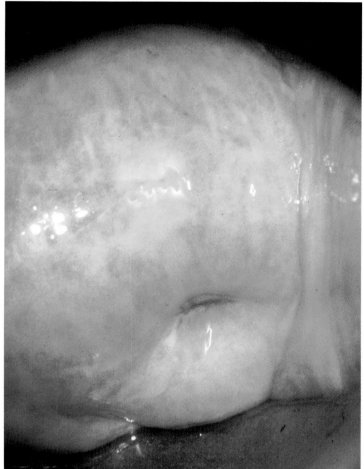

Fig. 11.**88a   Rather irregular reddish stippling of the cervix** due to trichomonas infection

Fig. 11.**88b** The inflamed area becomes white to some extent after application of acetic acid; its margins are indistinct

Fig. 11.**89   The vague margins of the inflamed areas** are well seen with the Schiller test

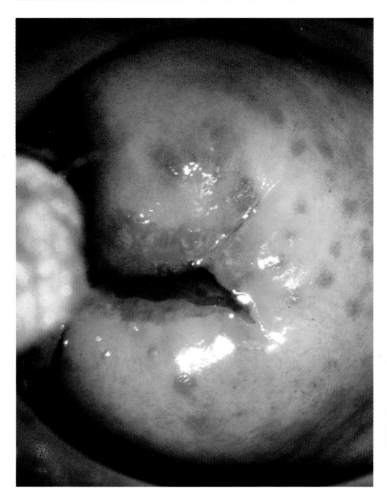

Fig. 11.**90 a** **The typical appearance of colpitis macularis,** with numerous round spots covering the cervix and vagina, due to focal round cell infiltration

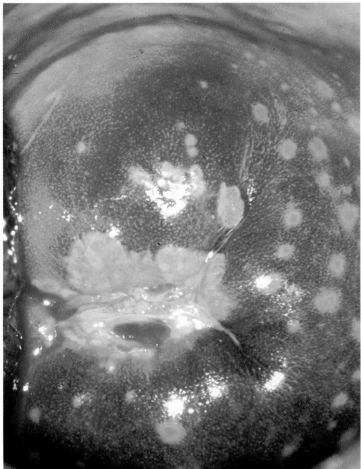

Fig. 11.**90 b** After the Schiller test, the inflamed areas in Fig. 11.**90 a** are poorly demarcated and are separated by fields showing so-called condylomatous colpitis

Polyps

Polyps can be easily seen colposcopically, even if they are situated farther up in the endocervical canal. The aim of colposcopic examination is not merely to detect them, but also to evaluate their surface configuration according to the usual criteria. In the first instance, a polyp may be invested by columnar epithelium only, in which case the typical grape-like appearance will be seen. More often, the polyp is covered by smooth squamous epithelium (Figs. 11.91 to 11.93). If the maturation of such histogenetically metaplastic squamous epithelium is irregular, then the various fields are clearly demarcated from each other (Fig. 11.92). Rarely, the squamous epithelium is atypical; in such cases, the colposcopic changes conform to those that occur elsewhere on the cervix. Polyps may be single or multiple, and may arise from ectopies, from transformation zones (Fig. 11.91), or from otherwise unremarkable cervices (Fig. 11.93).

11.91

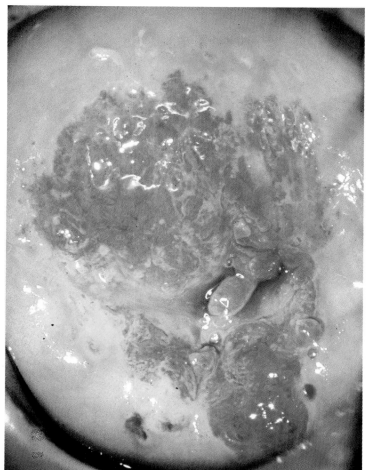

11.92

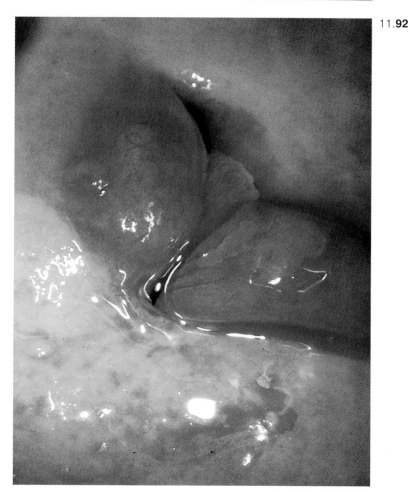

Fig. 11.**91 Cervical polyp in the transformation zone** covered by metaplastic squamous epithelium

Fig. 11.**92 Endocervical polyps** that have undergone metaplasia. A nabothian follicle has developed within one of the polyps. The lowermost polyp shows that the metaplastic process developed in separate, well-defined fields

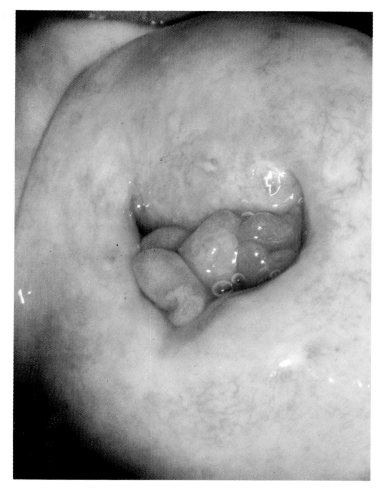

Fig. 11.**93 Multiple polyps arising from an atrophic cervix.** The metaplastic epithelium covering the polyps also arose in separate fields

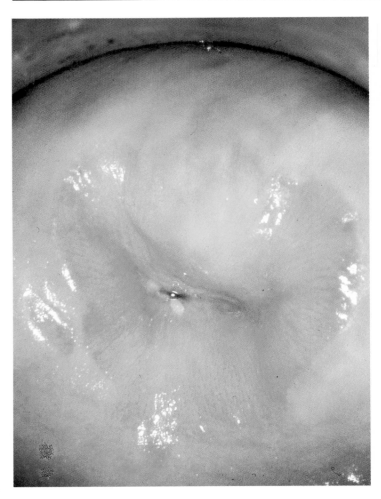

Fig. 11.**94 a**   **Cervix following conization.** The site of surgical removal can be identified by the scarring and the fine vasculature

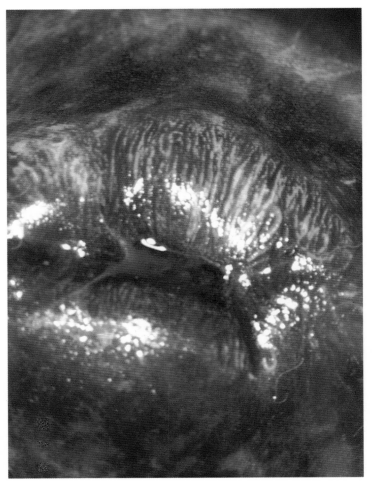

Fig. 11.**94 b**   Iodine staining reveals the uniform nature of the epithelium. The light yellow streaks correspond to scars

Postconization Changes

The cervix is usually smooth following conization and is covered by normal squamous epithelium. The squamocolumnar junction is again situated at the external os. Occasionally the operative scar clearly stands out from the residual cervix (Fig. 11.94 a) and may be mistaken for some other abnormality. The Schiller test will show, however, that the region in question stains brown in the same way as the rest of the cervix (Fig. 11.94 b). A nuance in color is merely due to the scar tissue under the epithelium. This is a good example of how the stroma may influence the colposcopic appearance.

Residual lesions due to incomplete excision by conization may be detected at follow-up colposcopy in the region of the reconstituted external os (Fig. 11.95) or farther out on the ectocervix when extensive (Fig. 11.96). The colposcopic appearance will vary according to the type of epithelium.

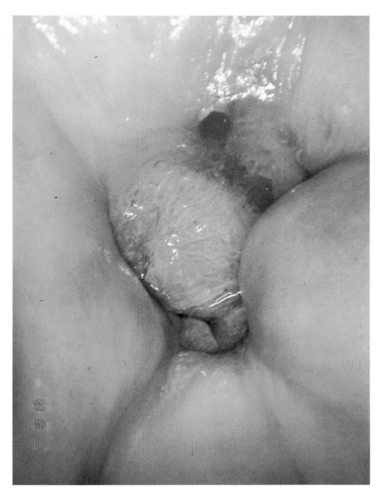

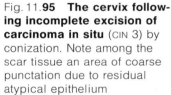

Fig. 11.**95** **The cervix following incomplete excision of carcinoma in situ** (CIN 3) by conization. Note among the scar tissue an area of coarse punctation due to residual atypical epithelium

Fig. 11.**96** **Extensive area of mild dysplasia** (CIN 1) left behind by inadequate conization

Changes due to Prolapse

Prolapse results in exteriorization of the squamous epithelium of the cervix and portions of the vagina so as to become part of the body surface. It is therefore open to outside influences. To be more protective, the glycogen-containing squamous epithelium changes and becomes skin-like. Histologically, there are acanthosis and hyperkeratosis.

This process proves that, according to demand, the non-keratinized glycogen-containing epithelium may become at any time like the epidermis. We designate this event alone as *epidermization*. As this type of epithelium is not native to the site, the term *abnormally maturing* was used. Glatthaar (8) referred to it as the *reactive form* of abnormally maturing (acanthotic) epithelium. This produces a diffuse uniform cover, as seen especially in cases of prolapse. Colposcopically, we encounter far more often the *regenerative form* of acanthotic epithelium that arises on a soil of metaplasia in clearly defined fields and, as often pointed out, is of great colposcopic significance. The important difference between the reactive and regenerative types is the reversible nature of the former: after the stimulus ceases, i.e., after repositioning of the prolapse, the epithelium resumes its original form. The well-circumscribed regenerative type of acanthotic epithelium, on the other hand, retains its position and contour for a lifetime. The regenerative type of acanthotic epithelium therefore corresponds to a morbid state and in this respect resembles chronic dermatoses.

The colposcopic appearance of the epidermized cervix is reminiscent of skin both in color and in its wrinkled surface contour (Fig. 11.97). It is obvious even with the naked eye that this type of epithelium is more durable and less vulnerable. A well-recognized complication of prolapse is ulceration of the extruded portion of the cervix or vagina, known as *decubitus ulcers*. These ulcers are punched out, their floor being flat and usually an angry red (Fig. 11.98), but it may be dirty gray if superinfected.

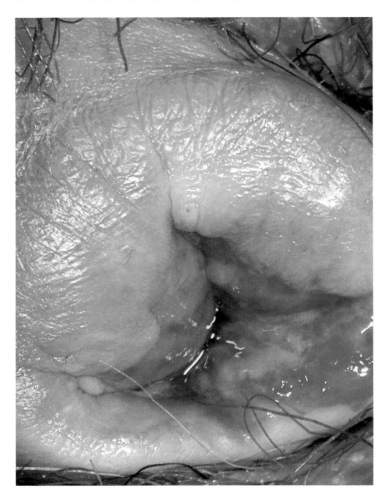

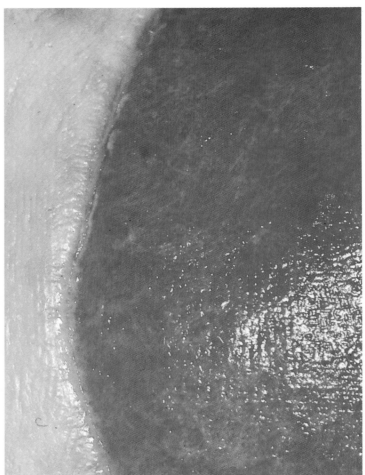

Fig. 11.**97   Typical appearance following epidermization of a prolapse.** The ectocervical epithelium assumes the character of wrinkled skin: this is due to various degrees of keratinization

Fig. 11.**98   Part of a decubitus ulcer associated with prolapse.** Note its typically flat floor and punched-out margin

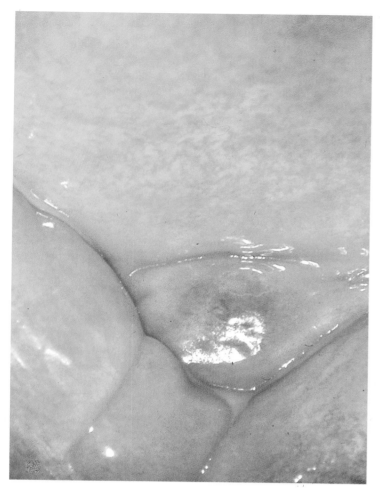

Fig. 11.**99** **Bluish endome-
triotic deposit** in the posterior
fornix of a 38-year-old woman,
on day 24 of the cycle

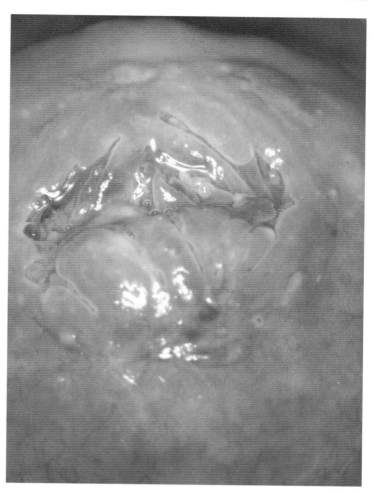

Fig. 11.**100** **Transformation
zone** with still recognizable
rugae of the ectropion. There
is a small bluish focus of endometriosis on the anterior lip

Endometriosis

Endometriosis of the cervix is rare (Figs. 11.**99** and 11.**100**),
the posterior vaginal fornix being more commonly involved.
The deposits appear as bluish spots shimmering through the
epithelium and are best seen prior to menstruation; they may
disappear altogether during the proliferative phase of the cycle.

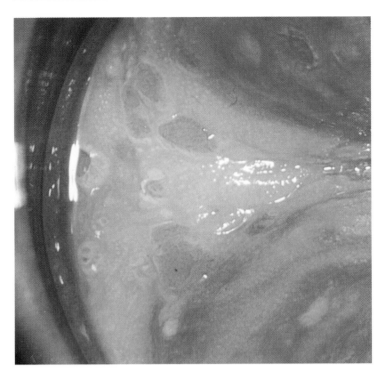

Fig. 11.**101   Vaginal adeno-sis.** The ectopy has undergone advanced transformation. Nabothian follicles have also developed. The red spots are due to residual glandular tissue

Vaginal Adenosis

Vaginal adenosis is defined as the presence of columnar epithelium in the vagina, and may be regarded as due to displacement to form an *ectopy, outside the cervix*. The colposcopic appearances are identical to those of the common cervical ectopy. The same applies to the transformation of vaginal adenosis, which usually "heals" by squamous metaplasia. The transformation zone may be typical or unusual, displaying all of the characteristics of either (Fig. 11.**101**); alternatively, epithelial types may arise that produce the colposcopic pattern of punctation or mosaic. Vaginal adenosis is rare in Europe.

The problem of vaginal adenosis has assumed special significance ever since American authors linked its development in female offspring to exposure to diethylstilbestrol (DES) in utero (10, 11, 21). Of even greater concern is the possible relationship of these changes to the development of clear-cell adenocarcinoma in young women and girls. Although direct transition of vaginal adenosis to clear-cell adenocarcinoma has been reported (2, 7), this previously theoretical consideration has prompted even radical therapy (24). The risk of development of clear-cell adenocarcinoma in exposed girls has been estimated as 0.14 to 1.4 per 1000 cases (9). It has also been postulated that women with vaginal adenosis run a higher risk of developing invasive squamous cell carcinoma (6, 26); this, however, has not been the experience to date. The incidence of carcinoma in situ in one study of 259 DES-exposed young women was 1.4%, 5 times the frequency in nonexposed subjects (25); other authors found the incidence of epithelial atypia to be much less common (5); still others believe the discrepancy is due to differing diagnostic criteria (5, 23). It is important to point out that punctation and mosaic produced by the transformation of vaginal adenosis are far less frequently associated with histologic CIN than similar colposcopic changes in the cervix (5).

It became appreciated later that, besides vaginal adenosis, DES-exposed subjects have a number of other abnormalities, including persisting "immature metaplasia" (15), cervical cockscombs, hoods, and cervicovaginal collars (1, 27). Similar deformities have been noted by Baader (4) in young non-DES-exposed women, and were associated in some cases with genital hypoplasia and subfertility (see p.195). The effect of DES appears to be primarily teratogenic and not carcinogenic, being exerted on the mullerian apparatus and the developing vagina of the embryo.

American authors recommend expectant management of vaginal adenosis (25). Treatment is needed only when epithelial atypia has developed.

References

1 Adam E, Decker DG, Herbst AL, Noller KL, Tilley BC, Townsend DE. Exposure in utero to diethylstilbestrol and related synthetic hormones. J Am Med Assoc 1976;236:1107.

2 Anderson B, Warting WG, Edinger DD Jr, Small EC, Netland AT, Safaii H. Development of DES-associated clear cell carcinoma: the importance of regular screening. Obstet Gynecol 1979;53:293.

3 Baader O. Kolpophotographische Studien, 1: Die Portio von Adoleszentinnen. Gynäkol Praxis 1982;6:101.

4 Burghardt E. Über die atypische Umwandlungszone. Geburtshilfe Frauenheilkd 1959;19:676.

5 Burke L, Antonioli S, Rosen S. Vaginal and cervical squamous cell dysplasia in women exposed to diethylstilbestrol in utero. Am J. Obstet Gynecol 1978;132:537.

6 Fowler WC, Edelman DA. In utero exposure to DES. Evaluation and follow-up of 199 women. Obstet Gynecol 1978;51:459.

7 Ghosh TK, Cera PJ. Transition of benign vaginal adenosis to clear cell carcinoma. Obstet Gynecol 1983;61:126.

8 Glatthaar E. Studien über die Morphogenese des Plattenepithelkarzinoms des Portio vaginalis uteri. Basle: Karger, 1950.

9 Herbst AL, Cole P, Norusis MJ, Welch WR, Scully RE. Epidemiologic aspects and factors related to survival in 384 registry cases of clear cell adenocarcinoma of the vagina and cervix. Am J Obstet Gynecol 1979;135:876.

10 Herbst AL, Kurman RJ, Scully RE, Poskanzer DC. Clear-cell adenocarcinoma of the genital tract in young females. N Engl J Med 1972;284:1259.

11 Herbst AL, Ulfelder U, Poskanzer DC. Adenocarcinoma of the vagina. N Engl J Med 1971;284:878.

12 Hinselmann H. Die Ätiologie, Symptomatologie und Diagnostik des Uteruscarcinoms. In: Veit J, Stöckel W, eds. Handbuch der Gynäkologie, vol 6:1. Munich: Bergmann, 1930:854.

13 Hinselmann H. Die Kolposkopie. Wuppertal: Girardet, 1954.

14 Hinselmann H. Kolposkopische Studien, vols 1–6. Leipzig: VEB Thieme, 1954–59.

15 Jordan JA. Vaginal and cervical neoplasia after exposure to stilbestrol in utero. Br J Obstet Gynecol 1975;82:588.

16 Meisels A, Fortin R, Roy M. Condylomatous lesions of the cervix, 2: cytologic, colposcopic and histopathologic study. Acta Cytol 1977;21:379.

17 Meisels A, Morin C, Casas-Cordero M, Roy M, Fortier M. Condylomatöse Veränderungen der Cervix, Vagina und Vulva. Gynäkologe 1981;14:254.

18 Meisels A, Roy M, Fortier M, et al. Human papillomavirus infection of the cervix: the atypical condyloma. Acta Cytol 1981;25:7.

19 Östör AG, Pagano R, Davoren RAM, Fortune DW, Chanen W, Rome R. Adenocarcinoma in situ of the cervix. Int J Gynecol Pathol 1984;3:179.

20 Pixley EC. Colposcopic appearances of human papillomavirus of the uterine cervix. In: Syrjänen K, Gissmann L, Koss LG, eds. Papillomavirus and human disease. Berlin: Springer, 1987:268–295.

21 Pomerance W. Post-stilbestrol secondary syndrome. Obstet Gynecol 1973;42:12.

22 Reid R, Stanhope CR, Herschman BR, Crum CP, Agronow SJ. Genital warts and cervical cancer, 4: a colposcopic index for differentiating subclinical papillomaviral infection from cervical intraepithelial neoplasia. Am J Obstet Gynecol 1984;149:815.

23 Robboy SJ, Prat J, Welch WR, Barnes AB. Squamous cell neoplasia controversy in the female exposed to diethylstilbestrol. Hum Pathol 1977;8:483.

24 Sherman AI, Goldrath M, Berlin A, et al. Cervical-vaginal adenosis after in utero exposure to synthetic estrogens. Obstet Gynecol 1974;44:531.

25 Stafl A, Mattingly RF. Vaginal adenosis: a precancerous lesion? Am J Obstet Gynecol 1974;120:666.

26 Stafl A, Mattingly RF. Diethylstilbestrol and the cervicovaginal epithelium. In: Jordan Ar, Singer A, eds. The cervix. Philadelphia: Saunders, 1976:28–331.

27 Townsend DE. The cervix and vagina of women exposed to synthetic nonsteroidal oestrogens. In: Coppleson M, Pixley E, Reid B, eds. Colposcopy. Springfield, IL: Thomas, 1978:14–341.

28 Treite P. Die Frühdiagnose des Plattenepithel-Karzinoms am Collum uteri. Stuttgart: Enke, 1944.

12

Comparative Colposcopy and Colposcopic Follow-up Studies*

* after O. Baader.

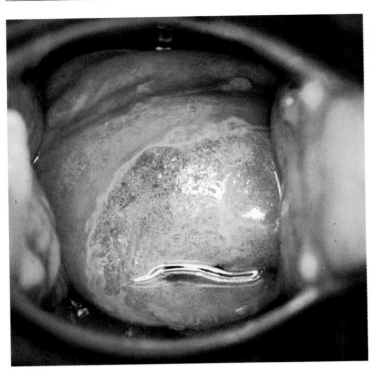

Fig. 12.1a Extensive ectopy with only a thin rim of transformation zone in a 14-year-old. The outer surface of the anterior lip and the fornix are corrugated

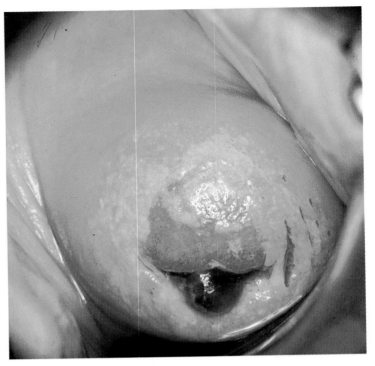

Fig. 12.1b After two years, the transformation is more advanced. The surface of the anterior lip is now smooth. (Courtesy of O. Baader.)

Functional Colposcopy

The term "functional colposcopy" was coined by Baader (5, 6). By this he meant the continued observation of the dynamics of cervical changes, as distinct from diagnostic colposcopy, which deals with the description, distinction between, and evaluation of the various colposcopic findings. The main thrust of colposcopy has been the study of cervical carcinogenesis, and little attention has been paid to the great variation that exists in the shape of the cervix between different women and in the same woman during different epochs of her life, the latter changes being related in all probability to her changing hormonal status. According to Baader (8), there are three ways in which the colposcopic appearance may be correlated with hormonal changes:

Short-Term Observations

These concern the scenario that occurs during a single menstrual cycle and include changes in the external os, in the consistency of the cervical mucus, and possibly in the everted portion of the endocervical mucosa.

Medium-Term Observations

These relate to certain hormone-induced changes during oral contraceptive therapy or during pregnancy. Foremost among these is hyperplasia of the endocervical mucosa, which is seen particularly in ectopy.

Long-Term Observations

Apart from the observations of Baader (7), some of which extended over a nine-year period, there are few such studies. He observed cervices from adolescence to well into reproductive life, paying particular attention to changes involving ectopic columnar mucosa. Ideally, such studies should begin by vaginoscopy in children and continue for several decades. This is a challenge for future researchers.

Fig. 12.3a Cocksomb-like lesion on the surface of the anterior lip and fornix in a 17-year-old. The polypoid structure around the external os is suggested only by the shallow notches

Fig. 12.3b Surprising stippling effect of iodine on the lesions in Fig. 12.3a. Only the posterior lip shows typical uniform mahogany-brown staining

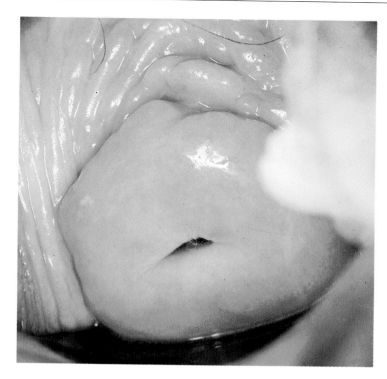

Fig. 12.**2** **Typical portio rugata** in a 29-year-old with primary infertility. (Courtesy of O. Baader.)

Shape and Size of the Cervix

Quite apart from the surprising variation in size, surface contour, and shape of the external os, the cervices of adolescent girls are of two basic types, related no doubt to genital function (3–5).

1. The normal cervix is cone-shaped, has a transverse os, and often displays a large ectopy. Its smooth surface extends to the vaginal fornix, where it merges with the corrugated vaginal mucosa (Figs. 12.1 a and b).

2. The hypoplastic cervix (portio rugata) is encountered especially in the newborn and during childhood (14). The cervix is dome-shaped, with a dimple-like os, but may be expanded distally to resemble a mushroom. Ectopy is not present during adolescence, nor does it arise later. The vaginal rugae often continue onto the cervix, especially anteriorly, and occasionally circumferentially, rather like a hood (Fig. 12.2). Sometimes the surface looks like a cockscomb (Fig. 12.3 b), and may resemble the appearances described in young girls with intrauterine exposure to diethylstilbestrol (DES) (1, 24). There is some evidence that this type of cervix, when it persists beyond adolescence, is associated

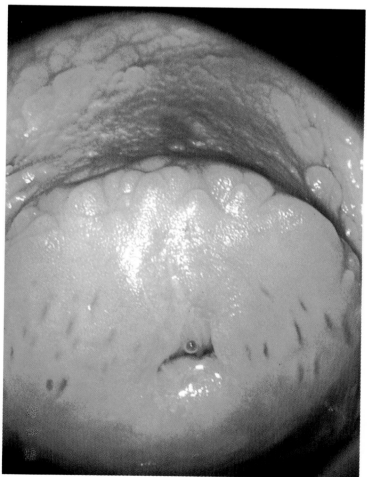

12.**3 a**

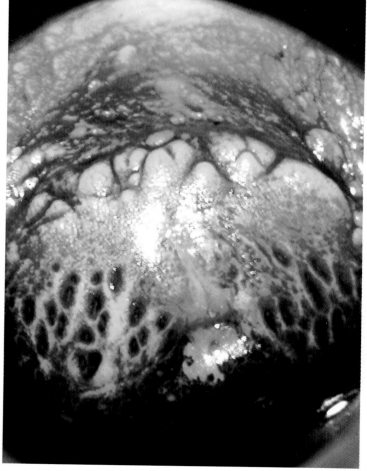

12.**3 b**

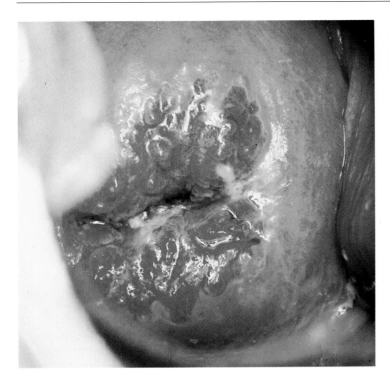

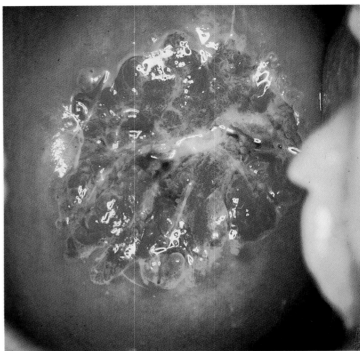

Fig. 12.**4 a** **Ectopy** in a
20-year-old who has never
taken oral contraceptives

Fig. 12.**4 b** Several months
later, after the patient had
been treated with levonorgestrel 0.15 mg and ethinyl
estradiol 0.03 mg, the ectopy
in Fig. 12.**4** has a strikingly
coarse papillary appearance

with reproductive dysfunction, in particular infertility and
increased fetal wastage (5, 7). These observations need confirmation.

Influence of Hormones on the Cervix

Ever since the work of Fischl (12) it has been known that approximately one in three female infants is born with an ectopy
of the endocervical mucosa, often referred to as Fischl's erosion. The incidence of congenital erosions has been stated to be
higher by other investigators (19, 20, 25). A more recent vagi-
noscopic study of newborn females has confirmed Fischl's figures (18). The same investigators found that a third of pubertal
girls also had an ectopy, yet congenital ectopies are known to
disappear (9, 10, 17, 18). In a study of 1483 vaginoscopies before the menarche, no cases of ectopy were found (22). The
question therefore still remains whether ectopy in puberty is
congenital or develops at that time by eversion of the endocervical mucosa.

Recent studies have emphasized cervical changes induced
by oral contraceptives. Baader (2−5) recognizes two kinds of
reactive changes that can be related to the types of cervix described above: *ectopic cervix*, which is hormone-induced, and
non-ectopic cervix, which remains unchanged, even with mas-
sive doses of hormones. Of the hormone-induced changes, hyperplasia of the endocervical mucosa is the best known; both
the ectopic and normally localized columnar epithelium may be
involved. The histologic changes have been described by a
number of authors (10, 11, 13−15, 21, 23), and are currently
designated as *microglandular hyperplasia*. The latter has been
confused with adenocarcinoma, or has at least been suspected
of being neoplastic (9, 14, 21, 23). Colposcopically, the most
pronounced change occurs in ectopic mucosa, which undergoes
striking hyperplasia and projects from the external os like a
polyp. On the whole, ectopies appear larger and coarser, even

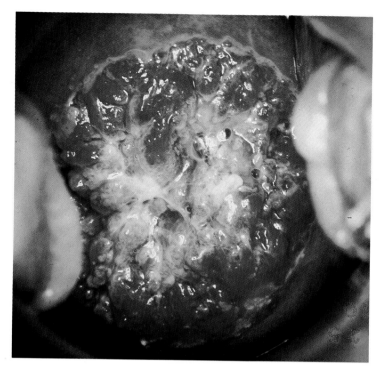

Fig. 12.**4c** Three years later, following childbirth, the same patient has been taking levonorgestrel 0.25 mg and ethinyl estradiol 0.05 mg for some months

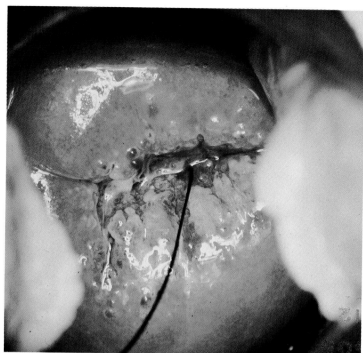

Fig. 12.**4d** A further year later, with an IUD in situ for 3 months. The transformation of the ectopy has been rapid. (Courtesy of O. Baader.)

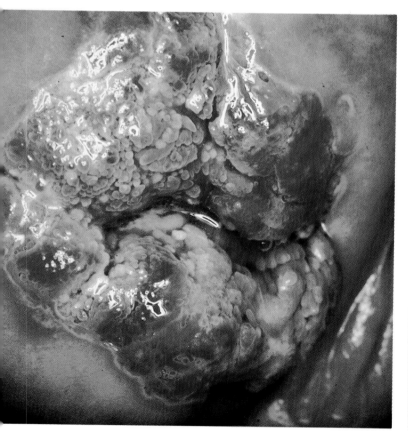

Fig. 12.**5a** **Partly polypoid ectopy** with coarse papillae after 4 years of oral contraception

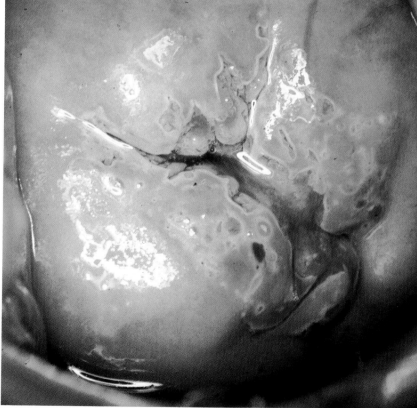

Fig. 12.**5b** Advanced transformation of the ectopy a year after insertion of an IUD in the same patient. (Courtesy of O. Baader.)

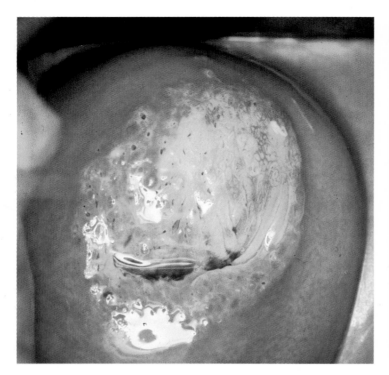

Fig. 12.**6 a** **Unusual transformation zone** and coarse mosaic in a 22-year-old nullipara. Note the clear line of demarcation between the

intensely white areas and the pale grayish-white areas with prominent gland openings

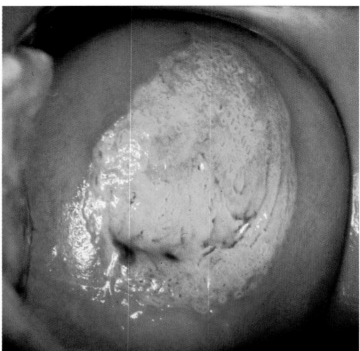

Fig. 12.**6 b** Four years later, the whole area is almost uniformly white and swollen after application of acetic acid.

Histologically, severe dysplasia and carcinoma in situ (CIN 3). (Courtesy of O. Baader.)

though no new territory has been gained (Fig. 12.4 a–d). It is remarkable how these changes revert to normal after cessation of hormone therapy (Fig. 12.5 a, b). Not only does the hyperplasia regress, but the process of transformation is initiated, occasionally producing a completely "healed" transformation zone. All the above processes have their counterparts in pregnancy-induced changes.

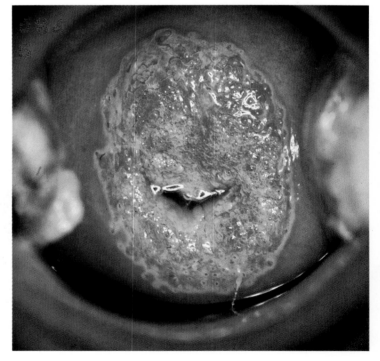

Fig. 12.**7** **Extensive ectopy** in a 29-year-old nullipara. There is little transformation at the periphery (Baader type 1)

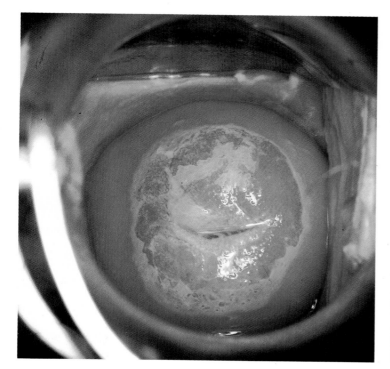

Fig. 12.**8a** **Active transformation** in 23-year-old nullipara, involving the periphery as well as a separate area on the anterior lip

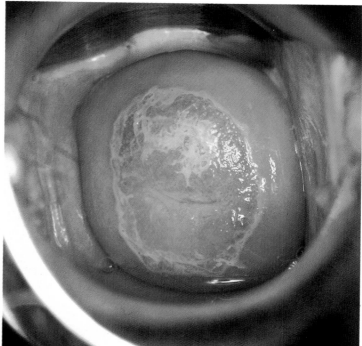

Fig. 12.**8b** Eight months later, the focus on the anterior lip is still separate, but has enlarged, and its contour has changed

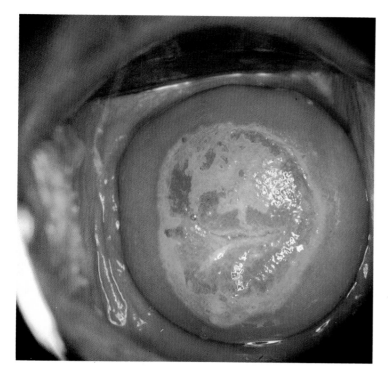

Fig. 12.**8c** Another 8 months later, transformation has progressed at the periphery and has established a connection with the enlarged focus on the anterior lip. (Courtesy of O. Baader.)

Colposcopic Follow-up Studies

As mentioned elsewhere, the development of atypical epithelium from a normal cervix (with or without ectopy) has never been documented. Baader has described a single case of apposition of a new field generated by atypical transformation to another preexistent atypical field (Fig. 12.6a, b). The illustration clearly shows how this may be interpreted as "progression" of CIN.

The process of transformation can be better studied by long-term observation of the same case over many years than by comparative studies between different cases (Figs. 12.1, 12.4, 12.5, 12.8). Baader (9) distinguished three types according to the tendency for transformation:

Type 1. Cases of ectopy that remain intact for a long time, with early arrest of transformation (Fig. 12.7; see also Fig. 11.9).

Type 2. This defines a group of adolescent girls in whom the transformation process is at its greatest activity. These cases are ideally suited for the study of the transformation process (Fig. 12.8a−c).

Type 3. The process of transformation is so intense in this type that one gets the impression that it will become atypical. Long-term follow-up, however, reveals that the distinctive, sharply demarcated aceto-white epithelium may in time become normal.

Future Prospects

These short remarks have merely skimmed the surface, and a whole host of questions remain unanswered. These relate not only to function, but also to carcinogenesis and the relationship between them. It is not known, for example, whether any particular type of cervix is more prone to develop cancer. Finding the solution to these problems is one of the challenges facing future generations of colposcopists.

References

1   Adam E, Decker DG, Herbst AL, Noller KL, Tilley BB, Townsend DE. Exposure in utero to diethystilbestrol and related synthetic hormones. A Am Med Assoc 1976;236:1107.

2   Baader O. Colposcopic findings in contraception. J Reprod Med 1974;12:186.

3   Baader O. Kolposkopische Befunde bei hormoneller Kontrazeption. Fortschr Med 1975;93:1303.

4   Baader O. Pilleneffekte an der Portio vaginalis uteri. Dtsch Ärztebl 1976;73:2851.

5   Baader O. Kann man aus dem Bild der Portio vaginalis uteri Hinweise für die Schwangerschaftsprognosen gewinnen? Fortschr Fertilitätsforschung 1977;5:118−127.

6   Baader O. Comparative and long-term colposcopic observation. In: Burghardt E, Holzer E, Jordan JA. Cervical pathology and colposcopy. Stuttgart: Thieme, 1978.

7   Baader O. Hormonell bedingte kolposkopische Befunde. Arch Gynäkol 1981;232:17.

8   Baader O. Probleme der Kolposkopie. Gynäkol Praxis 1982;6:91.

9   Baader O. Kolpophotographische Studien. Gynäkol Praxis 1982;6:101.

10 Breinl H, Gerteis W, Warnecke G. Kolposkopische und histologische Befunde am Epithel des Gebärmutterhalses nach langdauernder Behandlung mit Ovulationshemmern. Krebsarzt 1967;22:167.

11 Candy M, Abell R. Progesterone-induced adenomatous hyperplasia of the uterine cervix. J Am Med Assoc 1968;203:323.

12 Fischl W. Beiträge zur Morphologie der Portio vaginalis uteri. Arch. Gynäkol 1980;16:192.

13 Govan ADT, Black WP, Sharp JL. Aberrant glandular polypi of the uterine cervix associated with contraceptive pills: pathology and pathogenesis. J Clin Pathol 1969;22:84.

14 Graham J, Graham R, Hirabayashi K. Reversible "cancer" and the contraceptive pill. Obstet Gynecol 1968;31:190.

15 Haberich M. Histologischer Beitrag zum sog. Cervixfaktor der Ovulationshemmer [cited in Zentralbl Allg Pathol 1970;113:258].

16 Hamperl H. Die angeborene Pseudoerosion der Portio und ihr Schicksal. Arch Gynäkol 1965:200:299.

17 Hiersche HD. Funktionelle Morphologie des fetalen und kindlichen cervicalen Drüsenfeldes im Uterus. Ergeb Anat Entwicklungsgeschichte 1970;43:2.

18 Huber A, Zechmann W. Die zervikale Ektopie beim Kind und jungen Mädchen. Geburtshilfe Frauenheilkd 1974;34:97.

19 Linhartová A, Levý J. A quantitative approach to regression of congenital ectopy of the uterine cervix. Plzeň Lék Sborn 1973;39:5.

20 Pixley E. Morphology of the fetal and prepubertal cervicovaginal epithelium. In: Jordan JA, Singer A. The cervix. Philadelphia: Saunders, 1976:7−75.

21 Seidl S. Atypische endozervikale Hyperplasie bei hormoneller Kontrazeption. Geburtshilfe Frauenheilkd 1971;31:1006.

22 Sersiron D. A propos de 200 observations: 69 ectropions du col chez l'enfant. Gynécologie 1973;24:53.

23 Taylor HB, Irey NS, Norris HJ. Atypical endocervical hyperplasia in women taking oral contraceptives. J Am Med Assoc 1967;202:637.

23 Townsend DE. The cervix and vagina of women exposed to synthetic nonsteroidal oestrogens. In: Coppleson M, Pixley E, Reid B, eds. Colposcopy. Springfield, IL: Thomas, 1978.

25 Zeiguer BK de. Colposcopical findings in girls from birth to adolescence. In: Burghardt E, Holzer E, Jordan JA. Cervical pathology and colposcopy. Stuttgart: Thieme, 1978:10−32.

13

Colposcopy in Pregnancy

Introduction

No woman should go through pregnancy without at least one colposcopic examination, which is best performed at the time the pregnancy is confirmed. Normally, this will be during the first half of the first trimester. As with nonpregnant patients, a smear should be taken at the same time. A colposcopically suspect lesion can be safely biopsied during the first trimester, and one should proceed as in the nonpregnant patient. Should there have been no gynecological check-up in the years preceding the pregnancy, it would be a mistake to let another 40 weeks go by without assessing the cervix. If this rule is observed, the detection of cervical cancer will be avoided during the later stages of pregnancy or the puerperium. During the latter period, tumors often run a rapidly progressing course (7).

Pregnancy-Induced Cervical Changes

Pregnancy-related changes in the cervix have been described in detail by Stieve (11) and Fluhmann (3). Colposcopically, the most prominent features are the increase in size and number of the blood vessels and lymphatics, leading to hyperemia of the cervix. The stroma becomes softened and edematous, with a concomitant enlargement of the cervix, to which hyperplasia of the endocervical mucosa also contributes. Profileration of the columnar cells leads to enlargement and complex ramification of the glandular crypts, with the formation of numerous secondary clefts and tunnels (3). The endocervical mucosa thus becomes more plush, due to deeper extension into the stroma. The end result is a honeycomb appearance of the glandular field (Fig. 20.4).

A characteristic change is a decidual reaction of the stroma, which may be limited and focal, or may be quite extensive and may even produce polypoid lesions, referred to as "decidual polyps" (Fig. 13.8).

The concept of "erosion" during pregnancy is still controversial. Colposcopically, this corresponds to ectopy, with or without signs of a transformation zone. The frequency of this finding in advanced pregnancy (3) has led to the supposition that it is due to prolapse of the mucosa during the second half of the pregnancy (6). According to Fluhman (3), erosions during pregnancy may be preexistent, evolve during pregnancy, or come about during labor. Coppleson and Reid (1) found that both erosions and subsequent squamous epithelial metaplasia occur especially during the first pregnancy. In later pregnancies, there were no major changes. We are unable to support this view.

In our experience, an ectocervix completely covered by squamous epithelium need not undergo any change during the course of the pregnancy. It is also possible to produce "pseudo-erosion" during the later stages of pregnancy by everting the cervical lips during speculum examination.

The consistency and appearance of cervical mucus reflect hormonal changes, and have no relevance to the colposcopic detection of early cervical cancer. The cervical mucus undergoes characteristic changes during pregnancy, becoming viscous and cloudy, whitish or yellowish, and containing threads or particles (Figs. 13.2, 13.5). The significance for colposcopy lies in the fact that the mucus may be more difficult to remove with acetic acid than that of the nongravid patient.

Are There Pregnancy-Specific Changes?

The answer to this question must be negative. Apart from lesions such as decidual polyps (Fig. 13.8), the colposcopic appearances are not pathognomonic of pregnancy. Changes occurring during pregnancy are the same as those described in Chapters 3 and 4. The same applies to reactive changes, inflammation, and infections.

In the past, there has been lively debate as to whether dysplasia and carcinoma in situ can develop during pregnancy and regress after confinement (2, 10). It is, of course, well known that certain cases of dysplasia regress independently of pregnancy. A number of studies, on the other hand, have shown that carcinoma in situ detected during pregnancy has not regressed post partum (4, 5, 8, 9). Systematic examination of the cervices of aborting women has even shown a surprisingly high incidence of persisting carcinoma in situ (5). These results are not only of interest from the epidemiological point of view, but also underline the importance of screening during pregnancy.

Effects of Pregnancy on Colposcopic Appearances

Lividity in the cervicovaginal mucosa was one of the clinical signs of pregnancy long before biologic and immunologic tests were developed. This sign is due to the congestion of the lesser pelvis and its organs, especially involving the venous plexuses. Marked fluid retention gives the cervix a certain succulent consistency, and it becomes softer as the pregnancy advances. This development goes hand in hand with the increased lividity. Increased fragility, and a tendency towards contact bleeding, are observed not only during introduction of the speculum, but especially when taking a smear or biopsy (see below).

This lividity and succulence bring about background changes in the colposcopic appearances. In contrast to the nonpregnant state, these are coarse, and may give even benign changes a suspicious and alarming aspect (Figs. 13.3–13.7). This applies especially to the response to acetic acid.

Acetic Acid Test (see p. 114)

The effect of acetic acid is more pronounced during pregnancy, so that whitening even of benign lesions, may appear suspicious (Figs. 13.4, 13.5 b, 13.7 b). The response to acetic acid may therefore be difficult to interpret during pregnancy.

The Schiller Test (see p. 117)

The Schiller test is different during pregnancy only to the extent that the cervicovaginal mucosa turns a more intense brownish-black with iodine (Figs. 13.3 b, 13.10, 13.12 b). The Schiller test is particularly useful when an area that turns white after acetic acid displays a speckled, but not uniform, brown appearance with iodine (Fig. 13.7 c). Such a finding is not suggestive of atypia, but rather of a condylomatous lesion.

A particularly interesting finding is seen post partum, especially in breast-feeding mothers, when, after a normal colposcopy, several areas on the cervix and vagina do not take up iodine: that is, the epithelium is glycogen-free due to post-partum atrophy (Fig. 13.18 b). After cessation of breast-feeding, conditions revert to normal, with the usual uniform staining of the vagina and cervix with iodine.

Benign Changes in Pregnancy

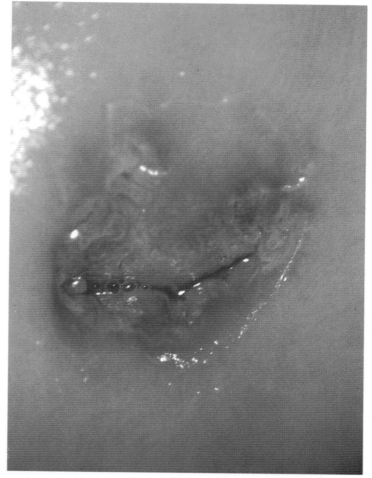

13.1

As already mentioned, the cervix may, at the beginning of pregnancy, be largely unchanged (Fig. 13.1), or may display a pre-existent lesion, such as the coarse grape-like appearance of an ectopy. The longitudinal folds of the cervical mucosa are particularly distinctive (Fig. 13.2). Such appearances once more recall the likelihood that they are caused merely by everting the endocervical canal with the speculum. The coarsening of the surface contour of the transformation zone may occur very early in pregnancy (Fig. 13.3 a). The Schiller test may bring out other diagnostic features, including islands of mature, glycogen-rich epithelium. The indistinct border between the transformation zone and the surrounding iodine-positive cervix is also in favour of a benign lesion (Fig. 13.3 b). After acetic acid is applied in pregnancy, a normal transformation zone often turns more intensely aceto-white than usual, with more prominent gland openings (Fig. 13.4). When transformation is complete, one can see retention cysts and gland openings shining through the lucid epithelium (Fig. 13.2).

Clearly delineated areas within a normal transformation zone may appear suspicious, especially when they display an intense reaction to acetic acid (Fig. 13.5 a, b). In pregnancy, this applies especially to acanthotic epithelium, which may also be clearly demarcated from original squamous epithelium and may show mosaic, or punctation or both (Fig. 13.6). In such cases, of course, the small size and regular appearance of the mosaic, or delicate and regular punctation, provide helpful diagnostic hints. In the case of some coarser-looking lesions, and certain combinations of changes, it may be difficult, if not impossible, to make an exact colposcopic diagnosis (Fig. 13.7 a–c).

Decidual reaction can hardly be seen colposcopically, as it manifests itself in the deeper cervical stroma. Decidual polyps, however, can be easily distinguished from the usual types of endocervical polyps, the latter often being covered by smooth, pink metaplastic squamous epithelium (Fig. 11.93), or displaying the typical grape-like pattern of columnar epithelium. Decidual polyps, on the other hand, are yellowish, and not covered by epithelium (Fig. 13.8).

Condylomatous lesions are relatively common in pregnancy. Except for a certain succulence, they are essentially similar to those which occur in the nonpregnant patient (Fig. 13.9). Inflammatory lesions look the same as they do outside pregnancy. Since the normal epithelium has a deeper brown color, they stand out strongly after iodine (Fig. 13.10; see also Fig. 11.90 b).

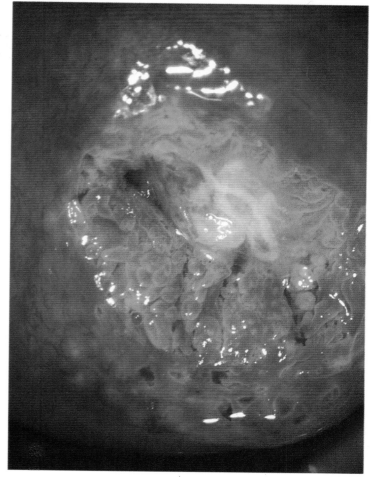

13.2

Fig. 13.1 Gravida 5, 10th week of gestation. Narrow transformation zone around the external os, slight lividity

Fig. 13.2 Gravida 3, 17th week of gestation. Ectropion of the cervical mucosa, with a coarsened texture and deep longitudinal folds. On the posterior lip, the transformation is complete, with gland openings and small cysts shining through. Livid coloration of the entire cervical mucosa. In the os, there is viscous mucus with whitish threads and granules, typical of pregnancy

13.**3 a**

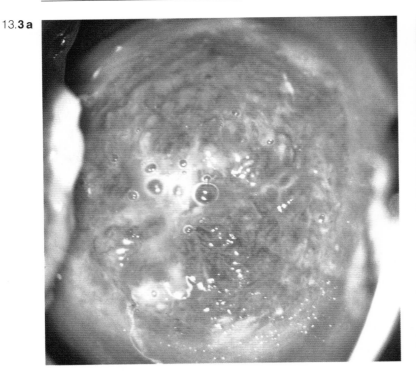

13.**3 b**

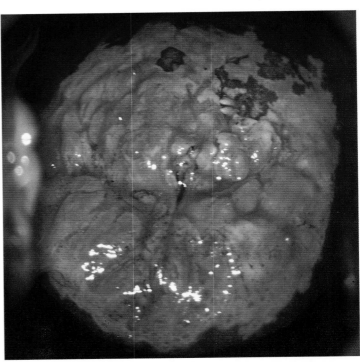

Fig. 13.**3 a**   **Gravida 2, 11th week of gestation. Preexistent transformation zone** with a slightly coarse surface and increased vascularity. Slightly livid coloration of the original cervical epithelium

Fig. 13.**3 b**   After the Schiller test, the squamous epithelium is stained dark brown. Within the transformation zone, there are islands of a mature and therefore glycogen-containing metaplastic epithelium

13.**4**

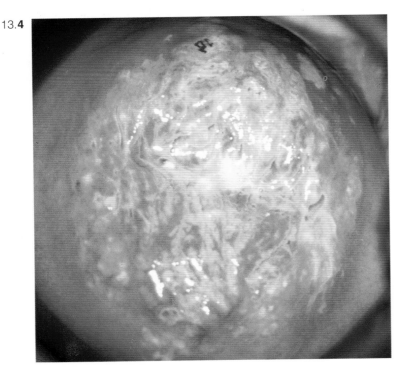

Fig. 13.**4**   **Gravida 1, 8th week of gestation. Typical transformation zone,** with a whitish reaction to acetic acid. Cuffed gland openings. Flat condylomatous lesions between the 12-o'clock and 2-o'clock positions at the edge of the transformation zone and just outside it

13.**5a**

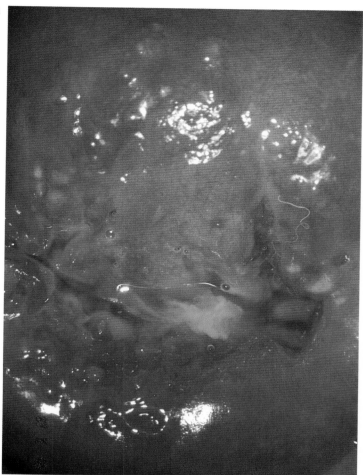

13.**5b**

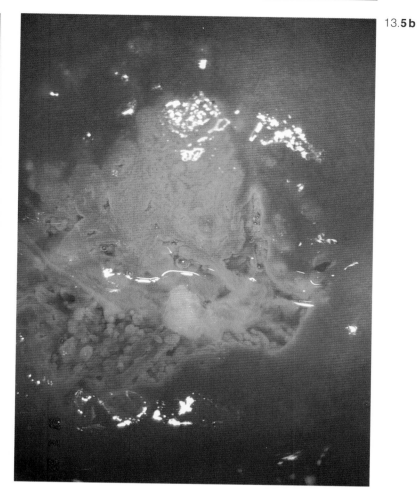

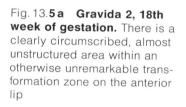

Fig. 13.**5a Gravida 2, 18th week of gestation.** There is a clearly circumscribed, almost unstructured area within an otherwise unremarkable transformation zone on the anterior lip

Fig. 13.**5b** A few gland openings and a discrete mosaic appear within the area described after application of acetic acid. Histology showed acanthotic epithelium with mild nuclear irregularities

13.**6**

Fig. 13.**6 Gravida 1, 11th week of gestation.** After acetic acid application, a white area with fine mosaic and punctation appears on the anterior lip and on the posterior lip outside an ectopy. The border with the slightly livid original epithelium is sharp. Histology showed acanthotic epithelium

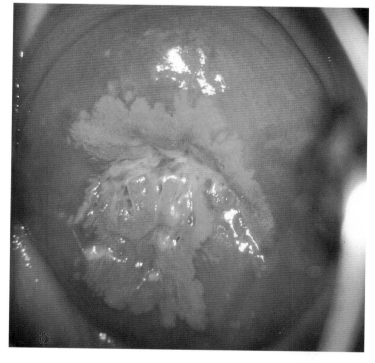

13.**7a**

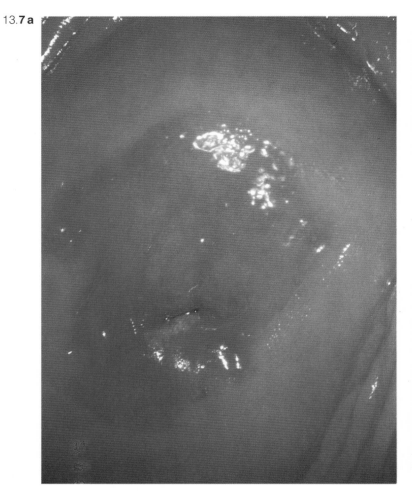

13.**7b**

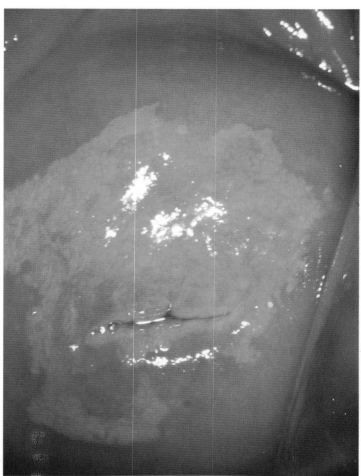

13.**7c**

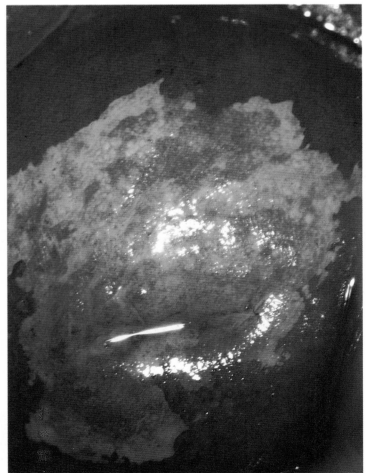

Fig. 13.**7a**   **Gravida 1, 11th week of gestation. Shiny red spot** within the livid squamous epithelial covering of the cervix

Fig. 13.**7b**   After acetic acid application, the entire area turns white, but without swelling. There are small areas of fine mosaic. An isolated field can be delineated between the 11-o'clock and 12-o'clock positions. Histology showed acanthotic epithelium

Fig. 13.**7c**   After staining with iodine, there is a patchy, partly brown coloration of the previously completely white area

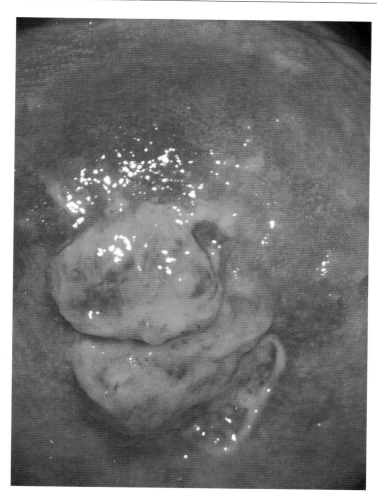

Fig. 13.**8**   **Gravida 3, 20th week of gestation. Grayish, solid polyps** at the external os. They show no epithelial covering, or any other superficial structure. Histology showed a decidual reaction

Fig. 13.**9**   **30th week of gestation.** The vagina and cervix are highly congested. A papillary area around the external os corresponds to flat condylomatous lesions. Within this lesion, and at its edge, there are condylamatous excrescences which have also assumed a livid red color

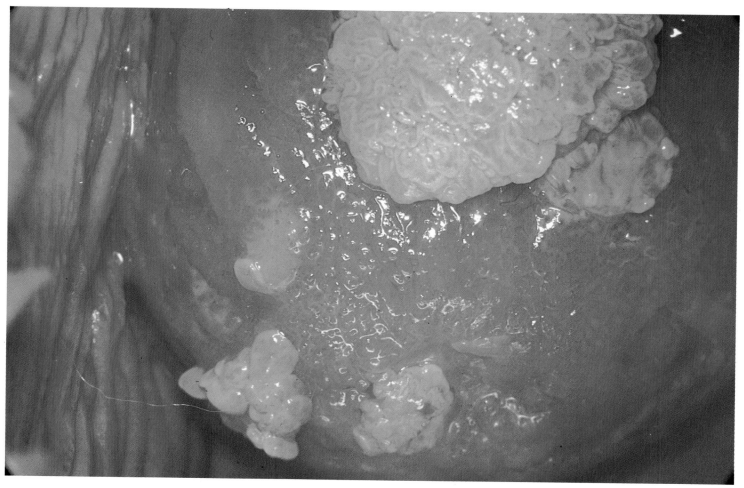

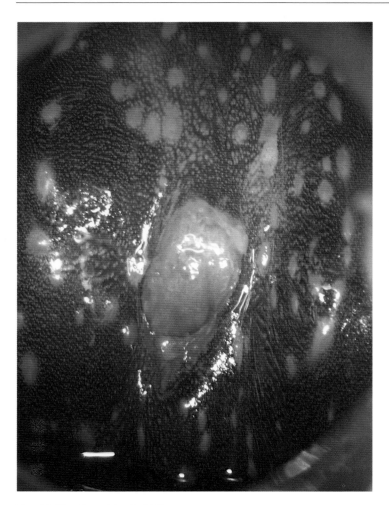

Fig. 13.**10 Gravida 8, 20th week of gestation. Cervix following conization.** The external os is slitlike; the mucosa on the anterior lip is slightly everted. The plaques of a macular colpitis are distinct from the dark brown cervical epithelium

Suspicious Changes

The appearances corresponding to atypical epithelium or cervical intraepithelial neoplasia are also rather uniform in pregnancy. The distinction between minor atypia (CIN 1) and acanthotic epithelium is always difficult (Figs. 13.11, 13.5–13.7). However, the irregular, coarser appearance of mosaic, for example, suggests high-grade atypia in pregnancy as well. The lesions often occur at the periphery of the transformation zone, and in parts also involving the original squamous epithelium (Figs. 13.12 a, b, 13.13). Lividity may give an atypical transformation zone a particular hue (Fig. 13.14) that may be overlooked or interpreted as harmless. In other cases, one may find an atypical appearance with intense white coloration of the sharply circumscribed transformation zone (Fig. 13.15). Colposcopic lesions, which are bright red and stand out against the livid surroundings, are particularly striking. These are always suspicious, and in cases of high-grade atypia, also respond characteristically to acetic acid (Fig. 13.16 a, b).

Atypical, flat condylomas lose their typical pearly-white appearance (Fig. 11.85) during pregnancy. They may even assume a livid undertone, which makes them difficult to recognize as condylomata (Fig. 13.17 a). An important diagnostic aid in such cases is the Schiller test, which shows a distinctive brown coloration, with sparing of small clear patches producing a speckled appearance (Fig. 13.17 b). This appearance corresponds to the iodine-positive mosaic in Figure 11.85 b. If one has an opportunity to observe the lesion during the course of the pregnancy, it can be seen to become coarser, more livid, and more succulent (Fig. 13.17 c, d). After confinement, one can observe time and again the regression of condylomatous lesions, leaving a new transformation zone (Fig. 13.17 e) which merely displays islands of brown-staining epithelium at the periphery (Fig. 13.17 f).

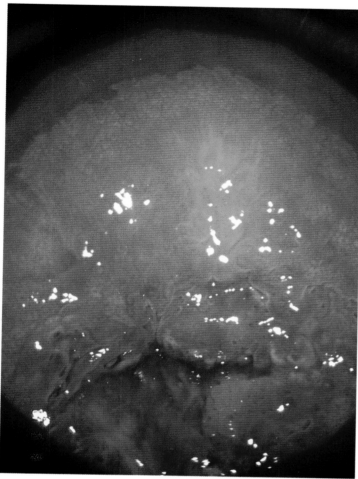

Fig. 13.**11   Gravida 1, 20th week of gestation.** Acetic acid has been applied. Outside the transformation zone, on the anterior lip of the external os, there is a fairly fine mosaic, sharply demarcated from its surroundings. Histology showed mild dysplasia (CIN 1)

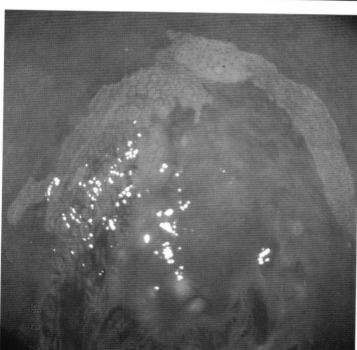

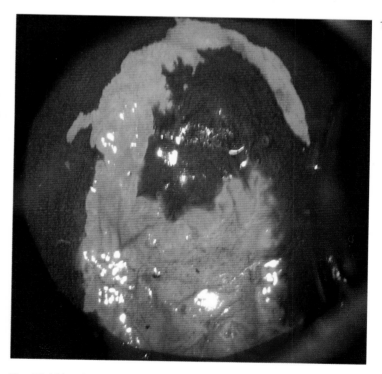

Fig. 13.**12 a   Gravida 2. A livid transformation zone** on the anterior lip, with mature epithelium and retention cysts shining through. The transformation zone is semicircularly surrounded by a narrow band of fairly coarse, irregular mosaic. Histology showed moderate dysplasia (CIN 2)

Fig. 13.**12 b**   At a lower magnification, and after the Schiller test, the narrow band with the mosaic is sharply demarcated. The epithelium in the completed transformation zone on the anterior lip is stained dark brown. On the posterior lip, there is an early transformation zone with a diffuse border

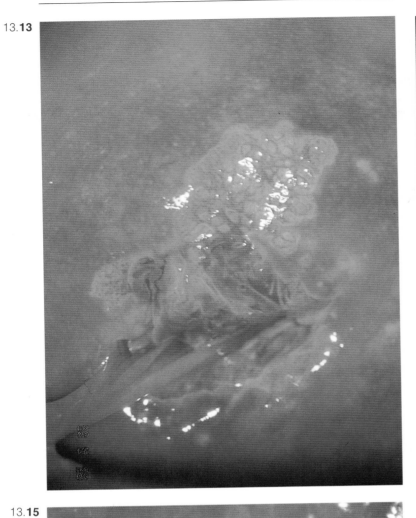

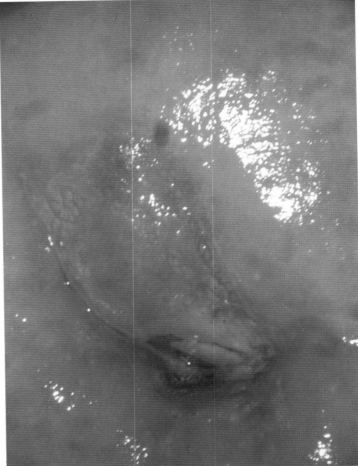

Fig. 13.**13   Gravida 1, 16th week of gestation.** After application of acetic acid, an irregular, coarse mosaic appears at the edge of, and outside, a small ectopia. Histology showed moderate dysplasia (CIN 2)

Fig. 13.**14   Gravida 2, 10th week of gestation.** After application of acetic acid, a deeply livid tongue-like area appears on the posterior lip. Within this area, there are only isolated gland openings; at its edge, there is a narrow band with coarse mosaic. Histology showed moderate dysplasia (CIN 2)

Fig. 13.**15   Gravida 4, 40th week of gestation.** The unusual transformation zone with isolated gland openings is stained intensely white by acetic acid and is sharply demarcated. Histology showed severe dysplasia (CIN 3), which was followed closely over the entire pregnancy. The bleeding resulted from a smear taken with a wooden spatula

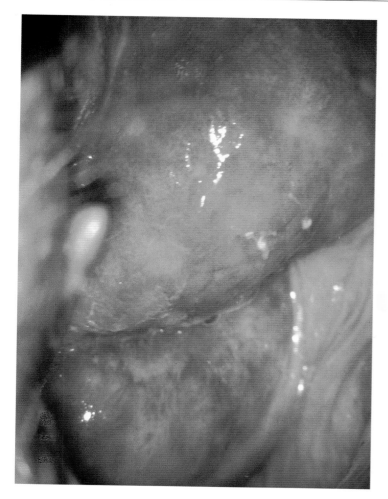

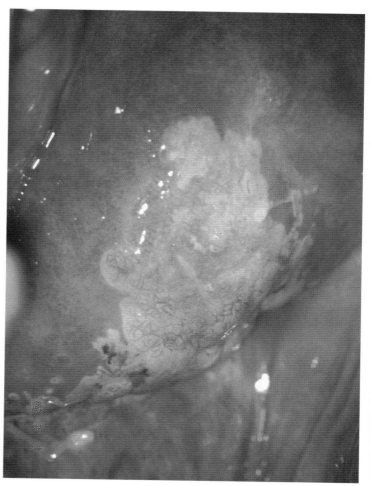

Fig. 13.**16 a** **Gravida 7, 29th
week of gestation.** Within the
deeply livid and succulent
epithelium, there is a sharply
demarcated red area without
any recognizable surface
structure

Fig. 13.**16 b** After application
of acetic acid, the area described swells, and coarse
mosaic appears. Histology
showed a carcinoma in situ
(CIN 3)

13.**17a**

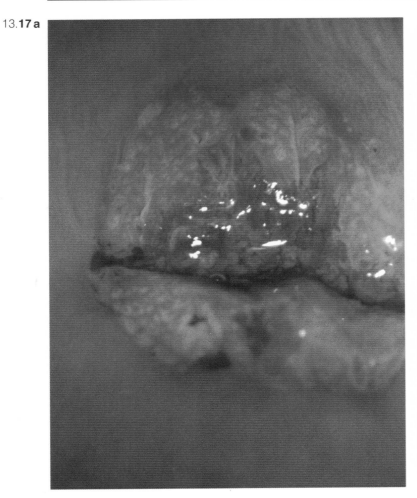

13.**17b**

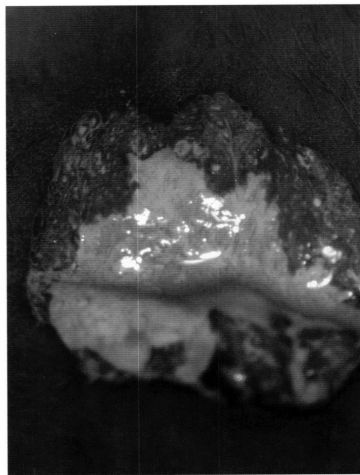

13.**17c**

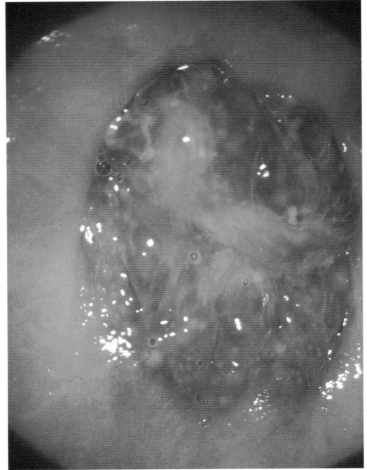

Fig. 13.**17a**   **Gravida 2, 8th week of gestation.** At the edge of an ectopy undergoing transformation, there is white-to-livid epithelium with cervical gland openings and white dots. The dots correspond to intraglandular squamous epithelium. Histology showed moderate dysplasia (CIN 2) with koilocytosis. HPV 16 and HPV 33 positive

Fig. 13.**17b**   The brown staining of the epithelium after application of iodine confirms the suspicion of a flat condyloma. The small, light spots could be termed iodine-positive punctation

Fig. 13.**17c**   By the 24th week of gestation, the lesion has become coarser and succulent

13.**17 d**

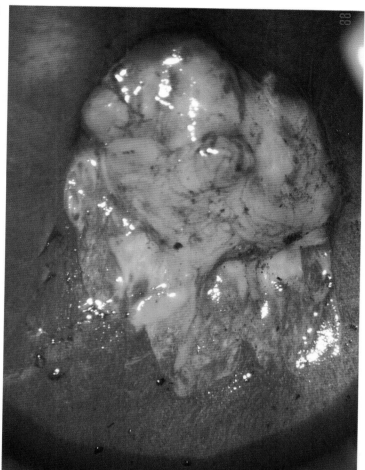

13.**17 e**

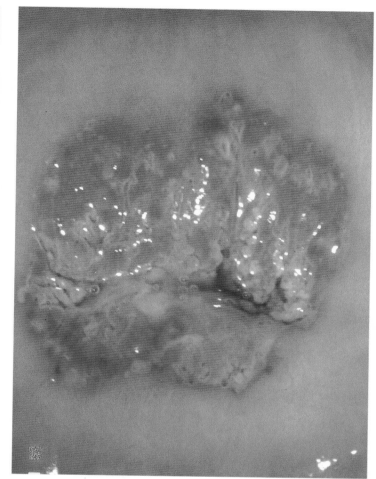

3.**17 f**

Fig. 13.**17 d**   After the Schiller test, the staining of the epithelium on the anterior lip is unchanged. Mucus prevents staining of the posterior lip

Fig. 13.**17 e**   Six weeks after delivery, the transformation zone appears normal and bright red. The lesion has become smaller. Histology showed acanthotic epithelium. HPV negative

Fig. 13.**17 f**   Application of iodine produces only patchy staining at the edge of the transformation zone

Puerperium

Lesions established during pregnancy remain essentially uchanged during the puerperium; they merely lose the characteristic features imparted by pregnancy (Fig. 13.17 a–f). Cases without any changes are often found at the time of the first colposcopic examination after confinement (Fig. 13.18 a). As mentioned at the outset, it is in such cases that the Schiller test may reveal surprising findings: parts of the cervix and varying lengths of the corrugated surface of the vagina remain unstained, that is, glycogen-free (Fig. 13.18 b). This applies especially to breast-feeding women. The appearances completely revert to normal after cessation of lactation. A satisfactory explanation for these phenomena is not yet forthcoming.

Biopsy During Pregnancy

It is quite possible to perform a punch biopsy during pregnancy (Fig. 7.6). Excessive bleeding can always be arrested with a tampon (Fig. 7.5), which should be left in for a few hours. Endocervical curettage may also be performed when indicated; naturally, this should not reach the upper confines of the endocervical canal, where lesions are rare during pregnancy. Conization during pregnancy is discussed on p. 274.

Fig. 13.**18 a**   Four weeks after delivery. The cervix is still slightly red and edematous, with a narrow transformation zone

Fig. 13.**18 b**   After the Schiller test, surprisingly large areas of the cervix and vagina are not stained, i.e., glycogen-free. Islands of brown staining appear within these areas

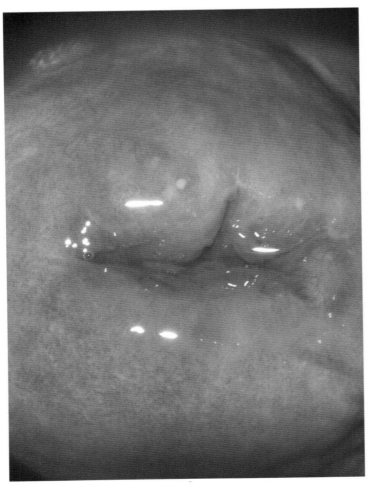

13.**18 a**

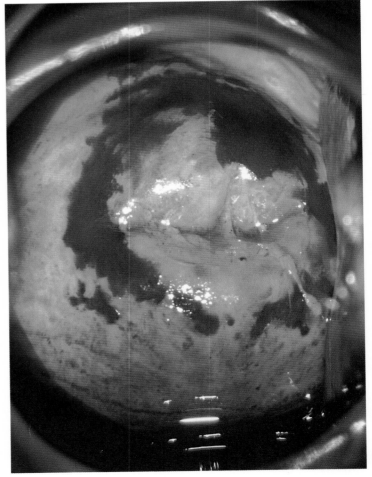

13.**18 b**

References

1 Coppleson M, Reid B. A colposcopic study of the cervix during pregnancy and the puerperium. J Obstet Gynecol Br Commonwealth 1966;73:575.

2 Epperson JWW, Hellman LM, Galvin GA, Busby T. The morphological changes in the cervix during pregnancy, including intraepithelial carcinoma. Am J Obstet Gynecol 1951;61:50.

3 Fluhmann CF. The cervix uteri and its disease. Philadelphia: Saunders, 1961.

4 Green RR, Peckham BM. Preinvasive cancer of the cervix and pregnancy. Am J Obstet Gynecol 1958;75:551.

5 Hamperl K, Kaufmann C, Ober KG. Histologische Untersuchungen an der Cervix schwangerer Frauen. Arch Gynäkol 1954;184:181.

6 Hamperl H, Kaufmann C, Ober KG, Schneppenheim P. Die "Erosion" der Portio. Die Entstehung der Pseudoerosion, das Ektropion und die Plattenepithelüberhäutung der Cervixdrüsen auf der Portiooberfläche. Virchows Arch [A] 1958;331:51.

7 Kottmeier HL. Carcinoma of the female genitalia. Baltimore: Williams and Wilkins, 1953.

8 Marsh M, Fitzgerald PJ. Carcinoma in situ of the human uterine cervix in pregnancy. Cancer 1956;9:1195.

9 Moore DB, Gusberg SB. Cancer precursors in pregnancy. Obstet Gynecol 1959;13:530.

10 Nesbitt REL Jr, Hellman LM. The histopathology and cytology of the cervix in pregnancy. Surg Gynecol Obstet 1952;94:10.

11 Stieve H. Der Halsteil der menschlichen Gebärmutter, seine Veränderungen während der Schwangerschaft, der Geburt und des Wochenbettes und ihre Bedeutung. Z Mikroanat Forschung 1927;11:291.

14

Assessment
of Colposcopic
Findings

Every colposcopist hopes to predict the histology from the colposcopic findings. This is relatively easy as far as original squamous epithelium, ectopy, or completely normal transformation zones are concerned. The task becomes more difficult when the colposcopic findings are abnormal: here the question arises whether the changes are benign or atypical.

These questions become particularly pressing when the colposcopic findings are similar, differing only in certain features which only an experienced colposcopist can recognize. If these diagnostic features were added to the list of colposcopic findings, the terminology of colposcopy could be expanded and would become the connecting thread for a kind of predictive colposcopy (see p. 135). For this to be useful, the individual criteria allowing a more accurate evaluation of the colposcopic appearances must be well known. It should be stated at the outset, however, that none of these features are pathognomonic of malignancy. They may be expressed to a variable degree, and may only facilitate the assessment of colposcopic changes. Any suspicious lesion should always be evaluated by cytology and biopsy.

In practice, the colposcopist must distinguish between two basic patterns:

nonsuspicious findings and
suspicious findings.

With increasing experience, the colposcopist will naturally succeed more and more in distinguishing between the two, thereby markedly reducing the number of biopsies. That colposcopic *suspicious findings* are not synonymous with colposcopic *abnormal findings*, and that the latter are not always due to premalignant lesions, are facts that can be understood only with knowledge of basic histomorphology.

Acanthotic and Atypical Squamous Epithelium

Regional, but widespread, variations in the interpretation of colposcopic findings are due to the fact that colposcopy is carried out all too often only for the evaluation of abnormal smears. Patient selection thereby ensures that abnormal colposcopic findings correspond to histologically atypical epithelia in the majority of cases. The few exceptions are so surprising and confusing that they require lengthy and elaborate explanations, rather like an exception to a rule.

Those who use colposcopy routinely take a diametrically opposed view. In their experience the histologic counterparts of leukoplakia, punctation, mosaic or unusual transformation zone are more often acanthotic than atypical epithelia. This has led to the use of the term *malignancy index* (18) in the German-speaking countries, which indicates the likelihood of an abnormal colposcopic finding having atypical epithelium as its cause. Table 14.1 shows the frequency of atypical epithelium or early stromal invasion in biopsies obtained from colposcopically suspicious lesions (1, 18). In cases of leukoplakia, the malignancy index was only 7.4%, while in cases of mosaic and punctation it was 18.6%. Biopsy evaluation of unusual transformation zones returned a malignancy index of 17% and of colposcopically inconspicuous iodine-negative areas (detected by the Schiller test) of only 1.7%. In such cases, more serious colposcopic findings were probably overlooked. It must be stressed that classical colposcopic abnormalities are not always due to precancerous epithelial lesions. This has been demonstrated most convincingly by studies of vaginal adenosis: no cases of epithelial atypia were found in 96 women with vaginal mosaic, and only 2 cases of dysplasia were found in 182 patients with "white epithelium" (4).

Table 14.**1**   Malignancy index

Findings at routine colposcopy	CIN or microinvasion
Leukoplakia	7.4%
Mosaic or punctation	18.6%
Leukoplakia + mosaic + punctation	31.0%
Unusual transformation zone	17.0%
Inconspicuous iodine-negative area	1.7%

(after Bajardi et al.)

The simple explanation for these observations is the so-called *acanthotic epithelium*, which Hinselmann called *simple atypical epithelium* and mistakenly believed to be premalignant. Classical European colposcopy has well recognized that eight out of ten cases of abnormal colposcopic findings are brought about by acanthotic epithelium (see p. 5). In the Anglo-American countries, however, the existence of acanthotic epithelium is little known and is referred to by a bewildering number of terms.

Acanthotic epithelium is a great imitator. Of great significance is the fact that it may arise in the transformation zone.

Thus, the metaplastic process may result in completely normal epithelium, atypical epithelium, or acanthotic epithelium (see Fig. 3.45). In analogy with epidermis, it is composed mostly of prickle cells, and shows at least parakeratosis (see p. 12). When arising from original squamous epithelium, it does so from the basal layer (3). It is important for colposcopic diagnosis, as acanthotic epithelium may develop in clearly demarcated fields. Normal glycogen-containing epithelium may, however, change to diffusely keratinizing acanthotic epithelium, as in prolapse (see p. 188).

If the distribution of acanthotic epithelium is focal, the individual areas have sharp borders. The surface usually shows various grades of parakeratosis or hyperkeratosis. Finally, acanthotic epithelium is very often peg-forming, being subdivided by tall stromal papillae. The pegs may appear as isolated columns or may be arranged in interlacing net-like ridges (see Figs. 4.9–4.11). Acanthotic epithelium may therefore appear in the transformation zone as leukoplakia, punctation, mosaic, or even aceto-white epithelium.

Recognition of the existence of acanthotic epithelium, and appreciation of its significance, are vital to the understanding of colposcopy. Without resorting to complicated explanations and theories, the problem is simply whether an abnormal colposcopic finding is due to disturbance of epithelial maturation or to neoplastic epithelial transformation.

Criteria for Differential Diagnosis

A number of features are of value in the differential diagnosis of similar colposcopic findings:
a sharp borders,
b response to acetic acid (white epithelium),
c surface contour,
d appearance of gland openings,
   blood vessels,
   surface extent (size),
   combination of abnormalities,
   iodine uptake, and
   keratinization.

Sharp Borders

Sharp borders are among the most important colposcopic findings. It is amazing how little appreciated this feature is in the colposcopic literature, and especially in work dealing with cervical pathology. The reason for this may be that the existence of pathologic atypia in well-circumscribed fields is not consistent with certain theories of carcinogenesis.

Almost all colposcopically significant lesions have sharp borders. Such borders are also found within large lesions, especially with the aid of the Schiller test.

Any sharply circumscribed epithelium must have formed by transformation; the process is not reactive, as such changes — like those induced by inflammation — are usually diffuse. Sharp borders are often recognizable by routine colposcopy. In any case, they become distinct following application of iodine (Fig. 14.1 a, b). As opposed to significant punctation and mosaic, which are always sharply circumscribed, punctation due to inflammation and mosaic simulated by chance arrangement of blood vessels have indistinct margins. In most cases, the sole criterion of sharp borders enables one to distinguish between significant and nonspecific colposcopic lesions. This feature, however, cannot be used to differentiate between acanthotic and atypical epithelia, as both possess sharp borders.

Response to Acetic Acid (White Epithelium)

As explained on page 114, acetic acid clarifies the colposcopic appearance by removing the mucus. Acetic acid also induces swelling of atypical epithelium, because of its poor intercellular cohesiveness. At the same time, the epithelium changes from red to white. If, in addition, the lesion displays punctation or mosaic, the white epithelial fields project above the surface. Vascular structures remain red and consequently become better contrasted. The unusual transformation zone remains unstructured except for the gland openings, and thus displays a white surface (Fig. 11.43). This feature is called "white epithelium" by those not familiar with the term "unusual transformation zone." The cohesiveness of the epithelium is directly proportional to its differentiation, the effect of acetic acid being maximal on undifferentiated epithelium. Thus, its effect on mildly dysplastic epithelium is considerably less than on epithelium showing anaplastic carcinoma in situ (Figs. 14.2, 14.3). Condylomata, especially flat ones, show a characteristic shiny white mother-of-pearl hue (Figs. 11.83, 11.85 a).

14.**1**a

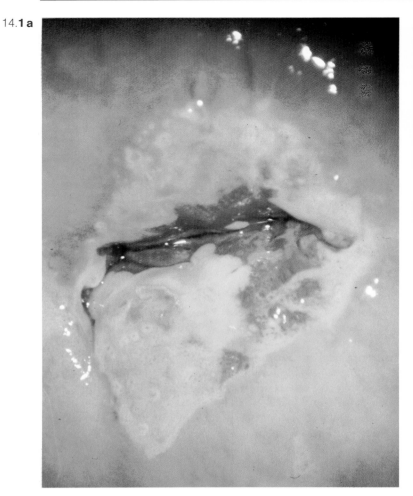

14.**1**

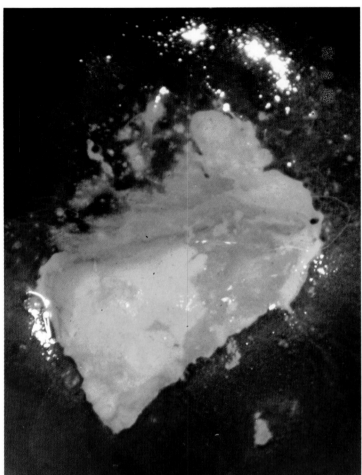

14.**2**

Fig. 14.**2** **Moderately coarse mosaic** with mild accentuation of the surface contour following application of acetic acid. Histologically, moderate dysplasia (CIN 2)

Fig. 14.**1**a **Unusual transformation zone** of quite uniform appearanc after acetic acid. Note the cuffed gland openings

Fig. 14.**1**b After application of iodine, it becomes clear that the typically yellowish discoloration is focal and the sharp border segmental. Between the 9-o'clock and 12-o'clock positions, the margin is quite indistinct. The iodine-yellow area was severely dysplastic histologically (CIN 3)

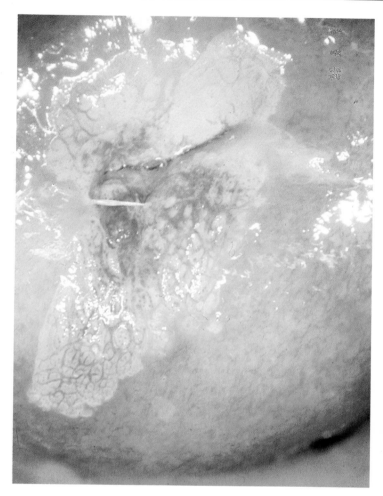

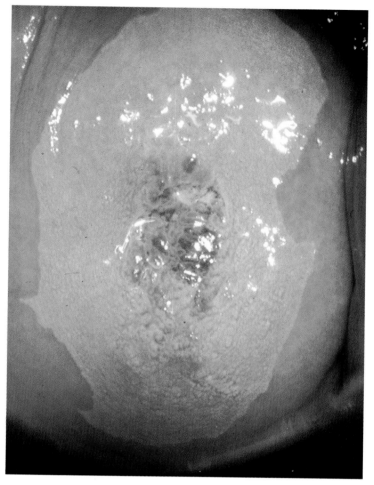

Fig. 14.**3**   **Coarse mosaic** with marked swelling and elevation of the epithelium after application of acetic acid. Histologically, carcinoma in situ (CIN 3)

Fig. 14.**4**   **Fairly fine mosaic.** The sharply circumscribed aceto-white epithelium re- mains in the same plane as its surrounds. Acanthotic epithe- lium histologically

Surface Contour

Punctation and mosaic produced by acanthotic epithelium re- semble a delicate sketch, the dots being small and the lines fine. The distance between the spots is not excessive, and the epithe- lial fields between the lines are small and regular. All these structures become more distinct following application of acetic acid (Fig. 14.4) but do not project from the surface. Punctation produced by atypical epithelium may appear in extreme cases as *elevated papillae* (Fig. 14.5) and the lines of mosaic as *coarse ridges* (Fig. 14.3). In contrast to acanthotic epithelium, the dots (or papillae) of atypical epithelium are more widely separated; similarly, the epithelial cobbles of a mosaic are larger. These structures become more prominent after application of acetic acid and become raised above the surface. In clear-cut cases, it is easy to differentiate between:

fine punctation and fine mosaic and between
coarse or papillary punctation and *coarse mosaic.*

There is a spectrum of appearances between the two extremes, the proper categorization of which depends on experience and on the evaluation of the remaining criteria.

Particularly coarse patterns of punctation and mosaic with an irregular surface configuration may be produced by *flat condylomas* (Fig. 14.6), which are essentially benign. Their pearly surface, however, may distinguish them from atypical le- sions, the surfaces of which are characteristically matt and opaque. A useful diagnostic feature is the presence of one or more spikes on or near the lesion, as flat condylomas may fre- quently coexist with papillary or spiked condylomas.

Cuffed Gland Openings

A characteristic feature of the transformation zone is the pres- ence of gland openings. They serve as visible proof that co- lumnar epithelium has been replaced by squamous epithelium, the metaplasia often being restricted to the rims of the gland outlets, leaving the mouths open. The metaplasia may, how- ever, also involve the glandular crypt. In such cases, the gland openings will be completely lined by squamous epithelium (Figs. 3.14, 4.13). Colposcopically, such events are evidenced by the development of white rings after the application of ace- tic acid (Fig. 11.13). If the epithelium is atypical, the ring will be wider and more pronounced after acetic acid (Fig. 11.43) than when the epithelium is normal or acanthotic (Figs. 11.13, 11.16). Such an appearance is referred to as a "cuffed gland opening."

14.**5**

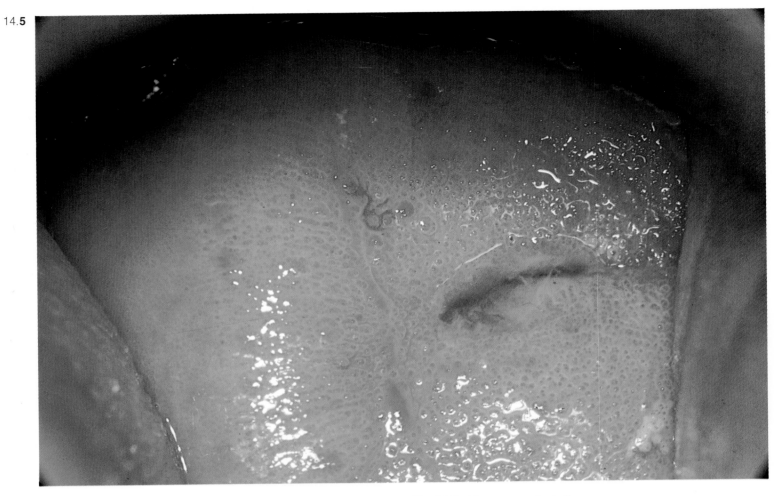

14.**6**

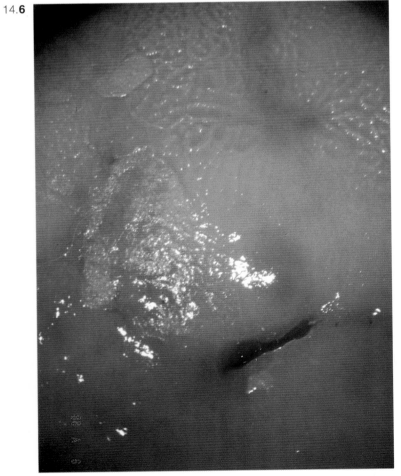

Fig. 14.**5 Pronounced papillary punctation:** histologically, carcinoma in situ (CIN 3) with early stromal invasion

Fig. 14.**6 Flat condylomatous lesions** with gyrated surfaces. In between, there are small, markedly cornified areas HPV negative

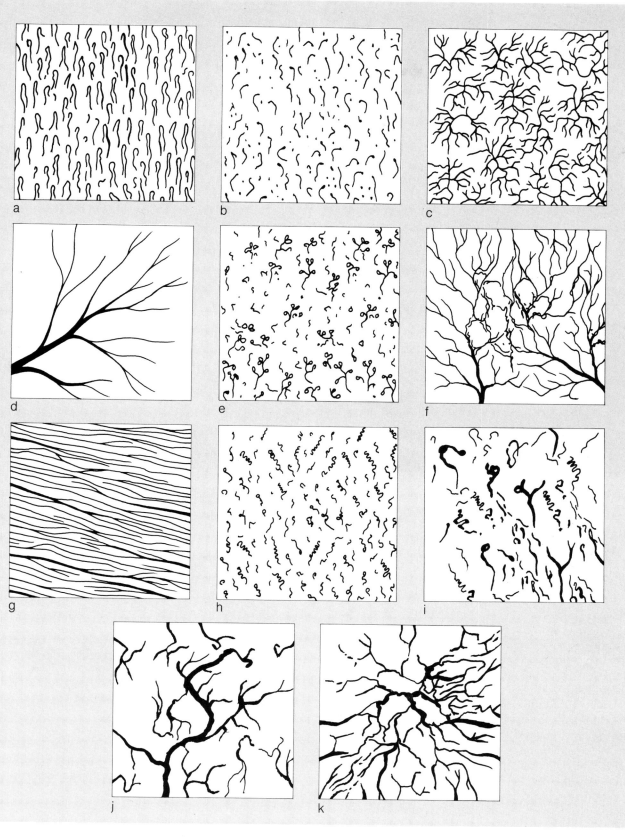

Fig. 14.**7a−k** Normal and atypical vascular patterns on the cervix. **a** Hairpin-shaped capillary loops. **b** Comma-shaped capillaries. **c** Blood vessels showing regular branching. **d** Long regularly branching vascular tree, with gradual decrease in caliber. **e** Staghorn-like vessels, seen especially in inflammation. **f** Regular vascular network, simultaning mosaic. **g** Long parallel-coursing blood vessels, showing some variation in caliber. **h** Irregular corkscrew vessels that vary only slightly in caliber. **i** Bizarre, tortuous, atypical vessels, showing marked variation in caliber. **j** Atypical blood vessels with gross variation in caliber and arrangement and abrupt changes in direction. **k** Irregular crazy vessels with great fluctuation in caliber

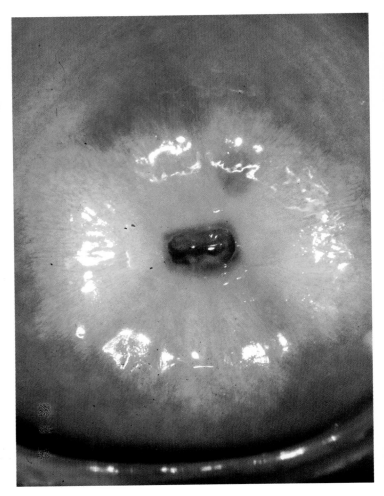

Fig. 14.**8 Thin atrophic squamous epithelium** allows the fine radial network of blood vessels to shine through; the vascular pattern is not suspicious (compare with Fig. 14.**12**)

Fig. 14.**9 Typical vascular tree** of a nabothian follicle; note the regular branching

Blood Vessels

Right from the start, Hinselmann (5, 7) attributed a great deal of importance to the vascular pattern, which became the subject of numerous subsequent studies (9, 10, 13, 16, 17, 19, 20). The nature of the blood vessels provides an important diagnostic clue. The vasculature of the thick and well-developed squamous epithelium of reproductive life is not always visible. The same applies to that of an intact ectopy. The vascular pattern, however, is enhanced by inflammation and by the attenuation of the covering epithelium, and is a prominent feature of well-circumscribed epithelial lesions.

The blood vessels are best observed at the beginning of the colposcopic examination. Acetic acid may suppress the vasculature to the point that it almost disappears (see Fig. 11.30). Applying a solution of the vasopressin derivative ornipressin (5 IU diluted with 2 ml physiologic saline) induces a reactive dilatation and makes the vessels become more prominent (8). Using a green filter, which screens out red and makes the vessels appear dark, the vascular appearance can be enhanced. Like other authors (14, 17, 20), we distinguish between various vascular patterns.

Nonsuspicious Vascular Pattern

The course and branching of the vessels are regular, with gradual reduction in caliber, the distance between the regular terminal capillary loops, the so-called *intercapillary distance*, being normal (Fig. 14.7 a–f). The distribution of these vessels is usually diffuse, and they do not appear in lesions that are clearly circumscribed.

Such vessels are characteristic of diffuse inflammation, when the cervix assumes a stippled appearance. On higher magnification, the capillary loops are hairpin or, when not seen in their entirety, comma-shaped. Diagnostic difficulties may arise if the inflammatory foci are not regularly disposed, as in colpitis macularis, but vary in size and distribution (see Fig. 11.88). The blood vessels in such lesions may be particularly clearly etched out and may be fork-shaped or antler-shaped; the intercapillary distance, however, remains normal. The appearances may mimic punctation. These lesions, however, are always poorly circumscribed, a feature seen especially well after application of iodine.

The neat, finely-knit meshwork of blood vessels of atrophic, postmenopausal squamous epithelium may be distinctive (Fig. 14.8).

14.**10**

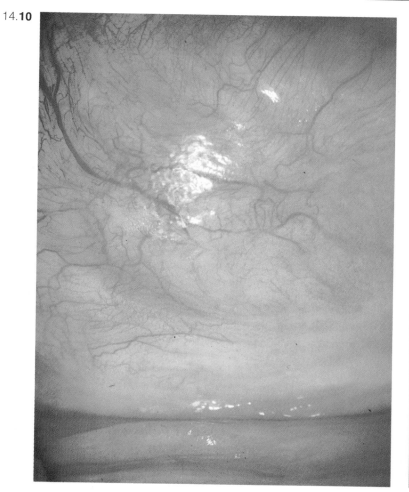

14.**11**

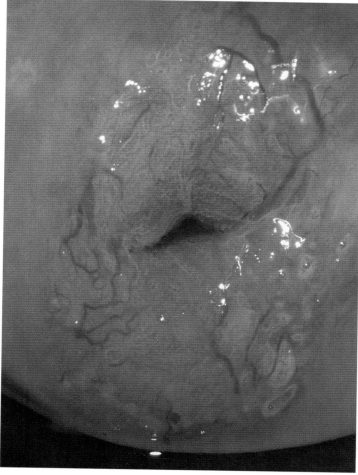

14.**12**

Fig. 14.10 Long, regularly branching blood vessels coursing over the surface of a deep-seated nabothian follicle; note the gradual decrease in their caliber

Fig. 14.11 Unusual transformation zone. Long vessels with slight variation in caliber and some abrupt changes in direction. Histology showed mild dysplasia with koilocytosis (CIN 1)

Fig. 14.12 Detail of an unusual transformation zone with various types of atypical vessels. Histology showed carcinoma in situ (CIN 3)

The individual blood vessels belonging to the vascular network of the normal transformation zone tend to be long and regularly arborizing, with no abrupt change in direction or in caliber. The vessels decrease in caliber as they ramify. Nabothian follicles classically display normal vascular patterns. The long blood vessels that traverse these yellowish structures are relatively large and exhibit regular branching and gradual loss of caliber (Fig. 14.9). They are so characteristic that the presence of deep-seated and otherwise invisible nabothian follicles can be deduced (Fig. 14.10).

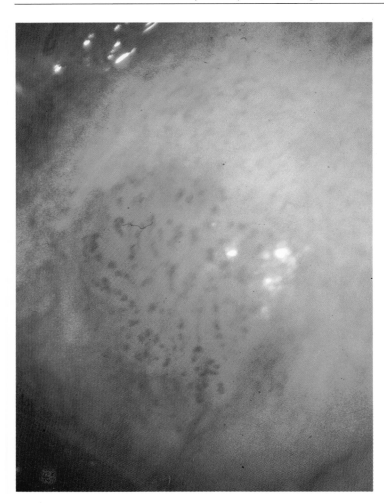

Fig. 14.**13 Coarse tortuous comma-shaped and cork-screw-shaped vessels** that vary distinctly in caliber. The intercapillary distance is markedly increased. Histologically carcinoma in situ (CIN 3) with early invasion

Suspicious Vascular Pattern

The first hint of pathologic atypia is the confinement of blood vessels to sharply circumscribed areas (especially with iodine) (Fig. 14.7 g, **h**). The blood vessels in punctation may be fine to coarse and hairpin, comma, or tortuous (corkscrew) in shape, but still regularly arranged. Within this pattern, the appearances may show wide variation. The capillary loops in punctation due to acanthotic epithelium are delicate and regular, with no increase in the intercapillary distance (see Fig. 11.25). The tortuous corkscrew and comma-shaped vessels associated with atypical epithelium are coarser, show haphazard branching, and display great variation in caliber; the intercapillary distance is increased (Fig. 14.11).

A similar range of apearances is seen in the various expressions of mosaic. The delicate mosaic pattern associated with acanthotic epithelium is produced by small, evenly distributed epithelial fields subdivided by thin red ridges (Fig. 14.4). In coarse mosaic, the dividing lines are more definite, the resulting fields being larger and more irregular (Fig. 14.3).

Even relatively regular and more or less parallel vessels may appear suspicious when they are wider (compare Figs. 14.8, **14.14**) and display an abrupt change in caliber (Fig. **14.11**).

The vascular pattern may on occasion mimic the appearance of mosaic. Closer inspection, however, will reveal that the vessels in these circumstances display tree-like branching and uniform reduction in caliber, and appear in poorly circumscribed areas (Fig. 14.7 f).

Atypical Vessels

Atypical vessels show a completely irregular and haphazard disposition, great variation in caliber, and abrupt changes in direction, often forming acute angles (Fig. 14.7 i−k). The intercapillary distance is increased, and tends to be variable (Fig. 14.15).

Highly atypical vessels are characteristic of invasive carcinomas (Figs. 11.61 b, 14.16, 14.17), especially when these are clinically overt. When flattish lesions display focal collections of such vessels, microinvasion should be suspected (Fig. 14.18).

14.**14**

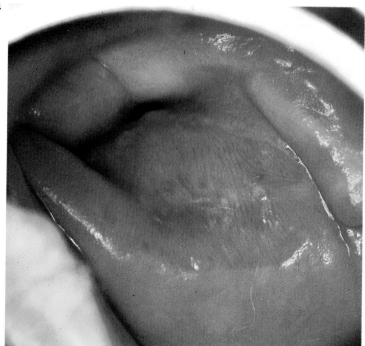

14.**15**

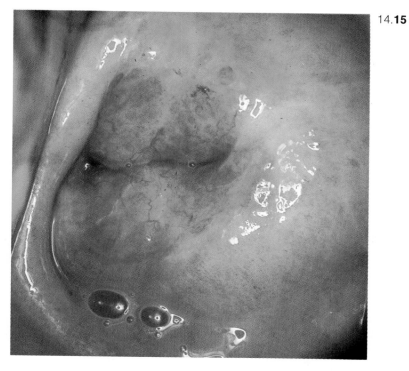

Fig. 14.**14** **Coarse parallel vessels** showing great variation in caliber, skirting an invasive squamous cell carcinoma

Fig. 14.**15** **Atypical vessels** showing gross fluctuation in width and abrupt change in direction at the margin of a squamous cell carcinoma within the canal

Fig. 14.**16** **Highly atypical vessels** on the anterior lip in a case of partly exophytic and partly endophytic squamous cell carcinoma. Note the complete irregularity and great variation in their width

Fig. 14.**17** **A great variety of atypical vessels** in an invasive squamous cell carcinoma

14.**16**

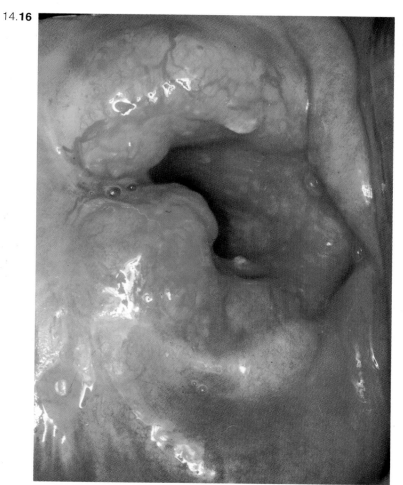

14.**17**

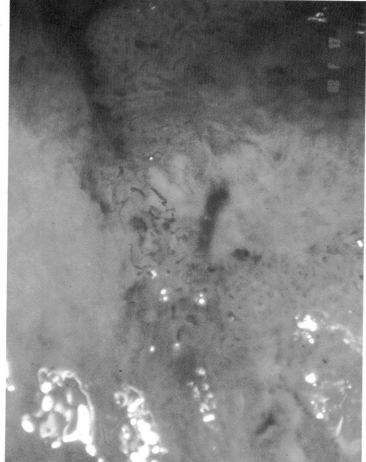

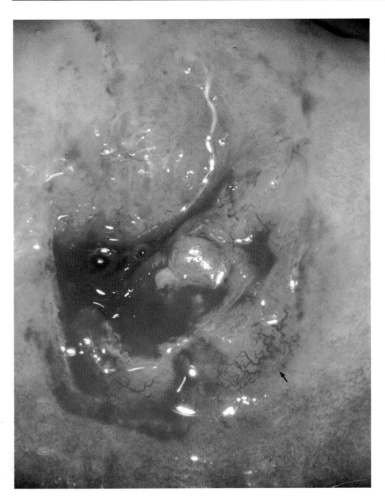

Fig. 14.**18   Focal collection of atypical vessels** running over the surface of a microcarcinoma on the posterior lip *(arrow)*

Surface Extent (Size)

Morphometric investigations of conization specimens have shown that the surface extent of atypical epithelium varies according to its nature, i.e., dysplasia, carcinoma in situ, or early stromal invasion (3, 11). Thus, lesions due to early stromal invasion are larger than those due to carcinoma in situ, which in turn are larger than those due to dysplasia (see Fig. 3.66). The same applies even to the various grades of dysplasia. This does not mean that fields of carcinoma in situ are larger than those of dysplasia per se, but that the former are more likely to be combined with the latter, the total area thus being larger. The marked increase in the surface extent of early invasive lesions is also due to coalescence of dysplastic fields and fields of in situ carcinoma (see Figs. 3.67–3.70). These observations are further detailed in Table 14.2), while Table 14.3 shows that the same is true for both cervical lips. In this way, a direct relationship between size and likelihood of invasion can be demonstrated (see Fig. 3.66).

The same conclusions apply to colposcopic lesions. Colposcopically suspicious but small lesions are rarely of histologic significance. Conversely, colposcopically highly suspicious lesions are always extensive. Small lesions are much more likely to be dysplastic than carcinomatous (in situ or invasive). This does not contradict the principles of evaluation of intraepithelial lesions as detailed previously (Chapter 3). On the contrary, the coexistence of different epithelia shows that invasive potential is acquired by their coalescence and not by progression of one type to another.

These statements do not apply to acanthotic epithelium, which may involve only small areas but may also cover the whole cervix and even parts of the vagina.

Consequently, size alone must never be considered as a diagnostic criterion; size should be considered only in concert with all other criteria. If the latter point to atypia, large size should further raise the colposcopic index of suspicion.

Table 14.**2**   Percentage of different types of atypical epithelia within a colposcopic lesion (n = 703)

Maximal diagnosis	Mild dysplasia only	All grades of dysplasia	Moderate to severe dysplasia only	Mild dysplasia and C.I.S.	Moderate to severe dysplasia and C.I.S.	All grades of dysplasia and C.I.S.	C.I.S. only
	%	%	%	%	%	%	%
Mild dysplasia (n = 60)	100	–	–	–	–	–	–
Moderate to severe dysplasia (n = 108)	–	81.5	18.5	–	–	–	–
C.I.S. (n = 489)	–	–	–	8.4	35.2	40.5	15.9
Early stromal invasion (n = 46)	–	2.2	–	–	50.0	19.6	28.3

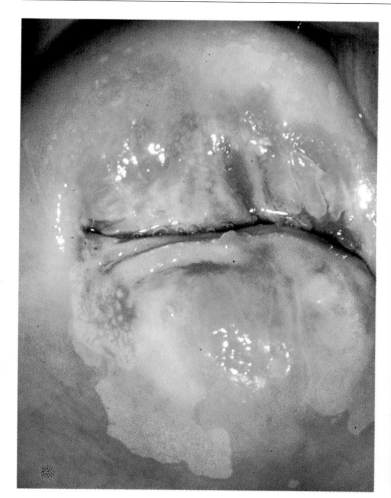

Fig. 14.**19a** **Acetic acid reveals a raised lesion with a variegated appearance** between the 6-o'clock and 8-o'clock positions. Note the moderately coarse mosaic between the 8-o'clock and 9-o'clock positions

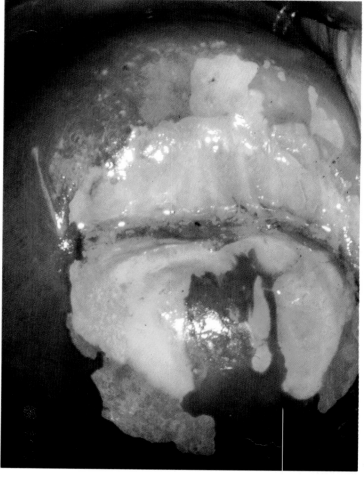

Fig. 14.**19b** Iodine staining allows a more detailed analysis of an already complex colposcopic picture. The area first referred to in Fig. 14.**19a**, now brownish, the epithelium of which contains glycogen and is supported by tall stromal papillae, is probably a flat condyloma. The brown area on the posterior lip represents fully mature transformed epithelium. The equally well demarcated iodine-yellow area at the 12-o'clock position is due to acanthotic epithelium. The remaining yellow patches are severely dysplastic (CIN 3)

Table 14.**3** Surface extent of atypical epithelium on the cervical lips

	Cases	One lip n	(%)	Both lips n	(%)
Mild dysplasia	27	21	(77.8)	6	(22.2)
Moderate to severe dysplasia	30	17	(56.7)	13	(43.3)
Carcinoma in situ	87	36	(41.4)	51	(58.6)
Early stromal invasion	66	10	(15.2)	56	(84.8)

Combination of Abnormalities

Table 14.1 (p. 218) lists the *malignancy index* of the various suspicious colposcopic findings. It is clear that no single lesion exceeds the 20% mark. If, however, the patterns of leukoplakia, mosaic, and punctation are combined, the chance of finding a histologically atypical epithelium climbs to 31%. These facts are entirely in agreement with the observation, detailed above, that significant lesions are a patchwork of several epithelial types, including those showing various degrees of atypia. Combination of different colposcopic patterns is simply due to combinations of different epithelial types (see Figs. 3.64, 3.65, 15.1–15.4).

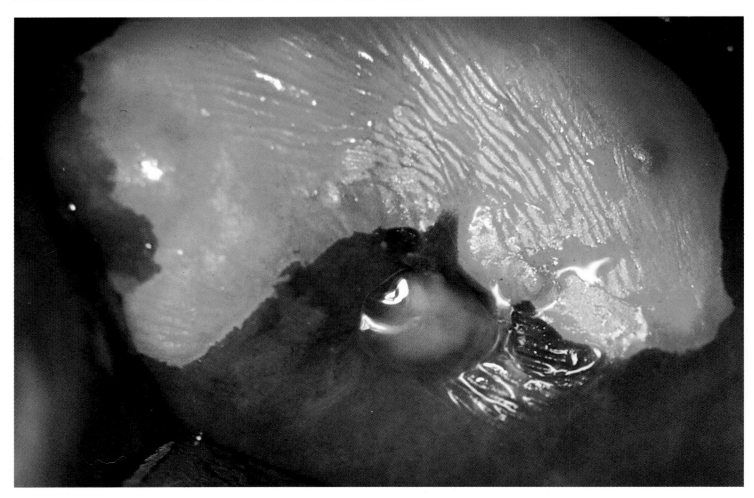

Fig. 14.**20 Shaprly circumscribed, smooth, iodine-yellow lesion** due to acanthotic
epithelium

Iodine Uptake

Quite apart from enhancing the abruptness of epithelial borders, the staining of colposcopic lesions with iodine is variegated (see also p. 117). A brownish or brown staining due to
glycogen should diminish one's suspicions (Fig. 14.19 a, b). An
area that does not take up iodine at all, or is merely covered by
it, may be due to columnar epithelium or thin, regenerating,
nonspecific epithelium (see Figs. 8.6 and 8.7). Well-developed
acanthotic epithelium characteristically stains uniformly canary-yellow, and remains flat (Fig. 14.20). Atypical epithelium
also stains canary-yellow, but it becomes mottled, and its surface is not so smooth. In cases of punctation and mosaic, the
surface contour remains more clearly visible when the epithelium is atypical and not acanthotic, as the latter is essentially
flat; the same applies when the Schiller test is used.

Keratinization

Keratinization is not a particularly useful diagnostic criterion.
All grades of keratinization, from mild parakeratosis to pronounced hyperkeratosis, may be shared by acanthotic and
atypical epithelia, both of which appear colposcopically as leukoplakia. However, a mild degree of kreatinization often corresponds to acanthotic epithelium, while flaky keratin suggests
epithelial atypia.

The keratin layer obscures not only the surface contour but
eventually also the margins, and inhibits the effect of acetic
acid. There is poor uptake of iodine, resulting in a light yellow
color. If the keratin layer can be peeled off, features of diagnostic importance may emerge. All cases of leukoplakia should be
evaluated by biopsy or at least by repeated cytologic study.

Evaluation of the Differential
Diagnostic Criteria

The diagnostic features described above may be expressed to
varying degrees, and may be found singly or in combination.
*The more distinct a feature is and the greater the variety of fea-
tures seen in combination, the higher the index of suspicion.* All
lesions must be viewed with a high degree of suspicion by the
beginner, who should evaluate his or her findings by biopsy as
part of the learning process. Quality control may also be
achieved by repeating the smear if this was initially negative.
With increasing practice, the colposcopist will be able to distinguish between *benign* and *suspicious findings* with a certain
degree of confidence. Attempting to differentiate between the
various grades of dysplasia and carcinoma in situ colposcopically is more questionable, as these lesions are regarded now as
forming a spectrum of the same biologic process (see p. 52).

References

1   Bajardi F, Burghardt E, Kern H, Kroemer H. Nouveaux résultats de la cytologie et de la colposcopie systématiques dans le diagnostique précoce du cancer du col del'utérus. Gynécol Prat 1969;5:315.

2   Burghardt E. Über die atypische Umwandlungszone. Geburtshilfe Frauenheilkd 1959;19:676.

3   Burghardt E. Early histological diagnosis of cervical cancer. Philadelphia: Saunders, 1973.

4   Burke L, Antonioli D, Rosen S. Vaginal and cervical squamous cell dysplasia in women exposed to diethylstilbestrol in utero. Am J Obstet Gynecol 1978;132:437.

5   Hinselmann H. Die Ätiologie, Symptomatologie und Diagnostik des Uteruscarcinoms. In: Veit J, Stöckel W, eds. Handbuch der Gynäkologie, vol. 6.1. Munich: Bergmann, 1930:854.

6   Hinselmann H. Einführung in die Kolposkopie. Hamburg: Hartung, 1933.

7   Hinselmann H. Der Nachweis der aktiven Ausgestaltung der Gefäße beim jungen Portiokarzinom als neues differentialdiagnostisches Hilfsmittel: Zentralbl Gynäkol 1940;64:1810.

8   Horcajo M. Über den Wert der Anwendung eines vasokonstriktorischen Peptids als Zusatzuntersuchung der Kolposkopie. Geburtshilfe Frauenheilkd 1976;36:388.

9   Ganse R. Atypische Gefäßentwicklung beim Portiokarzinom. Zentralbl Gynäkol 1952;74:749.

10 Ganse R. Die atypische Gefäßneubildung bei Karzinom. Zentralbl Gynäkol 1957;79:519.

11 Holzer E. Die Ausdehnung des atypischen Plattenepithels der Zervix. Arch Geschwulstforschung 1975;45:79.

12 Kishi Y, Inui S, Sakamoto Y. Colposcopic findings of gland openings in cervical carcinoma: their histological backgrounds. Int J Gynecol Obstet 1987;25:223.

13 Koller O. The vascular pattern of the uterine cervix. Oslo: Universitetsforlaget, 1963.

14 Kolstad P,. Stafl A. Atlas of colposcopy. Oslo: Universitetsforlaget, 1982.

15 Madej J. Significance of vascular changes in the colposcopic diagnosis of precancerous and early stages of cervical cancer. Geburtshilfe Frauenheilkd 1983;43:606.

16 Marsh M. Original site of cervical carcinoma: topographical relationship of carcinoma of the cervix to the external os and to the squamocolumnar junction. Obstet Gynecol 1956;7:444.

17 Mateu-Aragonés JM. Atlas de colposcopia. Barcelona: JIMS, 1973.

18 Navratil E. Colposcopy. In: Gray LA, ed. Dysplasia, carcinoma in situ and microinvasive carcinoma of the cervix uteri. Springfield, IL: Thomas, 1964.

19 Rieper JP, Marcones-Fonseca N. Patologia cervical. São Paolo: Manole, 1978.

20 Zinser HK, Rosenbauer KA. Untersuchungen über die Angioarchitektonik der normalen und pathologisch veränderten Cervix uteri. Arch Gynäkol 1960;194:73.

15

Colposcopic-Histologic Correlation

The real purpose of colposcopy is to correlate the colposcopic and the histologic findings. Ideally, each particular colposcopic appearance should have an exact histologic counterpart. Such a correlation, however, can never be fully achieved, and should not be attempted during routine colposcopy. In daily practice, it is enough to distinguish between entirely normal and suspicious findings comprising all grades of severity.

The colposcopist, however, who intends to explain the development of the various cervical lesions entirely by the findings, must make such a correlation the main goal. The colposcopic impression must be confirmed by target biopsies, which undoubtedly provide satisfactory information about the factors that govern colposcopic appearance (1). Once it is realized how heterogeneous in its composition a colposcopic lesion can be, it will become obvious how inadequate biopsy information may be (6). To analyze in detail each complex colposcopic lesion by innumerable biopsies is neither feasible nor fair to the patient.

For proper colposcopic-histologic correlation, it is necessary to take good colpophotographs and to evaluate the pathology by serial sectioning of conization specimens. We have carried out numerous such studies. The legends to the colpophotographs in this book repeatedly highlight details revealed by comparison between the colposcopic and histologic findings in conization specimens. In this chapter, a few examples have been chosen to illustrate the sort of information that can be obtained by careful analysis and comparison of a colpophotograph and serial sections from the corresponding conization specimen. For this purpose, cases with multiple pathologic findings were specially selected. Cases were also included in which at least some of the changes occurred *outside the transformation zone*, that is, outside the glandular field. The heavily dotted lines outline the borders of the glandular field, that is, the position of the *last gland* (see p. 38).

Borders within colposcopic lesions are not always easy to recognize. Nevertheless, it is quite surprising how distinct borders become on careful scrutiny of, and sketching from, colpophotographs. Further analysis of the photos will confirm the variety of findings already described in Chapters 3 and 4. First, it becomes obvious that all uniform epithelia arise in clearly circumscribed fields. Second, more differentiated lesions are found distal (toward the vagina) to those that are less differentiated. Carcinoma in situ lies proximal (toward the endocervical canal) to dysplasia, whereas acanthotic epithelium is the most peripheral (Figs. 15.1 to 15.3). Of particular importance is the relationship to the last gland. In the present cases, we found only dysplasia or acanthotic epithelium outside the last gland (Figs. 15.1 to 15.3). Inside the last gland, all kinds of epithelia are found, which nevertheless respect the topography described above (Figs. 15.1 to 15.4). Thus, dysplasia and acanthotic epithelium are found on either side of the last gland, and they often begin or end at the last gland. Hence colposcopy lends support to the significance of the histologic concept of the last gland in a most striking manner.

To complete the picture, Figure 15.3 illustrates the rare exception: histologically, a large area of the posterior lip is covered by dysplastic epithelium that is mostly outside the last gland, but some of it is inside, being entirely uniform and in continuity. If the corresponding colposcopic picture is closely studied, the somewhat coarse mosaic is seen to consist of two different fields, clearly separated from each other (*arrows*). It is obvious that in this case the two epithelia, which can hardly be distinguished from each other histologically, have arisen on either side of the last gland quite independently. It must be

pointed out that in this case the border of the glandular field at the 2-o'clock position is covered by normal squamous epithelium that must have arisen in the glandular field by metaplasia. Figure 15.4 is particularly instructive, as it shows a focus of invasive carcinoma especially well, without striking diagnostic features.

It has been often stated that cervical carcinoma can arise only in the transformation zone. Convincing histologic proof of the development of CIN outside the transformation zone, in original squamous epithelium, has met with considerable skepticism by colposcopists, who contend that colposcopic lesions appear uniform. This view ignores the fact that even uniform lesions may occur simultaneously both inside and outside the glandular field. Although the combination of different colposcopic changes is well known, it is little appreciated that they exist in clearly defined areas and that their sharp borders can be seen colposcopically. Naturally, there are lesions that arise completely outside the transformation zone, some exclusively from orginal squamous epithelium (Figs. 11.24, 11.25, 11.32, 11.35 and 11.51). Even these findings are dismissed by some, who maintain that glands must have existed there before. Yet an ectopic endocervical mucosa, as adenosis, will usually become covered by squamous epithelium via metaplasia. The glands beneath the new squamous metaplastic cover, however, remain there forever, as is the case in "occult (vaginal) adenosis" (5). For the same reason, the argument that the last gland is not really the last, some having disappeared, is not valid. If this were so, the position of the last gland would, by necessity, be haphazard. The unique topographic relationship of the last gland to epithelial abnormalities, seen both histologically (Figs. 3.57, 3.58) and colposcopically, (15.1, 15.4) is incontestable proof of the validity of the concept of the last gland (2–5).

It is easy to see how our interpretation of the significance and natural history of colposcopic lesions is based on colposcopic-histologic correlation. One can only a hope that other colposcopists will reach the same conclusion by carrying out their own correlative studies.

References

1   Bajardi F. Colposcopic findings and their histologic correlates. Geburtshilfe Frauenheilkd 1984;44:84.

2   Burghardt E. Gibt es ein Flächenwachstum des intraepithelialen Carcinoms an der Cervix? Arch Gynäkol 1973;215:1.

3   Burghardt E. Premalignant lesions of the cervix. Clin Obstet Gynecol 1976;3:257.

4   Burghardt E. The importance of the last cervical gland in the natural history of cervical neoplasia. Obstet Gynecol Surv 1979;34:862.

5   Burghardt E. Östör AG. Site of origin and growth pattern of cervical cancer: a histomorphological study. Obstet Gynecol 1983;62:117.

6   Homesley HD, Jobson VW, Reish RL. Use of colposcopically directed, four-quadrant cervical biopsy by the colposcopy trainee. J Reprod Med 1984;29:311.

7   Johnson LD, Driscoll SG, Hertig AT, Cole PT, Nickerson RJ. Vaginal adenosis in stillborns and neonates exposed to diethystilbestrol and steroidal estrogens and progestins. Obstet Gynecol 1979;53:671.

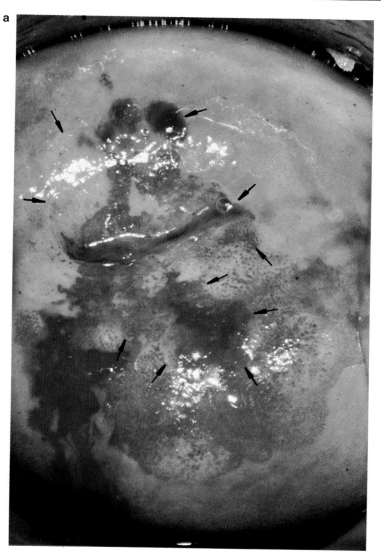

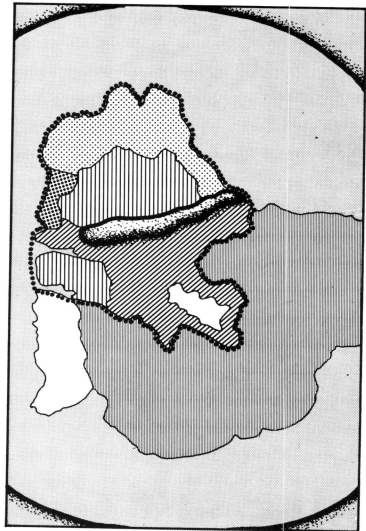

Fig. 15.1 a, b Correlation of the colposcopic picture with reconstruction of the histologic findings in serial step sections from the corresponding conization specimen. The arrows point to borders between colposcopic lesions

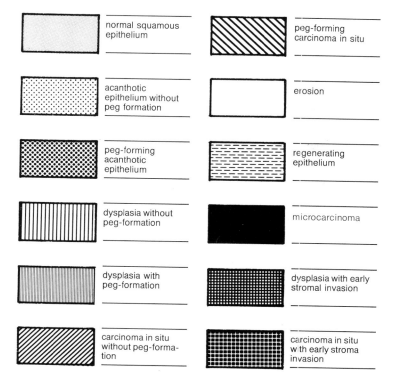

normal squamous epithelium

peg-forming carcinoma in situ

acanthotic epithelium without peg formation

erosion

peg-forming acanthotic epithelium

regenerating epithelium

dysplasia without peg-formation

microcarcinoma

dysplasia with peg-formation

dysplasia with early stromal invasion

carcinoma in situ without peg-formation

carcinoma in situ with early stroma invasion

●●●●●●●●●●●●● border of the glandular field

a

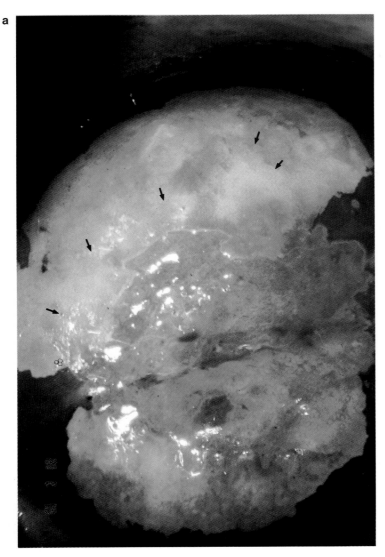

b

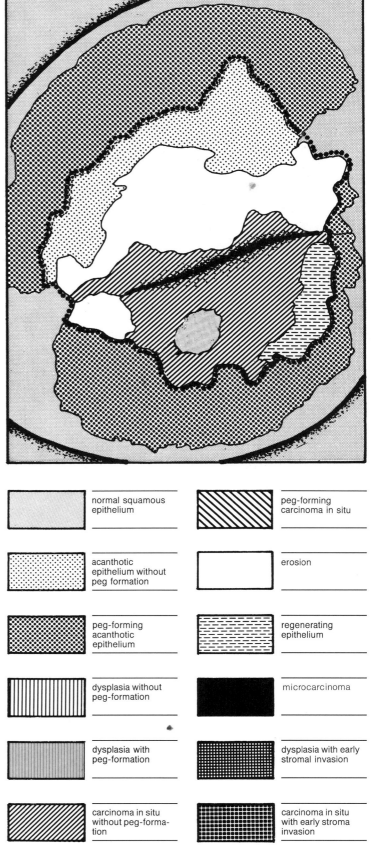

Fig. 15.**2a**, **b   Correlation of the colposcopic picture following the Schiller test with reconstruction of the histologic findings** in serial step sections from the corresponding conization specimen. The arrows point to discrete borders between colposcopic lesions

normal squamous epithelium

peg-forming carcinoma in situ

acanthotic epithelium without peg formation

erosion

peg-forming acanthotic epithelium

regenerating epithelium

dysplasia without peg-formation

microcarcinoma

dysplasia with peg-formation

dysplasia with early stromal invasion

carcinoma in situ without peg-formation

carcinoma in situ with early stroma invasion

•••••••••••••••   border of the glandular field

a

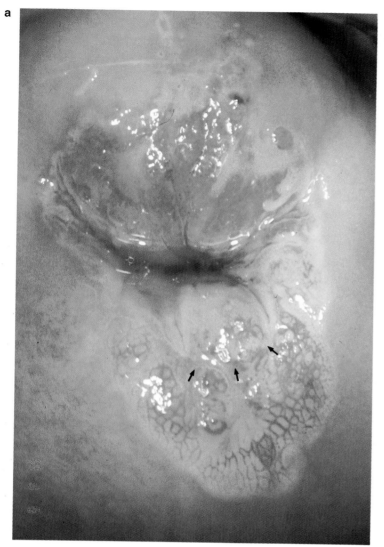

b

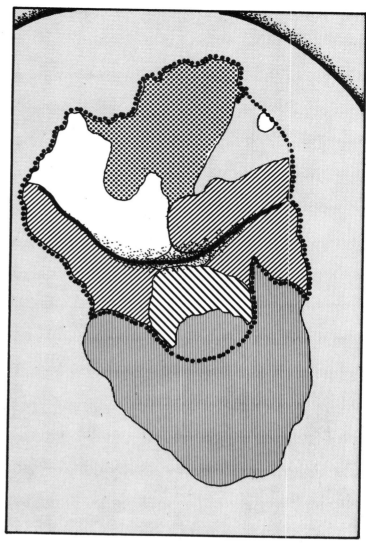

Fig. 15.3 a, b Correlation of the colposcopic picture with reconstruction of the histologic findings in serial step sections from the corresponding conization specimen. The arrows point to discrete borders between colposcopic lesions

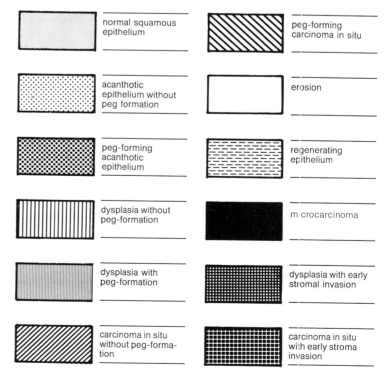

normal squamous epithelium	peg-forming carcinoma in situ
acanthotic epithelium without peg formation	erosion
peg-forming acanthotic epithelium	regenerating epithelium
dysplasia without peg-formation	microcarcinoma
dysplasia with peg-formation	dysplasia with early stromal invasion
carcinoma in situ without peg-formation	carcinoma in situ with early stroma invasion

••••••••••••••• border of the glandular field

a

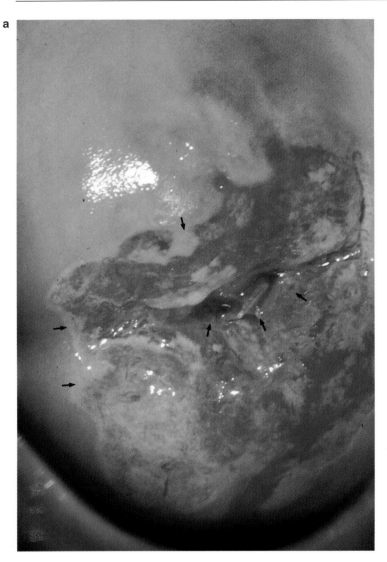

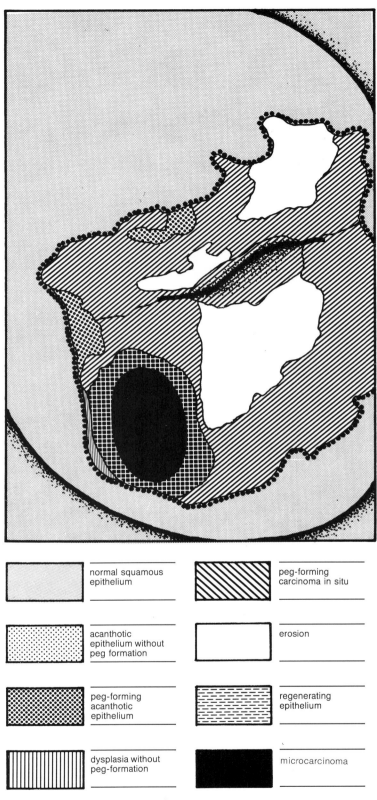

b

Fig. 15.4 a, b   Correlation of the colposcopic picture with reconstruction of the histologic findings in serial step sections from the corresponding conization specimen. The arrows point to discrete borders between colposcopic lesions

normal squamous epithelium

peg-forming carcinoma in situ

acanthotic epithelium without peg formation

erosion

peg-forming acanthotic epithelium

regenerating epithelium

dysplasia without peg-formation

microcarcinoma

dysplasia with peg-formation

dysplasia with early stromal invasion

carcinoma in situ without peg-formation

carcinoma in situ with early stroma invasion

••••••••••••••••• border of the glandular field

16

Documenting Colposcopic Findings

The value of accurate documentation of colposcopic findings cannot be overestimated, as it enables precise correlation of the colposcopic and histologic topography. Such comparisons, based on examination of properly processed conization specimens (see p.275), are particularly useful for the analysis of colposcopic appearances. On the other hand, long-term observation of patients in whom each finding has been fully documented allows the dynamics of all the benign and atypical changes that take place on the cervix to be documented. Such studies are still in their infancy. The evaluation of long-term follow-up studies is a challenge for future generations of colposcopists. To date, there is no well-documented case, for example, of the development of intraepithelial neoplasia from an ectopy or original squamous epithelium while under observation. It is to be expected that such studies will contribute significantly to the understanding of the genesis of cervical carcinoma.

When documentation is discussed, colpophotography immediately springs to mind. With the current state of the technique, however, it is not suitable for routine use. Consequently, one must also become familiar with graphic representation.

Colpophotographic Documentation

Most colposcopes are fitted with photographic equipment (see Fig. 5.3). The technical details are fully described in the instructions from the manufacturer. The camera is so constructed that the plane of the film coincides with that of vision. Fine focusing for the colposcopic examination serves the same purpose for photography. The flash used for illumination makes possible the shortest exposure time and the greatest depth of field. New developments, such as halogen lamps, ultrasensitive film, and automatic light meters, attempt to produce higher-quality pictures.

The technique of colpophotography is not completely reliable at the moment. The quality of the picture cannot be predicted, and depends to a large extent on the know-how and experience of the colposcopist. Although the pictures that appear in textbooks or in slide sets are satisfactory, they usually represent selections from much larger collections. Furthermore, they often show only a detail, and do not reflect the technical difficulties that may be encountered if larger lesions or the whole cervix are to be reproduced. It is not possible to portray faithfully each and every colposcopic lesion, so an accurate colposcopic diagnosis cannot be made merely from a colpophotograph. This problem, however, has been solved by other means (see below).

A special difficulty pertaining to colpophotography is the imperfect depth of field in the photograph. If we think of the cervix as hemisphere, it becomes understandable how difficult it is to telescope into the one plane the images of lesions that cover the entire surface. The larger a lesion, the more difficult it is to photograph.

Another troublesome feature of colpophotography is the ubiquitous presence of highlights. They appear in the most unexpected places, especially if a flash is used. Using specula with nonreflective surfaces was unsuccessful in eliminating this.

Stereocolpophotography has not overcome these problems; this technique, however, is eminently suitable for teaching purposes. A three-dimensional representation can be obtained by using a stereoviewer that depicts the surface relief of colposcopic lesions particularly well. Unfortunately, the picture can be seen by only one person at a time, and cannot be used in lectures.

Colpophotography normally employs color film. Black-and-white photography is useful to highlight certain details such as blood vessels. A green filter is particularly good for constrasting blood vessels. Fine-grained, orthochromatic film is recommended.

Other Photographic Equipment

The Kolpophot

The difficulties described above have led to the construction of a camera that can photograph the cervix directly and not through the colposcope. In 1953, Ganse (4) developed, in conjunction with the Dresden firm Ihagee, the Kolpophot for this purpose. It is possible to obtain very good pictures of cervical lesions with this technique, as is obvious from Ganse's two-volume publication *Kolpophotogramme* (4).

A further technical advance in this field was made by Baader (1, 3) from Freiburg, who started off with 35-mm photography but later replaced it with 60-mm (Rollei SL66). A combination of Zeiss-Planar S 120 and ring flash with pilot light achieved excellent results. Magnification of 1.5 times was used, allowing reproduction of areas measuring up to 4 by 4 cm, which meant that even large cervices up to 4 cm in diameter could be reproduced (Fig. 16.1). With use of a light-sensitive lens and a small aperture, a most satisfactory depth of field was achieved (Fig. 16.2).

The pictures produced by Baader cannot be bettered even by very high magnification. Using this technique, Baader could address the problem of comparative colposcopy and colposcopic follow-up studies (3) better than anyone else. His incredible collection comprises, among others, adolescents who have been observed photographically over many years (3). A problem with this method is its clumsiness: as opposed to colpophotography, which can be performed at the same time as the colposcopic examination, Baader's method is a completely separate procedure and is an extra imposition on the patient. If, however, the patient is given a proper explanation of its value, there should be no difficulties.

Cervicography

This technique was pioneered by Stafl (6, 7). According to Stafl, cervicography is not a substitute for colposcopy, only for colposcopic screening. This statement reinstates colposcopy to its original place. Colposcopy has always been regarded as part of the routine gynecological examination, and as a screening method it should contribute to the early detection of cervical carcinoma. After the widespread adoption of cytology, colposcopy was relegated in many places to the visualization and localization of atypical changes suspected by cytology. Elsewhere, especially in Europe, cytology was always combined with colposcopy, as described in Chapter 17. This practice requires each gynecologist to be his or her own colposcopist.

Cervicography has a place in countries where the gynecologists do not have sufficient colposcopic training. The camera devised by Stafl (National Testing Laboratories, St. Louis, Missouri) should enable anybody to take excellent photographs.

Cervicography had to overcome the technical problem of achieving satisfactory magnification from a working distance of at least 15 cm. A system was devised using a 100-mm macrolens attached to a 35-mm camera body with a 50-mm extension ring. To achieve constant magnification, the focusing ring of the lens is permanently fixed to 0.9 m. A ring strobe light is attached to the front lens of the objective. The cervicograph is focused by moving the entire system back and forth.

The cervicogram should be interpreted by experts. The cervicograph slide is projected on a screen 3 m or greater in

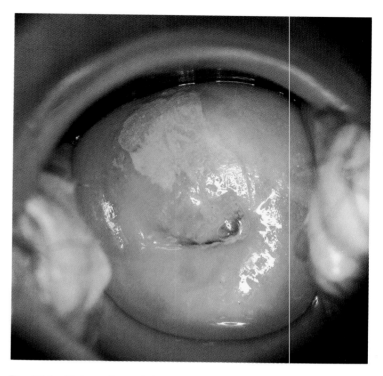

Fig. 16.**1**   Using of special photography, the entire cervix can be reproduced. (Courtesy of O. Baader.)

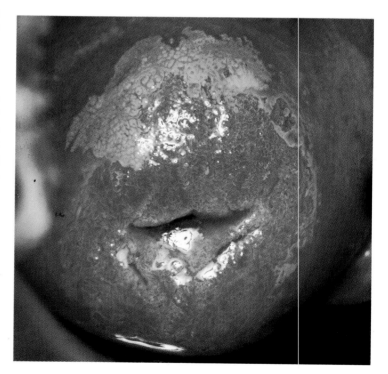

Fig. 16.**2**   The depth of field provided by special techniques allows photography not only of the cervix but even of the fornix. (Courtesy of O. Baader.)

width and observed from a distance of approximately 1 m. The apparent magnification is comparable to direct visual colposcopic magnification of 16 times.

Publications on the results of cervicographys have shown that cases of CIN were detected by this method, that were missed by cytology (8). However, the reported discrepancy between cervicography and cytology is unduly wide (see Table 17.2).

Graphic Representation of Colposcopic Findings

Because of the difficulties with photography described above the colposcopist needs a simple method of recording findings. This may be achieved by a simple sketch to accompany the written description. The use of a form with a schematic representation of the cervix, which can be easily inserted into the history, is of particular value. The cervix is shown as a circle with a small horizontal oval in the center to signify the external os (Fig. 16.3). Either a preprinted form or a rubber stamp may be used. The lesions can then be drawn in detail.

The various colposcopic findings are represented by symbols agreed on by most authors (Fig. 16.3). The findings are further designated by abbreviations (Table 16.1). The various phases of transformation can be conveniently represented by several combinations of letters. The drawing itself may be annotated with the abbreviations, with arrows pointing to each area (Fig. 16.3). Such drawings are particularly impressive when the result of the Schiller test is added (Fig. 16.3); if a red pencil is used, even the various shades of brown can be indicated.

References

1 Baader O. Colposcopic findings in contraception. J Reprod Med 1974;12:186.
2 Baader O. Probleme der Kolposkopie. Gynäkol Praxis 1982;6:91.
3 Baader O. Kolpophotographische Studien. Gynäkol Praxis 1982;6:101.
4 Ganse R. Kolpophotogramme zur Einführung in die Kolposkopie. 2 vols. Berlin: Akademie, 1953.
5 Ganse R. Über die Gefäßdarstellung kolposkopischer Befunde mit der Quecksilberdampflampe und dem Kolpophot. Zentralbl Gynäkol 1954:76:81.
6 Stafl A Cervicography: a new approach to cervical cancer detection. Gynecol Oncol 1981;12:292.
7 Stafl A. Cervicography: a new method for cervical cancer detection. Am J Obstet Gynecol 1981;139:815.
8 Tawa K, Forsythe A, Cove JK, Saltz A, Peters WH, Watring WG. A comparison of the Papanicolau smear and the cervigram: sensitivity, specificity, and cost analysis. Obstet Gynecol 1988;71:229.

Table 16.**1** Abbreviations for colposcopic findings

Diagnosis	Abbreviation
Ectopy	E
Transformation zone	TZ
Ectopy with early transformation	EET
Transformation zone with ectopic rests	TZER
Gland openings	GO
Nabothian follicles	NF
Inconspicuous iodine-negative area	IINA
Leukoplakia	L
Mosaic	M
Coarse mosaic	CM
Punctation	P
Coarse punctation	CP
Unusual transformation zone	UTZ
Cuffed gland openings	CGO
Atypical vessels	AV
True erosion	TE
Condyloma	C

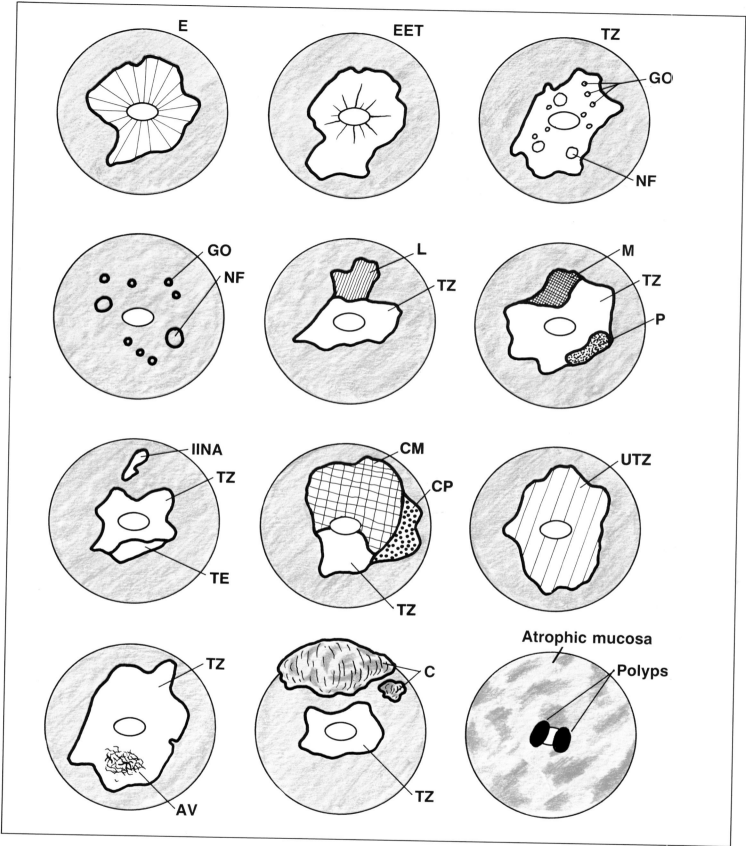

Fig. 16.3 Graphic documentation of colposcopic findings. It is easy to draw the contours of the various changes on a preprinted form and to indicate their nature using symbols and cross-hatching. Abbreviations can also be added (Table 16.1). Finally, the result of the Schiller test can be indicated with a red pencil

17

Uses of Colposcopy

Applications of colposcopy include (a) using it as an integral part of every gynecologic examination in concert with cytology, (b) using it to display and localize lesions suspected cytologically, and (c) using it to clarify the nature of clinically suspicious lesions.

Routine Colposcopy

This is by far the most appropriate application of colposcopy. It is indisputable that inspection of the cervix, vagina, and vulva forms an essential part of the gynecologic examination to detect and assess any visible abnormality. It stands to reason that such lesions are better seen when magnified and optimally illuminated. This applies to the detection not only of preinvasive and early invasive lesions but also inflammatory lesions, polyps, and small fistulas.

Like any technique that has been properly taught and practiced, colposcopy should not be too time-consuming. Selective use of the colposcope does not make sense to the physician accustomed to its routine use, any more than does naked eye "prescreening" of a spatial object to an astronomer.

Colposcopy must therefore be regarded as a modern diagnostic tool that *aids naked eye examination, particularly of the cervix, but also of the vagina.*

Colposcopy to Evaluate the Abnormal Smear

This selective use of colposcopy has several drawbacks.
1. The appearances the colposcopist is likely to encounter will be nonrepresentative. There will be a number of missing links hindering understanding of the physiologic and pathologic events taking place on the cervix.
2. There is no opportunity to pick up colposcopically any abnormality missed by cytologic screening.
3. Because colposcopy will be regarded as clumsy and time-consuming, its reputation will suffer.

To elaborate:

1. Routine colposcopy allows observation of the various dynamic processes that occur on the cervix throughout a woman's life. Of greatest interest is the observation of the same patient over many years. Alternatively, a large number of different patients may be examined, the various findings fitting together like a jigsaw puzzle and providing a complete picture of all the physiologic and pathologic events. At the same time, the colposcopist will become familiar with the morphogenesis of CIN. It is obvious that ignorance of even single pieces of the puzzle may lead to the wrong conclusions and to misconceptions.
2. The accuracy of cytologic diagnosis can be determined only by routine histology or by a second screening method. It is impractical to subject a large number of women to cervical biopsy just to check the cytologic prediction. It is quite possible, on the other hand, to combine every smear test with a colposcopic examination, and vice versa. The diagnostic accuracy of cytology and colposcopy may then be checked by biopsy of every colposcopically suspicious lesion (Table 17.1). In the absence of such quality control, the accuracy of cytology will be overestimated. Even a respected cytology laboratory may have a false-negative rate of 20%, at least

partly due to the taking of poor smears (2, 6, 9, 13, 15–19). A higher false-negative rate would be expected overall. Only a second screening method can compensate for these failures. If routine use of colposcopy is abandoned, it will be impossible to detect a good percentage of abnormalities missed by cytologic screening.

Table 17.1 Colposcopic and cytologic findings in 838 cases of histologically proven carcinoma in situ and microinvasive carcinoma*

Method of detection	Cases (%)
Colposcopy	663 (79.1)
Cytology	729 (87.0)
Colposcopy and cytology	828 (98.9)

* after Navratil (10)

3. Routine colposcopy enables the experienced colposcopist to reach a quick and exact diagnosis of visible lesions. Experienced colposcopists never cease to be amazed at the ado created at institutions where colposcopy is performed only in selected cases. It is through such practice that colposcopy attracts the reputation of being costly, cumbersome, and time-consuming. Only vigorous education and training can obtain for colposcopy the status that it should enjoy worldwide.

Colposcopy to Clarify the Nature of Clinically Suspicious Lesions

When colposcopy is used to clarify the nature of suspicious lesions, only changes seen with the naked eye are examined colposcopically: this practice is superior to colposcopy restricted to the evaluation of abnormal smears, because it is possible to detect lesions that may have been missed by cytology. The method is not as valuable as the routine use of colposcopy, since macroscopically invisible lesions will remain undetected, and there is no opportunity to inspect the lower portions of the canal. If we bear in mind that only 15–20% of lesions are purely endocervical (3–5, 7, 11, 12, 14), then not too much time is wasted by examination in these cases. If colposcopy is limited to evaluations of macroscopically suspicious lesions, then its role is merely to avoid unnecessary biopsies.

Cytology and Colposcopy

Both cytology and colposcopy are primarily screening methods for the detection of early cervical cancer. Cytology provides a snapshot of the changes taking place in the cervix at any one time. Colposcopy also allows observation of the natural history of physiologic processes in the cervix and assessment of the subsequent development of any given abnormality. Both methods are associated with a certain margin of error. Mistakes in cytology may result from taking poor smears or from misinterpreting them. Colposcopic failures are due to misinterpretation of the changes by the physician and to the fact that lesions in the canal may be out of reach of the colposcope. As the diagnostic principles of the two methods are quite different, it is unlikely that a lesion will be missed if both methods are used in concert (1, 4, 10, 11, 19).

Cytology is undoubtedly more accurate, and should be the method of choice if only one method is available. As its success does not depend on the location of a lesion, well-taken smears should reveal abnormalities in the canal at the same rate as those on the ectocervix. Cytology, of course, has its own failure rate, the reasons for which are not always clear. The false-negative rate is stated to be between 5% and 30% (see above). The wide range cannot be attributed merely to differing degrees of competency among the various observers. It also results from the type of quality control. Colposcopy is particularly suitable as a second screening method to compensate for cytologic failures (1, 4, 10, 11, 20).

The colposcopic failure rate must be higher than that of good cytology screening, simply because 10–15% of atypical lesions are situated in the canal, out of range of the colposcope (see above). To this must be added a further 5% due to misinterpretation of ectocervical changes. It is therefore reasonable to regard colposcopy as 80% accurate in the detection of early cervical carcinoma (1, 4, 8, 10, 11, 16).

Table 17.2 shows how the two methods complement each other in the diagnosis of carcinoma in situ and microinvasive carcinoma. In only 220 of 306 cases were both positive. Conversely, in only 4 cases (1.3%) were both colposcopy and cytology negative. Although cytology detected 51 more cases than colposcopy, 31 cases would have been missed had colposcopy not been performed.

These are the best results that can be achieved. The cytologic examinations referred to above were performed only by cytopathologists. With the widespread application of cytologic screening by personnel with less training, the failure rate must be higher. If colposcopy is reserved only for evaluation of abnormal smears, the failure rate is built in, and the detection rate cannot be improved. The usefulness of colposcopy is thereby diminished.

Table 17.**2** Cytologic and colposcopic findings in 306 cases of histologically proven carcinoma in situ and microinvasive carcinoma*

Finding	Cases	(%)
Cytology positive – colposcopy positive	220	(71.9)
Cytology negative – colposcopy positive	26	(8.5)
Cytology unsatisfactory – colposcopy positive	5	(1.6)
Cytology positive – colposcopy negative	51	(16.7)
Cytology negative – colposcopy negative	4	(1.3)
Detected by both methods	302	(98.7)

* after Navratil (10)

Colposcopically Directed Cytology

In contrast to cytology, colposcopy allows localization of suspicious lesions. Even if the ectocervix is colposcopically normal but the cytology is positive, an endocervical lesion may be safely predicted, provided the vagina and fornices have been excluded as the source of the abnormal cells. In this way, cytology can select patients for biopsy.

Conversely, it is possible to direct the cytology smear under colposcopic control. Thus, a colposcopic lesion can be scraped directly by an Ayre's spatula, or the endocervical canal can be carefully sampled when there are no lesions on the ectocervix. The reliability of cytology under these circumstances must be much greater than random sampling with the naked eye. There is no doubt that the quality of cytology can be improved by the simultaneous use of colposcopy.

Routine Combination of Colposcopy and Cytology

To achieve the best possible diagnosis of early cervical cancer, colposcopy may be routinely combined with cytology in two different ways:

1. A smear is taken at the time of colposcopy, and biopsy of any suspicious lesion is done at the same time without waiting for the result of cytology. In this way a false-negative cytologic result is compensated by colposcopy and biopsy. This practice may have several outcomes:

– *Colposcopy and biopsy positive, cytology positive*
– Colposcopy and biopsy positive, cytology negative
– Colposcopy positive, biopsy negative, cytology positive

(In this case, another area must undergo biopsy. If the latter is again negative, which is unusual, and the cytology is unequivocal, conization is indicated.)

– *Colposcopy positive, biopsy negative, cytology negative*

(In such cases, colposcopic and cytologic follow-up, and even repeat biopsy, are recommended.)

2. In spite of colposcopically suspicious lesions, one waits until the result of cytology is known. If it is normal, repeat smears should be taken, and the cytologist warned of the colposcopist's findings. In the rare instance of persistently normal cytologic findings in association with highly suspicious colposcopy, biopsy in indicated.

One final combination may result from the simultaneous application of colposcopy and cytology:

– *Colposcopy negative, cytology positive*

(In such a case, colposcopy should be repeated, and even a suspicious lesion at the ectocervix should be biopsied. In addition, the endocervical canal should be thoroughly curetted. If histology is normal and cytology remains abnormal, the biopsy should be repeated, or conization carried out. It must be remembered, however, that the vagina may also be the source of abnormal cytologic findings.)

References

1 Bajardi F, Burghardt E, Kern H, Kroemer H. Nouveaux résultats de la cytologie et de la colposcopie systématiques dans le diagnostique précoce du cancer du col de l'utérus. Gynécol Prat 1969;5:315.

2 Bayrle W. Kritische Betrachtungen zur Rate der "falsch negativen" Befunde in der gynäkologischen Zytologie. Geburtshilfe Frauenheilkd 1977;37:864.

3 Burghardt E. Early histological diagnosis of cervical cancer. Philadelphia: Saunders, 1973.

4 Burghardt E, Bajardi F. Ergebnisse der Früherfassung des Collumcarcinoms mittels Cytologie und Kolposkopie an der Univ.-Frauenklinik Graz 1954. Arch Gynäkol 1956;187:621.

5 Burghardt E, Holzer E. Die Lokalisation des pathologischen Cervixepithels, 1: Carcinoma in situ, Dysplasien und abnormes Plattenepithel. Arch Gynäkol 1970;209:305.

6 Coppleson LW, Brown B. Estimation of the screening error rate from the observed detection rates in repeated cervical cytology. Am J Obstet Gynecol 1974;119:953.

7 Kern G. Carcinoma in situ. Berlin: Springer, 1964.

8 Kolstadt P. Colposcopic diagnosis of cervical neoplasia. In: Jordan AJ, Singer A. The cervix. Philadelphia: Saunders, 1976:36−411.

9 Naujoks H, Leppien G, Rogosaroff-Fricke R. Negativer zytologischer Abstrich bei Carcinoma in situ der Cervix uteri. Geburtshilfe Frauenheilkd 1976;36:570.

10 Navratil E. Colposcopy. In: Gray LA, ed. Dysplasia, carcinoma in situ and microinvasive carcinoma of the cervix uteri. Springfield, IL: Thomas, 1964:10−228.

11 Navratil E, Burghardt E, Bajardi F, Nash W. Simultaneous colposcopy and cytology used in screening for carcinoma of the cervix. Am J Obstet Gynecol 1958;75:1292.

12 Ober KG, Bontke E. Sitz und Ausdehnung der Carcinomata in situ und der beginnenden Krebse der Cervix. Arch Gynäkol 1959;192:55.

13 Pederson E, Hoeg H, Kolstadt P. Mass screening for cancer of the uterine cervix in Ostfold County, Norway: an experiment. Second report of the Norwegian Cancer Society. Acta Obstet Gynecol Scand 1971; suppl 11.

14 Reagan JW, Pattern F Jr. Dysplasia: a basic reaction to injury in the uterine cervix. Ann NY Acad Sci 1962;97:662.

15 Rylander E. Negative smears in women developing invasive cervical cancer. Acta Obstet Gynecol Scand 1977;56:115.

16 Seidl S. Praktische Karzinom-Frühdiagnostik in der Gynäkologie. Stuttgart: Thieme, 1974.

17 Seybolt JF, Johnson WD. Cervical cytodiagnostic problems: a survey. Am J Obstet Gynecol 1971;109:1089.

18 Shingleton WP, Rutledge R. To cone or not to cone: the cervix. Obstet Gynecol 1968;31:430.

19 Stafl A, Friedrich EG, Mattingly RF. Detection of cervical neoplasia: reducing the risk of error. Clin Obstet Gynecol 1973;16:238.

20 Walker EM, Dodgson J, Duncan ID. Does mild atypia on a cervical smear warrant further investigation? Lancet 1986;11:672

18

Histopathologic Evaluation of the Abnormal Smear and Colposcopy

MEDICAL LIBRARY
ODSTOCK HOSPITAL
SALISBURY SP2 8BJ

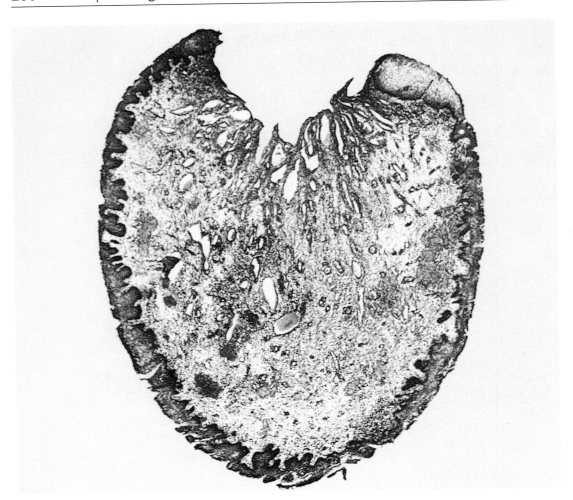

Fig. 18.1 Histologic preparation from a punch biopsy. The surface is covered by peg-forming acanthotic epithelium. Note the junction with normal squamous epithelium

In evaluating an abnormal smear or colposcopy, it is important to distinguish between a provisional and a definitive diagnosis. First we must establish whether we are dealing with atypia that requires confirmation by colposcopically directed target biopsy. Conization provides the definitive diagnosis. Such a two-step procedure is rejected by some, who prefer to proceed directly to conization, a disadvantage of which is that, in a number of cases, conization will fail to confirm the presence of atypia. The value of preliminary biopsy lies in prevention of unnecessary conization.

Initial Biopsy

This comprises punch biopsy, loop diathermy excision, and endocervical curettage. The technique is described in Chapter 9. Punch biopsy and diathermy excision are more informative since they contain the underlying stroma as well as epithelium (Fig. 18.1). Consequently, even invasive carcinoma can be diagnosed in some cases. Only tissue fragments are obtained in endocervical curettage, and the relationship between epithelium and stroma is often lost (Fig. 18.2). Exceptionally, fragments derived from frankly invasive carcinoma will be diagnostic (Fig. 18.3).

Quite the opposite problem arises when superficial destructive therapy is performed without a firm diagnosis. If the strict criteria (see p. 260) are not observed, mistakes can be made, as can be seen from Table 18.1, which shows the discrepancy between the findings on target biopsy and the definitive diagnosis on conization.

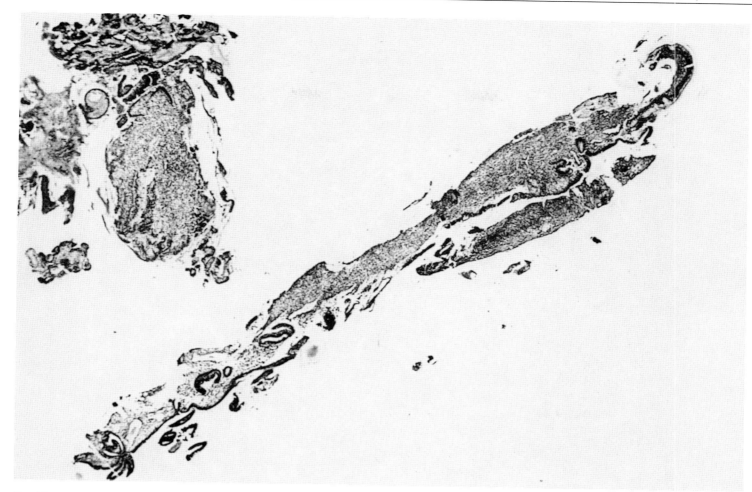

Fig. 18.**2** **Material obtained at endocervical curettage,** consisting of fragmented endocervical mucosa and strips of thin squamous epithelium

Table 18.**1** Correlation between colposcopically directed target biopsy and conization findings, University of Graz Dept. of Obstetrics and Gynecology*

Indication for conization	Total	Findings in the conization specimen							
		Nonsuspicious	Mild dysplasia	Moderate to severe dysplasia	Carcinoma in situ	Early stromal invasion	Microcarcinoma	More advanced invasive carcinoma	Adenocarcinoma
		n (%)	n (%)	n (%)	n (%)	n (%)	n (%)	n (%)	n (%)
Dysplasia	44	9 (20.5)	15 (34.1)	11 (25)	7 (15.9)	2 (4.5)			
Moderate to severe dysplasia	394	34 (8.6)	35 (8.9)	92 (23.3)	178 (45.2)	31 (7.9)	15 (3.8)	6 (1.5)	3 (0.8)
Carcinoma in situ	212	8 (3.8)	8 (3.8)	19 (8.9)	124 (58.5)	24 (11.3)	22 (10.4)	6 (2.8)	1 (0.5)
Suspicious of invasion	33				8 (24.3)	10 (30.3)	11 (33.3)	4 (12.1)	
Early invasive carcinoma	3					1 (33.3)	1 (33.3)	1 (33.3)	
Total	686	51 (8.4)	58 (9.1)	122 (17.5)	317 (45.5)	68 (9.6)	49 (6.9)	17 (2.4)	4 (0.6)

* after Neubert (7)

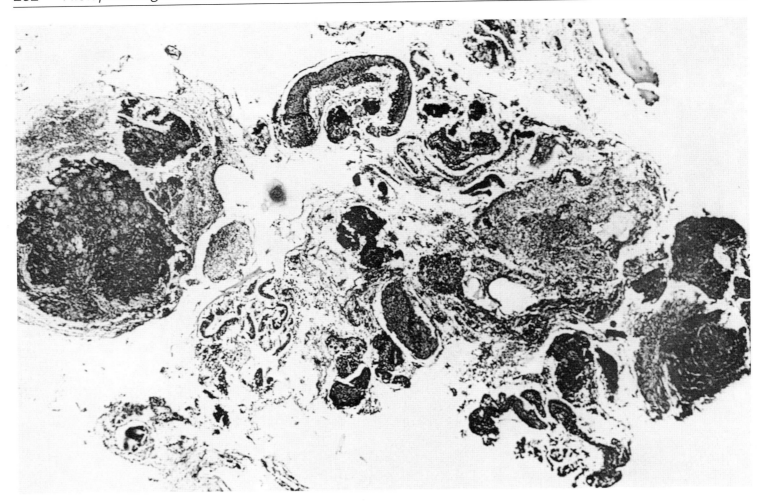

Fig. 18.**3 Larger fragments of malignant tissue,** together with strips of atypical squamous epithelium, the relationship of which to the underlying stroma is unclear

Punch biopsy, diathermy loop excision, or endocervical curettage should not be used to make a definitive diagnosis. Each is nonrepresentative, sampling merely part(s) of usually larger lesions. Not even early stromal invasion in a small target biopsy specimen can be regarded as conclusive, as there is no indication of its real extent. As current thinking favors individualization of treatment based on the size of the tumor (see p. 264), establishment only of the presence of invasion is not sufficient. This does not apply, of course, to clinically or colposcopically overt cancer. It is to be appreciated that larger lesions are comprised of several different epithelial components (Figs. 3.69, 3.70, Table 14.2), which explains the not uncommon discrepancy between repeat biopsies and the definitive diagnosis based on the conization specimen (1, 2, 6–8, 9). Table 18.1 shows that the diagnostic accuracy of target biopsy exceeds 50% only in cases of carcinoma in situ. The table also illustrates how misleading the result of the initial biopsy may be. In 650 cases of intraepithelial neoplasia initially diagnosed by target biopsy, subsequent full evaluation detected 110 cases of invasion, including 12 lesions larger than microinvasive carcinoma and 4 adenocarcinomas.

Final Histologic Diagnosis

Histology is the final arbiter of any cytologic or colposcopic abnormality. Presently there is a tendency to predict the histology from cytology and colposcopy, and to base therapeutic decisions on such "diagnoses." Such an approach is only partly valid, and above all only when the lesion is confined to the ectocervix (in range with the colposcope), and its relatively delicate surface configuration and limited extent (Fig. 3.66) do not raise any suspicion of invasion. A really precise evaluation demands complete excision of an abnormality and careful histologic examination. This can be achieved only by conization (see Chapter 20). In exceptional cases, local excision of a lesion colposcopically confined to the outer surface of one lip may be acceptable, especially when not too close to the os. If the lesion is circumoral, and the squamocolumnar junction can be visualized, flat conization may be carried out.

There are strict *indications for conization* (see Chapter 20). It must be carried out only if one knows that one is dealing with high-grade dysplasia, carcinoma in situ, or persisting dysplasia of any grade. Conization is also indicated for histologically proven or colposcopically suspected microinvasion, as it is desirable to determine the extent of the invasion (see p. 263). It is currently fashionable to avoid conization at all cost. It is certainly true that a number of unnecessary conizations were carried out in the past, mostly on the basis of abnormal cytology only. Similarly, local excision of small lesions on the ectocervix under direct colposcopic control has also been advocated. It is, however, erroneous to believe that epithelial atypia can be characterized so precisely by cytology and colposcopy that histologic confirmation becomes unnecessary (see p. 257). To do so would be to take a risk that, in the final analysis, the patient must bear.

References

1 Ahlgren M, Ingemarsson I, Lindberg LG, Nordquist SRB. Conization as treatment of carcinoma in situ of the uterine cervix. Obstet Gynecol 1975;46:135.
2 Bjerre B, Eliasson G, Linell F, Söderberg H, Sjöberg NO. Conization as only treatment of carcinoma in situ of the uterine cervix. Am J Obstget Gynecol 1976;125:143.
3 Burghardt E. Early histological diagnosis of cervical cancer. Philadelphia: Saunders, 1973.
4 Burghardt E. Östör AG. Site of origin and growth pattern of cervical cancer: a histomorphological study. Obstet Gynecol 1983;62:117.
5 Holzer E. Die Ausdehnung des atypischen Plattenepithels der Zervix. Arch Geschwulstforschung 1975;45:79.
6 Jones HW III, Buller RE. The treatment of cervical intraepithelial neoplasia by cone biopsy. Am J Obstet Gynecol 1980;137:882.
7 Neubert C. Restbefunde nach diagnostischen Konisationen. Geburtshilfe Frauenheilkd 1968;28:428.
8 Sprang ML, Isaacs JH, Boraca CT. Managment of carcinoma in situ of the cervix. Am J Obstet Gynecol 1977;129:47.
9 Van Nagell JR Jr, Parker JC, Hicks LP, Conrad R, England G. Diagnostic and therapeutic efficacy of cervical conization. Am J Obstet Gynecol 1976;124:134.

19

Therapeutic Implications of Atypical Colposcopic Appearances

Treatment of suspicious colposcopic findings without knowledge of their histopathologic basis should not be acceptable. Evaluation must be based at least on colposcopically directed target biopsy (see Chapter 18). This is complemented by cytology, which, however, can indicate only whether epithelial atypicality is present or not. "Predictive cytology" (predicting the exact histology from smears) is of further help, but it must be viewed with caution. Under no circumstance may cytology be the sole determinant of cancer therapy.

Management of Benign Colposcopic Findings

Ectopy

A large ectopy may produce unpleasant symptoms during the reproductive period, such as mucous discharge due to hypersecretion. Quite apart from the annoying secretions, the alkaline mucus also changes the pH of the vagina. This disturbs the normal vaginal flora and allows proliferation of pathogenic microorganisms, which in turn produces a discharge. Furthermore, the delicate columnar epithelium is subject to contact bleeding, and even spontaneous bleeding, which may alarm the patient. Finally, ectopy may be regarded as the soil for transformation that may lead to malignant change.

Therefore, treatment of ectopy may be *purely therapeutic* or *prophylactic.*

Only selected cases are suitable for the *purely prophylactic* approach, which is absolutely contraindicated in girls and young women in whom ectopy may be unusually large as a result of use of hormonal contraceptives. In symptomatic women, any hormone therapy should be stopped in the first instance. Prophylactic treatment is indicated, particularly for large ectopies, in women who have completed their families.

An ectopy may be physically destroyed or removed by shallow excision. *Electrocoagulation diathermy* is particularly effective. Alternatively, *cryosurgery* or *laser* may be used. We prefer to perform *flat conization* using a diathermy loop, removing the papillary endocervical mucosa together with a good portion of the glandular field.

Irrespective of the method employed, the end result should be reepithelialization by normal glycogen-containing squamous epithelium. In favorable cases, the squamocolumnar junction will lie at the external os.

Normal Transformation Zone

It is rarely necessary to treat the transformation zone per se. Therapy may be required for discharge, or contact bleeding as in ectopy, or for prophylactic intervention in cases of delayed maturation of the transforming epithelium. The treatment is the same as for ectopy.

Acanthotic Epithelium Producing Leukoplakia, Punctation, or Mosaic

Colposcopic findings due to acanthotic epithelium tend to be stable. Long-term observations reveal little change in the contours or cytologic makeup (see p. 5), and consequently they need no treatment. It is therefore important to evaluate the above colposcopic changes by cytology or biopsy, or both. If the findings are conclusively normal, both the patient and physician may feel reassured. Follow-up need not be any more stringent than for colposcopically nonsuspicious findings.

If one does embark on treatment for one reason or another, this should be superficial ablative therapy only. It must be borne in mind, however, that the regenerated squamous epithelium may resemble the one that was there before.

Condylomatous Lesions

First, we must distinguish between papillary and spiked condylomas and endophytic and flat ones.

First-line treatment for *papillary* and *spiked* condylomas should consist of surgical-ablative methods. Papillary lesions, and also extensive lawn-like ones, may be removed with the diathermy loop with a current setting not so high as to damage the underlying tissues. Flat condylomas in the neighborhood of papillary lesions may be removed with a diathermy loop in the same way, or cauterized, but only after biopsy evaluation. Electrocoagulation diathermy of the base of the lesion is important, as it may prevent recurrences due to residual virus-infected tissue.

Cryosurgery has also been used with success. Spontaneous regression has been observed of spiked condylomas adjacent to lesions destroyed by cryosurgery, presumably due to immune response to freezing (19).

Laser ablation is the treatment of choice for condylomas (5, 24). Laser can destroy condylomas of the cervix, vagina, or vulva under direct colposcopic control in a most elegant manner.

The therapy of *flat condylomas* requires caution, insofar as one must be sure of the diagnosis. For the treatment of pure flat condylomas the destructive and surgical methods described above should be considered. If the surface of a lesion is particularly coarse, then it may have an endophytic component, and, to prevent recurrence, the depth of destruction should be increased. Should the biopsy indicate some degree of atypia, the treatment should be as for intraepithelial neoplasia (see below).

Because of the danger of recurrence, adjuvant therapy may be necessary after surgery. Local application of interferon α 2c hydrogel has proved best (22, 63). Topical treatment of the lesion with interferon α 2b is possible, also as an adjuvant measure. Systemic interferon therapy is somewhat less effective, but does not delay wound healing (20, 23, 62). Single-agent treatment with podophyllin or 5-fluorouracil is complicated, and has a number of side effects (18, 38, 52, 55, 64).

Treatment of Atypical Squamous Epithelium (CIN)

Diagnostic Requirements

This section comprises treatment of dysplasia and carcinoma in situ, that is, all CIN lesions. Mild dysplasia (CIN 1) can and should be managed merely by careful short-term follow-up, as such lesions may regress, especially if poorly circumscribed colposcopically. If a well-defined lesion persists for at least a year, then it must be regarded and treated as carcinoma in situ. The aim of therapy is to remove or destroy the atypical epithelium in its *entirety*. Definitive therapeutic intervention should be based on *precise definition* of the lesion, the criteria being set out in Table 19.1.

Table 19.**1**   Diagnostic criteria for CIN

1 Histologic appearance of the atypical epithelium
2 Magnitude of surface spread, including extension into the endocervical canal
3 Depth of involvement of cervical glands or crypts
4 Exclusion of invasion

As shown in Table 19.2, neither colposcopy nor cytology, or even target biopsy, should be relied upon for accurate diagnosis (see Chapter 14). It is clear that *colposcopy* can satisfy only the second requirement, and only when the changes are confined to the ectocervix. The endocervical speculum (see Fig. 7.4), of course, helps to visualize the lower portion of the canal. However, lesions may extend high into the endocervical canal, so that their upper edges are out of reach of the colposcope. Although the colposcopic criteria for evaluating epithelia are well known (see p. 218), they are not sufficiently accurate for therapeutic decisions. Furthermore, microinvasive carcinoma can be diagnosed colposcopically only when it has reached a certain size, is situated on the ectocervix, and is not too far under the surface. *Cytology* can satisfy only the first criterion. Cytologic features suggestive of early invasion have, of course, been described (42); to address this question, however, is not the aim of routine screening.

The success of target *biopsies* depends entirely on the sites from which they have been taken, which in turn is determined by the colposcopic impression. Detection by biopsy of glandular involvement or of invasion is not always guaranteed, and endocervical curettage shows only extension of CIN into the canal. In the fragmented material (see Fig. 18.3), it is not always possible to establish histologically whether there is invasion or not, nor is it possible to determine the extent of glandular involvement and the depth to which the crypts reach.

It must be stressed that none of the primary diagnostic methods, even in combination, can satisfy criteria 3 and 4. Consequently, definitive diagnosis of CIN cannot be reached from cytologic, colposcopic, or target biopsy evaluations.

A truly definitive diagnosis can be achieved only if the total abnormal area is excised and submitted to rigorous histologic examination; for this purpose, conization or wide diathermy loop excision are ideal.

Table 19.3 shows the extent to which treatment results in 1609 cases of carcinoma in situ depended on the initial diagnostic method (12, 30). In 390 cases where the primary diagnosis was made by colposcopically directed target biopsy or ring biopsy, eight women died with recurrent carcinoma of the cervix. The treatment schedules included Schauta's radical vaginal hysterectomy (1), simple hysterectomy (2), high cervical amputation (1), and irradiation (2); in only two women was ring biopsy the sole form of therapy.

Table 19.**2**   Diagnostic limitations of individual methods*

Diagnostic Criteria for CIN	Diagnostic method			
	Colpo-scopy	Cyto-logy	Target biopsy	Coni-zation
Histologic appearance	(+)	+	+	+
Surface extent	+ (only ecto-cervix)	−	−	+
Glandular involvement	−/+	−	−	+
Exclusion of invasion	−	−	−	+

* after Holzer (29, 30)

Table 19.**3**   Results of treatment in 1609 cases of CIS, 1950−1974

Treatment	Cases	Lost to follow-up	Recurrence		Died of cancer
			Pre-invasive n (%)	Invasive n (%)	n (%)
Hysterectomy after target biopsy	245	5	6 (2.5)	7 (2.9)	5 (2.1)
Hysterectomy after ring biopsy	82	4	3 (3.8)	1 (1.3)	1 (1.3)
Ring biopsy	63	1	6 (9.6)	5 (8.1)	2 (3.2)
Hysterectomy after incomplete conization	183		7 (3.8)		
Incomplete conization	317	33	27 (8.5)	7 (2.2)	
Complete conization	719	61	2* (0.3)		

* Mild dysplasia 4 and 11 years after conization

Superficial Ablative Therapy of CIN

With the worlwide acceptance of colposcopy, the idea arose that it should be possible to destroy lesions under direct colposcopic control (14, 16, 33, 44, 45, 53, 54, 58, 65). This would avoid conization, which in the past was often performed without proper indication.

To be sure, total destruction of atypical epithelium should achieve complete cure. If this result could be guaranteed, there would not be much to choose among electrocoagulation diathermy, cryosurgery, and laser therapy. The crux of the matter, however, is *how can one be sure that all the atypical epithelium has, in fact, been destroyed.*

Every responsible advocate of the above methods stresses that only cases in which the lesions are *predominantly ectocervical* and in which the entire squamocolumnar junction is seen are suitable for destructive therapy (31, 32, 54, 57, 59). Such selection ensures that lesions that reach high into the canal will not go undestroyed. The danger exists, however, that atypical epithelium may remain in deep-seated ectopic glands under the surface. In fact, study of 343 conization specimens has shown that involved glands extended to a maximum depth of 5.22 mm from the surface, whereas normal glands reached a maximum depth of 7.83 mm (2). However, we have also found glands at a depth of 10 mm and in unexpected places (Fig. 19.1), outside the range of destruction of superficial ablative methods. Finally, *microcarcinomas* may arise from the base of crypts, with no connection with any atypical epithelium on the surface. Such invasive tumors may extend deeper than 5 mm into the stroma and may also arise in unexpected places (see Fig. 4.40).

The likelihood of deep extension is no doubt related to the surface size of the lesion, and is less in cases of dysplasia than in carcinoma in situ. This is due to the fact that carcinoma in situ, as distinct from dysplasia, which is more peripheral, develops more often on a soil of squamous metaplasia within the glandular field and its crypts. Conversely, in cases of atypical transformation of original squamous epithelium, glandular involvement is impossible. Furthermore, there is a direct relationship between the colposcopic surface extent of a lesion and the likelihood of invasion, since in general only large lesions are invasive (see Fig. 3.66).

Table 19.**4**   Age distribution of 119 patients with CIN according to its location

	Under 25 years	26–40 years
Exclusively ectocervical	5	1
Ectocervical and visible portion of the canal	11	33
Upper portion of the endocervical canal	20	49

Destructive methods should be used only in the following circumstances:

(a) mild to moderate dysplasia,
(b) a small lesion,
(c) a smooth lesion,
(d) purely ectocervical location,
(e) when the squamocolumnar junction is visible.

We have determined the chance of finding cases of CIN that satisfy the above criteria by examining conization specimens (Table 19.4). Even including severe dysplasia and carcinoma in situ, we found only 6 in 119 cases (5%). If we add a further 44 cases (37%) in which CIN extended into the lower portion of the canal and the squamocolumnar junction might have been visible, the figure is 42% at best.

It is a grave misconception that *regular follow-up* after conservative therapy of CIN will detect any persistent or recurrent abnormality in good time. Of greatest concern is persistence of carcinoma in situ in glands or of a deep-seated microcarcinoma with no connection to the surface of the remodeled cervix. Neither cytology nor colposcopy can cater for these contingencies, as such lesions will become manifest only when the surface is breached by invasive tumor. Such a case has been reported (35).

Recurrence following superficial ablative therapy and three normal follow-up examinations is rare (46). On the other hand, residual, mostly preinvasive, disease following conservative therapy is frequent (15, 17, 21, 28, 34, 37, 41, 56, 61). Treatment therefore often has to be repeated. For this reason, cryosurgery is no longer deemed suitable for the treatment of grade 3 CIN (41). It has also been established that the recurrence rate is inversely proportional to the depth of destruction. The amount of tissue damage required is comparable to that excised by adequate surgery (24, 37). In practice, the difference between the two treatment methods is that the former can be an office procedure, whereas the latter requires admission to a hospital, albeit for a short time. Another significant difference is that conservative methods destroy the tissues, and consequently the opportunity to determine histologically the exact nature of the disease is lost.

More worrisome are the increasing reports of *all stages of invasive carcinoma and mortality following conservative therapy* of CIN (26, 27, 35, 50, 60). The stark reality is not improved by reports stating that some of the patients have been inadequately investigated and selected prior to therapy (35, 60). In the hands of experts, the results of superficial ablative therapy should be, and have been, reported as excellent. But only recently, a report appeared from an experienced group describing 9 cases of invasive recurrences after laser ablation, with one death to date. Four patients who developed a frankly invasive cancer had been treated for CIN 3, according to the initial histology report (1a). It is also disturbing when such methods, used for the treatment of a potentially fatal disease, are propagated on a commercial basis. An office procedure is of course tempting for both patient and physician. Such a desire, however, is often coupled with little appreciation of its limitations and poor understanding of cervical pathology. The above-mentioned therapeutic misadventures therefore proved to be inevitable.

Basing their views on the successes and failures of destructive techniques, Jordan (31) and Jordan and Mylotte (32) stated that, before such methods are considered, the following requirements should be met:

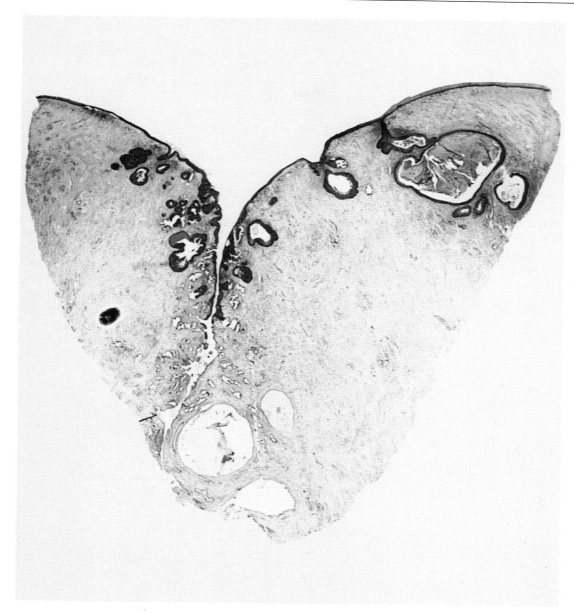

Fig. 19.**1 Conization specimen.** The surface of both lips is covered by carcinoma in situ (CIN 3). Note the abrupt change at the junction with normal squamous epithelium. The carcinoma in situ involves glands and extends into the lower portion of the canal. On the right there is extensive involvement of glands, which extend 10 mm under the surface. Such localization cannot be detected or suspected colposcopically

1. The patient is seen and assessed by an expert colposcopist.
2. The expert colposcopist can see the entire lesion, i.e., can see the squamocolumnar junction.
3. The expert colposcopist must exclude invasive carcinoma by colposcopically directed biopsy or biopsies.
4. The expert colposcopist must perform the destructive method himself or herself.
5. There must be good cytological and colposcopical follow-up.
   To this list, we would add:
6. The lesion should not be too large.
7. The colposcopist should have a detailed knowledge of cervical pathology.

Every physician who intends to use these treatment methods must therefore consider carefully to what extent he or she is able to fulfill the above requirements and whether his or her level of expertise is sufficient to carry out any procedure for the right indications. In the final analysis, the physician must bear the responsibility for any therapeutic misadventure.

Therapeutic Conization

Conization has become notorious because of its indiscriminate use, which has resulted in operations, many of which proved to be unneccessary. In addition, poor operative technique engendered complications that could have been avoided.

Conization cannot be regarded primarily as a therapeutic approach. Any further steps following diagnostic conization depend on the quality of the histologic examination and whether the lesion has been completely removed or whether some has been left behind in the residual cervix.

1. *Complete excision.* If the disease is purely intraepithelial or early invasive with virtually no metastatic potential, nothing further need be done. As with the management of any cancer, however, careful follow-up with periodic cytology and colposcopy is indicated. We have followed for at least 6 years 733 women with carcinoma in situ and 28 with microinvasive carcinoma in whom the lesion was completely excised (Table 19.5). In only three patients did carcinoma in situ and mild dysplasia recur after 2, 4 and 11 years respectively, and this may well have been new disease. Higher rates of recurrence noted by some investigators may have been due to inadequate histologic assessment resulting in uncertainty as to the completeness of excision.

Table 19.**5**   Results after conization with complete removal of lesions (1958—1975) and follow-up for at least 6 years

	Cases	Recurrences
Carcinoma in situ	733	3*
Microinvasive carcinoma	28	

* One case of CIS after 2 years; two cases of mild dysplasia 4 and 11 years after conization

2. *Incomplete excision.* We report incomplete excision if the margins pass through at least mildly dysplastic squamous epithelium. This, however, does not necessarily mean that major lesions have remained in the residual cervix, for (a) the margin of excision may pass very close to the edge of a lesion, and (b) small portions of residual atypical epithelium may be sloughed off during the healing process.

Before any further therapy is undertaken, a number of questions have to be answered:

1. At which margins are the lesions incompletely excised?
2. At what distance from the margins of excision are invasive foci found?
3. Is preservation of the uterus desired?

Easiest to manage are cases in which the ectocervical margin is involved. In such cases, a persistent abnormality can be reliably detected by colposcopy (Figs. 11.95 and 11.96). It is not so convenient if the apex of the cone is involved. Conservative management of such cases is risky. Cytologic follow-up should be supplemented by periodic endocervical curettage. The most difficult cases to manage are those in which the stromal (side) edges are concerned, with the margins running close to or throught atypical epithelium in endocervical crypts (Figs. 19.1 and 19.2). As with the destructive methods, malignant epithelium may be buried in residual crypts following healing and re-epithelialization of the surface. Such cases can be detected cytologically and colposcopically only when they have become in-

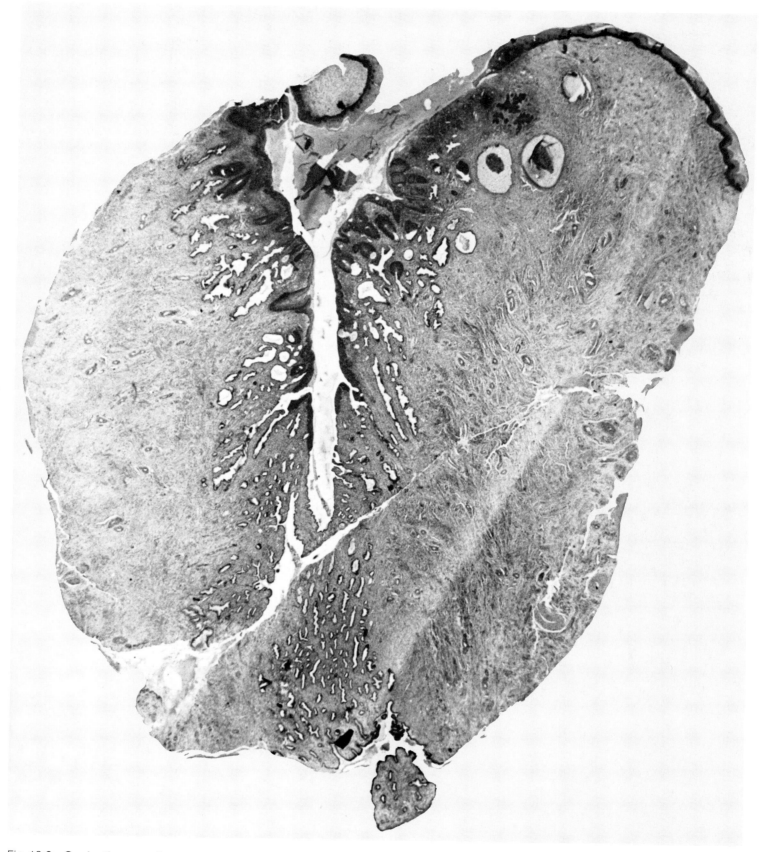

Fig. 19.**2 Conization specimen.** The right lip harbors a microcarcinoma, measuring 2 mm in diameter. The surface and the glands show carcinoma in situ (CIN 3). The carcinoma in situ on the left side extends to the margin of resection

Table 19.**6**   Findings in the uterus removed within a year after incomplete conization for CIS in 388 women (1958–1975)

	Cases	%
Preinvasive lesions	78	20.1
Microinvasive carcinoma	29	7.5
More advanced invasive carcinoma	8	2.1
Total	115	29.7

vasive and have breached the surface. This is also true of invasive nests close to the resection margins; similar foci may remain in the residual cervix.

Preservation of the uterus for fertility must be carefully weighed against the risks. The risk of expectant therapy for incompletely excised superficial lesions is not high, provided regular follow-up can be ensured. As seen in Table 19.6, the incidence of residual disease in uteri extirpated following inadequate conization is 30%; however, this includes cases of microinvasion and more advanced invasive carcinomas. Of 314 women treated by inadequate conization alone, regular cytologic and biopsy follow-up detected 35 cases (11%) of persistent disease, 7 of which, however, were either microinvasive or more advanced invasive carcinoma (Table 19.7). The lower incidence of residual disease in these 314 cases is no doubt due to the strict selection of patients.

Table 19.**7**   Results after conization with incomplete removal of CIS in 314 women (1958–1975)

	Cases	%
Preinvasive lesions	28	(8.9)
Microinvasive carcinoma	3	(0.9)
More advanced invasive carcinoma	4	(1.3)
Total	35	(11.1)

Repeat Conization

Residual atypical lesions can be completely removed by repeat conization following inadequate excision of an abnormality by the first cone, provided sufficient cervical tissue has remained. The technique is the same. We successfully treated a 35-year-old woman by conization following two previous conizations elsewhere; she subsequently became pregnant for the first time and later became pregnant again. The antenatal course of both confinements was uneventful. The two babies weighed 3550 g and 3110 g respectively, and were delivered spontaneously and without complication.

Hysterectomy

The objections to, and risks of, destructive methods also apply to *hysterectomy as the initial treatment* of inadequately evaluated CIN. The greatest danger is overlooking an invasive lesion. Mortality from cervical cancer following primary hysterectomy can only be explained by inadequate biopsy evaluation prior to the operation (see Table 19.3).

Should a primary hysterectomy be done at all, it must be based on stringent indications. *Vaginal hysterectomy* is far preferable to the *abdominal* route because, as Table 19.8 shows, the recurrence rate following the vaginal procedure is much lower. This is due to the fact that the cervix is excised during vaginal hysterectomy under direct vision, whereas in abdominal hysterectomy a lesion may be cut through.

Table 19.**8**   Results of hysterectomy within the first year after incomplete conization for CIS (1958–1974)

Procedure	n	Recurrence (%)
Vaginal hysterectomy	84	3
Vaginal hysterectomy with vaginal cuff	47	—
Total	131	3 (2.3)
Abdominal hysterectomy	33	3
Abdominal hysterectomy with vaginal cuff	13	1
Total	46	4 (8.7)

Treatment of Microinvasive Carcinoma

Ever since the introduction of the concept of microinvasive carcinoma, its definition and treatment have remained controversial. Even with the new FIGO definition (3), which is clear and reproducible, differences in opinion remain. The main difficulties lie with those who advocate a restrictive definition of microinvasive carcinoma (4) and who believe that the FIGO classification should be used as a guide to therapy. This belief, however, is blatantly false, since the purpose of the classification is not to dictate treatment, but to allow the results of treatment to be compared. Restricting the definition of microinvasion to a depth of penetration of 1 mm, for example (4), and using this as a guide to therapy, would leave little leeway in the treatment of somewhat larger tumors. It should also be borne in mind that, by assigning all tumors with a depth of invasion of more than 1 mm to Stage Ib would lead to a great watering-down of this category.

The idea of adding a second dimension to the definition of Stage Ia2 is based on the fact that a neoplasm which invades to 4–5 mm may measure up to 22 mm in width (36, 39, 49, 51). A tumor which measures 5×20 mm is not merely a microcarcinoma, but a carcinoma of distinct size, which should properly be put into the Stage Ib category.

Early Stromal Invasion (Stage Ia1)

(see p. 89)

The incidence of early stromal invasion in conization specimens removed for carcinoma in situ and examined by serial sectioning is 11% in our material. The tiny invasive foci have no apparent clinical significance and can be managed the same way as in situ disease. We must bear in mind, however, that the surface area, including extension into the endocervical canal, is significantly greater than in cases of dysplasia or carcinoma in situ (see Fig. 3.66). Glandular involvement is also more common and extensive. These facts become particularly clear when we examine the likelihood of complete excision of the various changes by conization (Table 19.9). When conization reveals early stromal invasion, hysterectomy is required much more often than in cases of preinvasive lesions.

During the last 31 years we have treated 344 women with early stromal invasion (Table 19.10). The treatment has varied considerably during this period. We have not resorted to any radical operations since 1971, during which time we have made increasing use of conization as the sole therapeutic procedure. During the last 7 years, conization alone has been employed in 73% of cases. The hysterectomy rate has declined pari passu. Hysterectomy was carried out only in cases of incomplete excision by conization, or if there were other gynecologic indications.

We have seen 6 patients with carcinoma in situ in the vaginal vault shortly after hysterectomy. These patients most likely had persisting disease (Table 19.11). One patient presented again with Stage IIb cervical cancer 12 years after conization. She had not gone to follow-up examinations in the interim. This patient apparently had a new cancer. There is only one report of invasive recurrence after adequately diagnosed early stromal invasion in the literature (6). This patient had an early invasive lesion in the vaginal vault 20 months after hysterectomy. Local disease was eradicated by radiotherapy, but the patient developed para-aortic metastases.

Table 19.**9** Removal of lesions by conization in 2522 cases (1958–1976)

Finding in cone	Complete removal		Incomplete removal	
	n	%	n	%
Mild dysplasia	186	86.1	30	13.9
Moderate dysplasia	352	75.5	114	24.5
Severe dysplasia or CIS	923	61.2	585	38.8
Early stromal invasion	83	35.9	148	64.1
Microcarcinoma	27	26.7	74	73.3

Table 19.**10** Treatment of 344 patients with early stromal invasion (Stage Ia 1)

	n	1958–1970		1971–1975		1976–1981		1982–1988	
		n	%	n	%	n	%	n	%
Radical vaginal hysterectomy	45	45	36.3	—		—		—	
Abdominal radical hysterectomy with lymphadenectomy	3	3	2.4	—		—		—	
Simple hysterectomy	170	59	47.6	60	68.2	40	44.0	11	26.8
Conization	124	15	12.1	28	31.8	51	56.0	30	73.2
Irradiation	2	2	1.6	—		—		—	
Total	344	124		88		91		41	

Table 19.**11**   Results of treatment of 309 patients with early stromal invasion (Stage Ia 1) followed up for at least 5 years, 1958–1983

	n	Persistent disease	Recurrence	Died of cervical carcinoma
Radical vaginal hysterectomy	45	2	–	–
Abdominal radical hysterectomy with lymphadenectomy	3	–	–	–
Simple hysterectomy	166	4	–	–
Conization	93	–	–	1
Irradiation	2	–	–	–
Total	309	6	–	1

Microcarcinoma (Stage Ia2)

(see p. 90)

Although the largest dimensions of these small tumors should not exceed 5×7 mm, their volume is incomparably larger than that of early stromal invasion. Nevertheless, the biologic behavior of microcarcinoma appears to be less aggressive than that of frank carcinomas.

A total of 17 fatal recurrences have been reported among 1429 microcarcinomas with up to 5 mm invasion (Table 19.**12**). The recurrences occurred independently of the size of the lesions, certain risk factors, and the type of treatment. One patient with a lesion showing only 1 mm of invasion and no vascular invasion died despite having undergone extended hysterectomy with lymphadenectomy. Several other cases showed invasion up to 3 mm, some also with no risk factors.

Of 89 women with microcarcinoma treated by surgery at our clinic between 1958 and 1983 and followed up for at least 5 years (Table 19.**12**), there were recurrences in 6 patients, 3 of whom died of the disease. The microcarcinoma was associated in 4 cases with capillary-like space involvement (Fig. 19.3). As we accumulated more experience, the treatment of microcarcinoma was changed (Table 19.**13**), resulting first in a significant

reduction in the number of radical operations. Following the first recurrence in 1976, microcarcinoma with capillary-like space involvement was again treated by radical hysterectomy and pelvic lymphadenectomy, but to date no lymph node metastases have been found in 29 cases. The rate of simple hysterectomy varied inversely with that of the radical precedure. Conization was used with increasing frequency as the sole therapeutic method. During the last 7 years, more than half of patients with microcarcinoma have been treated solely by conization.

A study of clinically invasive carcinomas has shed some new light on the significance of *capillary-like space involvement* (13). The incidence of lymph node metastases was significantly higher in cases associated with vascular invasion that in those without. Yet there was also a remarkable correlation between tumor volume and vascular invasion, on the one hand, and the incidence of lymph node metastases on the other; in spite of vascular involvement, the frequency of lymph node metastases was significantly lower with small tumors than with large ones (Fig. 19.4). Nevertheless, it may be assumed that the metastatic potential of microcarcinoma is significantly less than that of larger tumors. Because of the great variation in the *volume of microcarcinomas*, the maximal diameter of which may range from 1 to 7 mm, the question arises whether the

Table 19.**12**   Fatal recurrences after treatment of microcarcinomas with a maximal depth of 5 mm

Author	n	Dead of cancer	CIS involvement	Confluent pattern	Depth (size)	Primary treatment
Sedlis et al. 1978	133	2	2	1	3 mm 5 mm	Abdominal hysterectomy
Lohe et al. 1978	134	2	2	NS	3×4×5 mm 3×4×5 mm	Abdominal rad. hysterectomy Abdominal hysterectomy
Yajima & Noda 1979	188	2	0	0	1.2 mm 1.0 mm	Simple hysterectomy Extended hysterectomy with lymphadenectomy
Taki et al. 1979	115	1	0	NS	2 mm	Extended hysterectomy
van Nagell et al. 1983	32	2	2 (?)	2 (?)	3.1–5 mm	Radical hysterectomy with lymphadenectomy
Creasman et al. 1985	95	1	1	1	3.7 mm	Radiation
Kolstad 1989	643	4	2	NS	2 mm 4 mm 4 mm	Hysterectomy
Burghardt et al. 1991	89	3	3	2	5×7 mm 3×6 mm 2×6 mm	Hysterectomy Conization
Total	1429	17 (1.2%)				

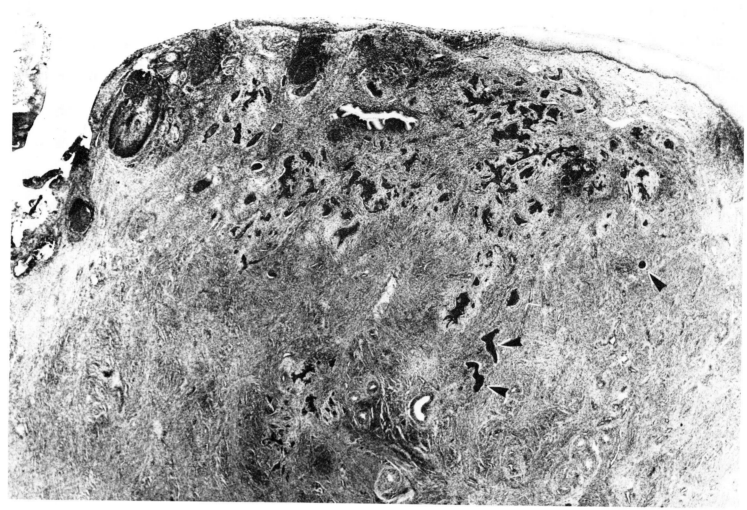

Fig. 19.**3** **Portion of a conization specimen** containing a microcarcinoma with depth of invasion of 5 mm and horizontal spread of 9 mm. Several foci of capillary-like space involvement are indicated by *arrows* (from Obstet Gynecol 1977;49:641

Table 19.**13** Results of treatment of 101 patients with microcarcinoma (Stage Ia 2); changes in treatment, 1958−1983

	n	1958−1970	1971−1975	1976−1981	1982−1988
Radical vaginal hysterectomy	35	29	6	−	−
Abdominal radical hysterectomy with lymphadenectomy	15	2	−	8	5
Hysterectomy	25	5	11	3	6
Conization alone	26	1	1	9	15
Total	101	37	18	20	26

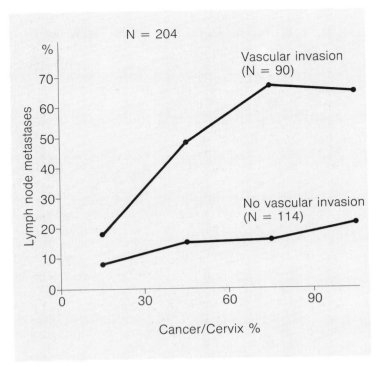

Fig. 19.**4   Correlation between tumor size, vascular invasion, and lymph node metastasis in cervical cancer.** The incidence of lymph node metastasis is significantly higher in tumors with vascular involvement than in tumors without. The size of the tumor is expressed as a percentage ratio of the total cervical size (from Clin Oncol 1982;1:323

presence of vascular invasion carries a different prognostic import even within this group. That this does not necessarily apply can be seen from Table 19.**14.** In any case, vascular invasion is a risk factor of great significance. The same is true for differentiation and a confluent growth pattern. But vascular invasion and poor differentiation were found in at least 25% and 60% of all Stage Ia2 cases, respectively, and are thus of low specificity.

Boyes et al. (6) were the first to suggest that confluent growth is an unfavorable factor with regard to metastasis. A number of authors subsequently adopted this assessment— without confluent growth ever having been precisely defined (1). Roche and Norris (47) saw no association between confluent growth and capillary-like space involvement; they doubt whether this pattern plays a role in tumors with less than 5 mm invasion. The classification of growth patterns proposed by Hamperl (25) is much more accurate, but has not received wide attention. Hamperl distinguished between *reticular infiltration* (as in Fig. 4.**42**) and *plump infiltration* (Fig. 4.**44**). Reticular infiltration, always associated with poorer differentiation, was suspected of having a poorer prognosis than the plump pattern.

There can be no strict guidelines as to the treatment of microcarcinoma. It is a great mistake to believe that the classification FIGO, by dividing microinvasive carcinoma into Stage Ia1 (early stromal invasion) and Stage Ia2 (microcarcinoma), should be the blueprint for standard treatment. The therapy of Stage Ia2 tumors must be individualized for each patient. Since this decision rests above all on histologic criteria, it is of paramount importance that there must be close consultation with a specialist in gynecological pathology. It is to be hoped that, with the help of the strict new FIGO definition, we will finally gain enough knowledge of the natural history of microcarcinomas of various sizes.

If the decision has been made not to treat microcarcinoma radically, there is little to choose between conization and simple hysterectomy. If a lesion that has not metastasized has been completely removed by conization, leaving behind the body of the uterus and outer portion of the cervix can have no deleterious effect.

References

1   Anderson MC. The pathology of cervical cancer. Clin Obstet Gynecol 1985;12:87.

1a   Ali SW, Evans AS, Monaghan JM. Results of laser cylinder vaporization of cervical intraepithelial disease in 1234 patients: an analysis failures. Br J Obstet Gynaecol 1986;93:75.

2   Anderson MC, Harteley RB. Cervical crypt involvement by intraepithelial neoplasia. Obstet Gynecol 1980;55:546.

3   [Anon.] FIGO news: changes to the 1985 FIGO report on the result of treatment in gynecological cancer. Int J Gynaecol Obstet 1987;25:87.

4   Averette HE, Nelson JH, Ng ABP, Hoskins WJ, Boyce JG, Ford JH Jr. Diagnosis and management of microinvasive (Stage Ia) carcinoma of the uterine cervix. Cancer 1976;38:414.

5   Baggish MS. Complications associated with carbon dioxide laser surgery in gynecology. Am J Obstet Gynecol 1981;139:568.

6   Boyes DA, Worth AJ, Fidler HK. The results of treatment of 4389 cases of preclinical cervical squamous carcinoma. J Obstet Gynaecol Br Commonwealth 1970;77:769.

7   Burghardt E. Early histological diagnosis of cervical cancer. Philadelphia: Saunders, 1973.

8   Burghardt E. Das Mikrokarzinom der Cervix uteri. Wien Klin Wochenschr 1978;90:477.

9   Burghardt E. Zur Frage der sogenannten konservativen Behandlung des atypischen Zervixepithels. Geburtshilfe Frauenheilkd 1981;41:330.

10   Burghardt E. Pathology of preclinical invasive carcinoma (microinvasive and occult invasive carcinoma). In: Coppleson M, ed. Gynecologic oncology. Edinburgh: Churchill Livingstone, 1981.

11   Burghardt E, Holzer E. Diagnosis and treatment of microinvasive carcinoma of the cervix. Obstet Gynecol 1977;49:641.

12   Burghardt E, Holzer E. Treatment of carcinoma in situ: evaluation of 1609 cases. Obstet Gynecol 1980;55:539.

12a Burghardt E, Girardi F, Lahousen M, Pickel H, Tamussino K. Microinvasive carcinoma of the uterine cervix. Cancer, 1991 (in press).

13   Burghardt E, Holzer E. Minimal invasive cancer (microcarcinoma). Clin Oncol 1982;1:1−2.

14   Chanen W, Hollyhock VE. Colposcopy and the conservative management of cervical dysplasia and carcinoma in situ. Obstet Gynecol 1974;43:527.

15   Charles EH, Savage EW, Hacker N, Jones NC. Cryosurgical treatment of cervical intraepithelial neoplasia. Gynecol Oncol 1981;12:83.

15a Creasman WT, Fetter BF, Clarke-Pearson DL, Kaufmann L, Parker RT. Management of stage Ia carcinoma of the cervix. Am J Obstet Gynecol 1985;153:164.

16 Crisp WE, Asadourian L, Romberger W. Application of cryosurgery to gynecologic malignancy. Obstet Gynecol 1967;30:668.

17 Edelmann WLA, Fowler DA, Photopulos WC. Cryosurgery for the treatment of cervical intraepithelial neoplasia during the reproductive years. Obstet Gynecol 1980;55:353.

18 Fisher AA. Severe systemic and local reactions to topical podophyllum resin. Cutis 1981;28:233–66.

19 Friedrich EG. Vulvar disease. Philadelphia. Saunders, 1976.

20 Geffen JR, Klein RJ, Friedman–Kien AE. Intralesional administration of large doses of human leucocyte interferon for the treatment of condylomata acuminata. J Infect Dis 1984;150:612.

21 Gray LA, Christopherson WM. The treatment of cervical dyplasias. Gynecol Oncol 1975;3:149.

22 Gross G. Interferone zur Behandlung von Condylomata acuminata. Dtsch Med Wochenschr 1987;112:571.

23 Gross G, Roussaki A, Schöpf E. Successful treatment of condylomata acuminata and bowenoid papulosis with subcutaneous injections of low-dose recombinant interferon-α. Arch Dermatol 1985;122:749.

24 Hahn GA. Carbon dioxide laser surgery in the treatment of condyloma. Am J Obstet Gynecol 1981;141:1000.

25 Hamperl H. Über das infiltrierende (invasive) Tumorwachstum. Untersuchungen am Carcinom und am sog. Carcinoma in situ. Virchows Arch [A] 1966;340:185.

26 Henriksen HM. The cryosurgical treatment of intraepithelial neoplasia. Acta Obstet Gynecol Scand 1979;58:271.

27 Hilgarth M, Hillemanns HG, Roll H. Der besondere Fall: Plattenepithelkarzinom der Cervix uteri nach Kryosation bei einer 23jährigen Patientin. Fortschr Med 1979;97:2145.

28 Hollyhock VE, Chanen W. Electrocoagulation therapy for the treatment of cervical dysplasia and carcinoma in situ. Obstet Gynecol 1976;47:196.

29 Holzer E. Die Behandlung des Carcinoma in situ, 1. Arch Gynecol 1979;227:205.

30 Holzer E. Die Behandlung des Carcinoma in situ, 2. Arch Gynecol 1979;227:225.

31 Jordan JA. CO₂ laser therapy. In: Coppleson M, ed. Gynecologic oncology, vol 2. Edinburgh: Churchill Livingstone, 1981:817.

32 Jordan JA, Mylotte J. Treatment of CIN by destruction: laser. In: Jordan JA, Sharp F, Singer A, eds. Pre-clinical neoplasia of the cervix. London: Royal College of Obstetrics and Gynaecology, 1982:205.

33 Kaufmann RH, Conner JS. Cryosurgical treatment of cervical dysplasia. Am J Obstet Gynecol 1971;109:1167.

34 Kaufmann RH, Irwin JF. The cryosurgical therapy of cervical intraepithelial neoplasia, 3. Am J Obstet Gynecol 1978;131:381.

34a Kolstad P. Follow-up study of 232 patients with stage Ia1 and 411 patients with stage Ia2 squamous cell carcinoma of the cervix (microinvasive carcinoma). Gynecol Oncol 1989;33:265.

35 Kranzfelder D, Mestwerdt W. Kollumkarzinom 3 Jahre nach kryochirurgischer Behandlung der Portio vaginalis uteri. Geburtshilfe Frauenheilkd 1978;38:289.

36 Larsson G, Alm P. Gullberg B, Grundsell H. Prognostic factors in early invasive carcinoma of the uterine cervix. Am J Obstet Gynecol 1983;146:145.

36a Lohe KJ, Burghardt E, Hillemanns HG, Kaufmann C, Ober KG, Zander J. Early squamous cell carcinoma of the uterine cervix: II. clinical results of a cooperative study in the management of 419 patients with early stromal invasion and microcarcinoma. Gynecol Oncol 1978;6:31.

37 Masterson BJ; Krantz KE, Calkins JW, Magrina JF, Carter RP. The carbon dioxide laser in cervical intraepithelial neoplasia: a five-year experience in treating 230 patients. Am J Obstet Gynecol 1981;139:565.

38 Montaldi DH, Giambrone JP, Courey NG, Taefi P. Podophyllin poisoning associated with the treatment of condyloma acuminatum: a case report. Am J Obstet Gynecol 1974;119:1130.

39 Mühlberger G. Morphologische Studie an 167 Wertheim-Operationspräparationen. Geburtshilfe Frauenheilkd 1975;35:27.

40 Nel WS, Fourie ED. Immunotherapy and 5% topical 5-fluorouracil jointment in the treatment of condylomata acuminata. S Afr. Med J 1973;47:45.

41 Ostergard DR. Cryosurgical treatment of cervical intraepithelial neoplasia. Obstet Gynecol 1980;56:231.

42 Patten SF Jr. Diagnostic cytopathology of the uterine cervix. Basle: Karger, 1978.

43 Powell LC Jr. Condylomata acuminata: recent advances in development, carcinogenesis and treatment. Clin Obstet Gynecol 1978;21:1061.

44 Renzienhausen K, Brandt M, Marzotko F, Altrock H. Über die Kryotherapie an der Cervix uteri (Untersuchungs- und Behandlungsergebnisse). Zentralbl Gynäkol 1974;96:1281.

45 Richart RM, Sciarra JJ. Treatment of cervical dysplasia by outpatient electrocauterization. Am J Obstet Gynecol 1968;101:200.

46 Richart RM, Townsend DE, Crips W, et al. An analysis of "long-term" follow-up results in patients with cervical intraepithelial neoplasia treated by cryotherapy. Am J Obstet Gynecol 1980;137:823.

47 Roche WD, Norris HJ. Microinvasive carcinoma of the cervix: the significance of lymphatic invasion and confluent patterns of stromal growth. Cancer 1975;36:180.

48 Schellhas HF. Laser surgery in gynecology. Surg Clin North Am 1978;58:151.

49 Sedlis A, Sall S, Tsukada Y, et al. Microinvasive carcinoma of the uterine cervix: a clinical-pathological study. Am J Obstet Gynecol 1979;133:64.

50 Sevin BU, Ford JH, Girtanner RD, et al. Invasive cancer of the cervix after cryosurgery. Obstet Gynecol 1979;53:465.

51 Simon NL, Gore H, Shingleton HM, Soong SJ, Orr JW, Hatch KD. Study of superficially invasive carcinoma of the cervix. Obstet Gynecol 1986;68:19.

52 Slater GE, Rumack BH, Peterson RG. Podophyllin poisoning: systemic toxicity following cutaneous application. Obstet Gynecol 1978;52:94.

53 Sonek MG, Acosta AA, Collins RJ, et al. Cryosurgery in treatment of abnormal cervical lesions: an invitational symposium. J Reprod Med 1971;7:147.

54 Stafl A, Wilkinson EJ, Mattingly RF. Laser treatment of cervical and vaginal neoplasia. Am J Obstet Gynecol 1977;128:128.

55 Stoehr GP, Peterson AL, Taylor WJ. Systemic complications of local podophyllin therapy. Ann Intern Med 1978;89:362.

56   Stromby EB. A study of cryosurgery for dysplasia and carcinoma in situ of the uterine cervix. Br J Obstet Gynaecol 1979;86:917.

56a   Taki I, Sugimori H, Matsuyama T, Kashimura Y, Yoshivo T. Treatment of microinvasive carcinoma. Obstet Gynecol Surv 1979;34:839.

57   Toplis PJ, Casemore V, Hallam N, Charnock M. Evaluation of colposcopy in the postmenopausal woman. Br J Obstet Gynaecol 1986;93:843.

58   Townsend DE. Cryosurgery. Obstet Gynecol 1975;4:331.

59   Townsend DE. Cryosurgery. In: Coppleson M, ed. Gynecologic oncology, vol 2. Edinburgh: Churchill Livingstone, 1981:809.

60   Townsend DE, Richart RM, Marks E, Nielsen J. Invasive cancer following outpatient evaluation and therapy for cervical disease. Obstet Gynecol 1981;57:145.

61   Tronstad SE, Kirschner R. Treatment of cervical intraepithelial neoplasia with local excisional biopsy and cryosurgery. Acta Obstet Gynecol Scand 1980;59:349.

62   Vance J. Bart BJ, Hansen RC, et al. Intralesional recombinant alpha-2 interferon for the treatment of patients with condyloma acuminatum or verruca plantaris. Arch Dermatol 1986;122:272.

62a   van Nagell JR, Greenwell N, Powell DF, Donaldson ES, Hanson MB, Gay EC. Microinvasive carcinoma of the cervix. Am J Obstet Gynecol 1983;145:981.

63   Vesterinnen E, Meyer B, Purola E, et al. Treatment of vaginal flat condyloma with interferon cream. Lancet 1984;1:157.

64   Ward JW, Clifford WS, Monaco AR, Bicherstaff HJ. Fatal systemic poisoning following podophyllin treatment of condyloma acuminatum. South Med J 1954;47:1204.

64a   Yajima A, Noda, K. The results of treatment of microinvasive carcinoma (stage Ia) of the uterine cervix by means of simple and extended hysterectomy. Am J Obstet Gynecol 1979;135:685.

65   Younge PA. Premalignant lesions of the cervix: clinical management. Clin Obstet Gynecol 1962;5:1137.

20

Technique of Conization and the Histologic Processing of the Cone

Indications for Conization

Conization concerns itself with the shape of the cervix and the topographic distribution of the various epithelial abnormalities. It is usually performed with a sharp scalpel (cold knife conization). Nowadays it can also be done with the laser. However, this is not a true conization, since only a cylindrical block of tissue can be removed (20), thereby loosing more of the fibromuscular stroma of the cervix than necessary.

Which technique should be used is difficult to say. According to the supporters of laser treatment, cold-knife conization has numerous disadvantages, poor operative technique being the foremost among these. One advantage of laser cones is perhaps the lower incidence of postoperative hemorrhage (20). A distinct disadvantage is the unduly large wound left after removal of the cylindrical tissue. The relative incidence of cervical incompetence following the two procedures is not yet known.

Diagnostic Conization

There is no question that conization provides definitive diagnosis of CIN, provided the lesion has been completely excised. If removal is incomplete, further procedures may be necessary. Conization is always indicated if atypical cervical lesions are to be diagnosed with the greatest degree of accuracy. Based on our knowledge of evaluation of CIN (see p. 52), the indications for conization are:

1. Persistent mild and moderate dysplasia (CIN 1 and 2), as these may be morphologic expressions of biologically well-differentiated carcinoma in situ.
2. Severe dysplasia and carcinoma in situ (CIN 3), as these lesions are unlikely to regress.
3. Established early stromal invasion, as the size of the invasive lesion, determined from the conization specimen, is of therapeutic importance.

Therapeutic Conization

Only histologic examination and diagnosis can decide whether conization is adequate therapy in individual cases (5). We must know whether the lesion has been completely excised. In cases of microinvasion, the question of lymph node metastases arises (see Chapter 19). Should conization be the sole mode of therapy, then the specimen must be examined in great detail histologically to answer these questions (5).

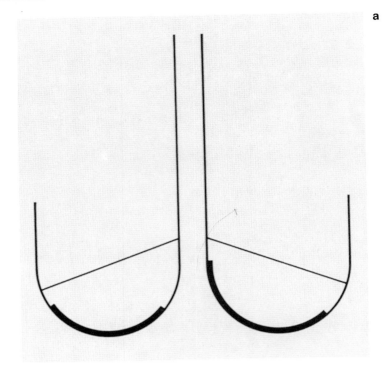

a

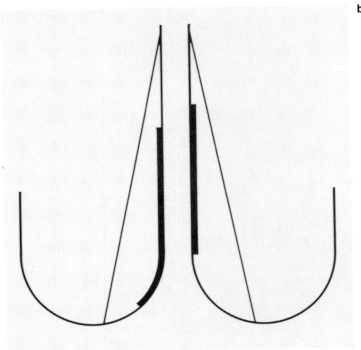

b

Fig. 20.**1 a**, **b**   **Different types of cones**

Fig. 20.**1 a**   If the lesion is primarily on the ectocervix, a shallow cone is sufficient

Fig. 20.**1 b**   If the lesion is mostly up the canal, a long, narrow cone reaching to the region of the internal os is required (from Clin Obstet Gynecol 1982;25:849)

Technique of Conization

Cold Knife Conization

Conization is not a simple operation. It is certainly not comparable to curettage, and should not be undertaken by the inexperienced. Thorough knowledge of the possible location and significance of atypical lesions is a prerequisite. By using a standard technique, on the other hand, conization allows the cervical epithelial abnormalities to be diagnosed with a high degree of accuracy.

The size and quality of the conization specimen are crucial; all too often pathologists complain that the cone is too small, morcellated, or hard to orientate. Excision may be technically difficult because of variable consistency of the tissue to be removed and excessive bleeding that may obscure the view. Such difficulties may be overcome by infiltration of the cervix with a hemostatic agent, such as 1:100000 solution of epinephrine in saline (15). An unpredictable rise in blood pressure is an undesirable side effect (5, 6, 11, 14). The use of synthetic agents such as ornipressin is preferable in a dilution of 5 IU/200 mL of physiologic saline (4, 6). Injecting larger amounts may also raise the blood pressure. Peripheral vasoconstriction may be detected by pallor of the skin, especially of the face. We have not encountered a single serious complication from the use of hemostatic agents in over 4000 operations. Pure physiologic saline can be used, but the hemostasis it provides is not as good as that of ornipressin.

In the past, in addition to any visible lesion on the ectocervix, approximately two-thirds of the endocervical canal was always removed. Now a shallow cone biopsy may be performed, provided the lesion is confined colposcopically to the ectocervix or lower portion of the canal (Fig. 20.1 a).

If the lesion extends up the canal out of range of the colposcope, approximately two-thirds of the canal should be excised (Fig. 20.1 b). Thus, the shape of the cone may be broad and shallow, or narrow and elongated, according to the site of the lesion.

Our technique (4, 6) is a modification of that described by Scott et al. (16), and is carried out in several steps: the cervix is grasped and brought into view with two tenacula, placed at the 3-o'clock and 9-o'clock positions outside any lesion; alternatively, the descending branches of the uterine artery are tied with catgut, which then serves to provide holding sutures.

The injection is made with a medium-gauge needle far from any visible lesions at 4 or 6 points (Fig. 20.2 a). According to the size of the cervix, 30 to 80 mL of solution is injected, enough to produce ballooning and blanching of the entire cervix (Fig. 20.2 b).

Next the cervix is bathed in Lugol's solution to delineate the margin of nonstaining abnormal tissue to be removed (Fig. 20.2 c).

Circumferential incision to outline the base of the cone now follows; ideally, there should be at least a 5-mm margin outside any lesion. If the lesion is very large, one is forced to cut close to the margin, or even cut through the iodine-negative area; this should be included in the operation notes, and the pathologist should be informed accordingly. Any lesion extending to the vaginal fornix, or even to the upper portions of the vagina beyond the margin of excision, should be subjected to multiple biopsies.

As the excision is deepened, the injected tissue will appear snow-white and will not bleed (Fig. 20.2 d). The soft, edematous tissue allows even excision. Incision is extended at an angle to achieve the required height of the cone or length of the canal to be removed. To avoid opening up the cone, a tangential cut running too close to the canal must be avoided. As the excision approaches the tip of the cone, a tenaculum may be introduced into the defect, the apex pulled into view, and the incision completed (Fig. 20.2 d).

The wound surface is whitish, and there may be several bleeding points (Fig. 20.2 e). The entire raw area is then electrocoagulated, particular attention being paid to the bleeding points. This not only helps in arresting the bleeding, but also allows contraction of the raw area as a result of evaporation of the injected solution (Fig. 20.2 f). Finally, the wound and the vagina are packed with gauze for 48 hours.

Stitches are not necessary. Sturmdorff sutures, in particular, lead to irregular healing and distortion of the cervix, which result in cervical stenosis. The cervix reconstitutes itself best in the absence of sutures.

Approximately 6 weeks after conization, the cervix resembles that of a nullipara (Fig. 20.3). Any shortening is detected only by palpation.

Laser Cone Biopsy

The ornipressin infiltration described above is also of value for laser cone biopsy. The borders of the lesion are identified with iodine solution. The laser is used in the cutting mode at the highest power and the smallest spot size. The lesion is first circumscribed with a margin of at least 3 mm. Cutting vertically, the incision is deepened as far as seems necessary with respect to the estimated intracervical extension of the lesion. The base of the circumcised cylinder is then cut with a knife. This is facilitated by grasping the stromal defect with a tenaculum (Fig. 20.2 d), pulling the tissue block outward. Cutting with a cold knife may produce severe bleeding which can be avoided by the preoperative infiltration of the cervix. By manipulating the specimen with a tenaculum, the cutting of the base can also be completed with the laser.

Loop Diathermy Cone Biopsy

The technique is the same as in loop diathermy excisions using a larger loop and making a deeper cut. We have used a triangular loop entering the cervical canal at an acute angle. The cone is formed by turning the loop around its axis and cutting with the hypothenusis. Cones obtained by diathermy excision are not as ideal histology as those obtained by other methods.

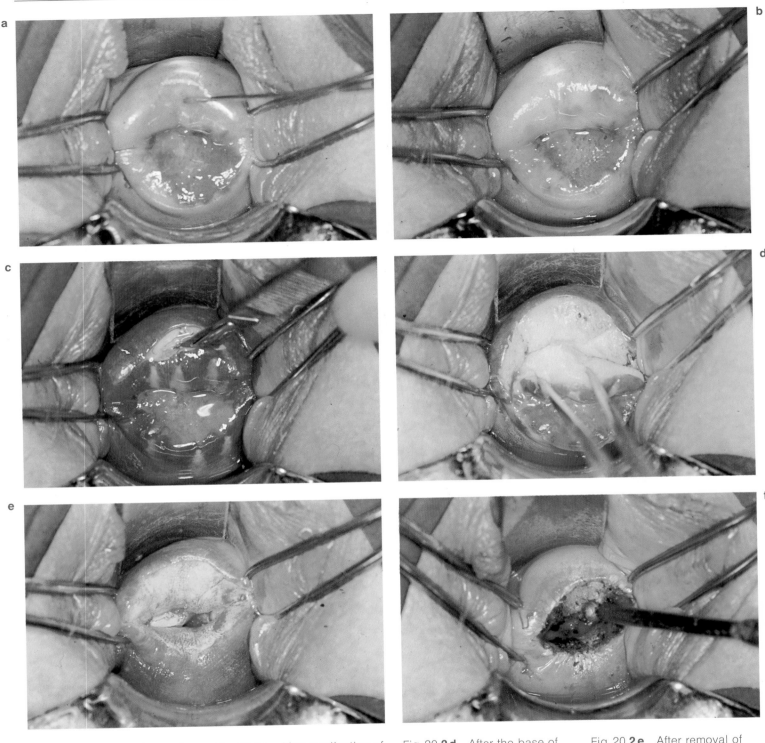

Fig. 20.**2 a–f**   **Technique of conization**

Fig. 20.**2 a**   The needle is inserted outside the lesion

Fig. 20.**2 b**   After injection at several points, the entire ectocervix shows ballooning and blanching

Fig. 20.**2 c**   After application of Lugol's iodine, excision can commence. The injected tissue appears snow white. The injection sites are indicated by the apices of the clear triangle, which are due to seepage of the injected solution and consequent dilution of Lugol's iodine

Fig. 20.**2 d**   After the base of the cone, which is still attached at its tip, is excised, the cone is grasped by a tenaculum placed peripheral to the epithelial surface. The tissue is quite bloodless

Fig. 20.**2 e**   After removal of the cone, several bleeding points appear

Fig. 20.**2 f**   The surface of the raw area is electrocoagulated. The cervix contracts as the solution evaporates; the wound surface is thus reduced

Complications of Conization

It is customary at the present time to stress the disadvantages and complications of conization. Publications are supported by selected references giving the operation an adverse bias. It is of course true that conization must be carefully performed, using a meticulous technique.

The most common complication is secondary hemorrhage, which occurs classically between the eighth and tenth postoperative day (6, 10). Excessive bleeding during and immediately after the operation is always due to poor technique, which may also increase the frequency of secondary hemorrhage. Although the incidence of secondary hemorrhage is cited as between 3% and 20% (1, 2, 3, 10, 17, 18), this was reduced from 23% to 4% in some series (2, 15) merely by preoperative cervical injection of a hemostatic agent. Our own experience is similar (Table 20.1). The use of Sturmdorff sutures makes no difference in the frequency of secondary hemorrhage (1, 17), but because it frequently results in stenosis (see above), it is best avoided. Ligation of the descending branch of the uterine artery does not reduce the incidence of secondary hemorrhage either (10, 15).

Infective complications may be prevented by clearing up associated vaginal infection prior to operating. The infection rate, in our hands, is about 0,3%. Other complications, such as perforation of the cervix, are distinctly rare (Table 20.1).

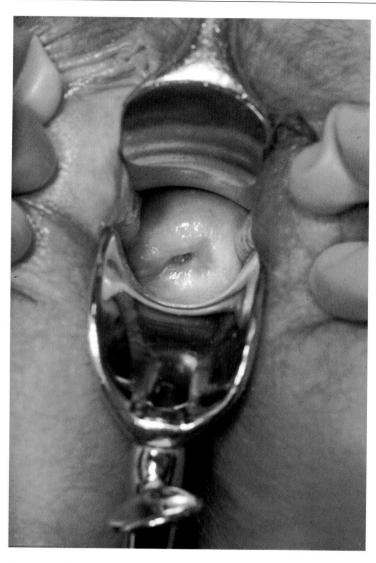

Fig. 20.**3**   The cervix, 2 months after conization. The external os resembles that of a nullipara

Table 20.**1**   Complications of 4452 cases of conization, 1958–1981

Complication	n	%
Perforation	2	0.04
Secondary hemorrhage	293	6.6
Blood transfusion	56	1.3
Infection	12	0.3
Stenosis	32	0.7

Conization during Pregnancy

In our experience, there is no essential difference between cold knife conization during pregnancy and conization at any other time (8, 9), provided it is not carried out after the 20th week. Because of eversion during pregnancy, lesions are usually ecto-cervical, and can often be excised by shallow conization. However, a lesion can extend relatively far into the cervical canal, or deep into the glands; occasionally, a microcarcinoma can be found (Fig. 20.4).

Some authors avoid conization during pregnancy, or perform it only in selected cases (18), while others do not regard pregnancy as a contraindication (7, 9, 19). In a study of 24 patients from our clinic who had conization during pregnancy, four aborted between 6 and 12 weeks after the operation. It should be pointed out, however, that these four women had also had abortions before conization. In three other cases, pregnancy terminated early at 30, 32, and 34 weeks respectively. The first two of these women had also had abortions previously. In the remaining 17 cases, the pregnancy was carried to term and, apart from a single cesarean section, labor was spontaneous and delivery uneventful.

Pregnancy after Cold Knife Conization

A technically good conization should have no influence on fertility or on the later course of pregnancy (8, 10, 12), in spite of reports of increased risk of late abortions and prematurity (2, 3). Of 376 women under the age of 40 years from our clinic, 128 (34%) became pregnant, some for the first time, following conization. The fertility rate was no different from that generally expected: 51.1% in those under 30 years of age and 23.8% in women between 31 and 40 years.

We observed the course and outcome of 174 intrauterine pregnancies following cold knife conization. There were 44 (25.3%) abortions. This compares favorably with a 19.5% incidence of abortions in the same group prior to conization. Furthermore, a higher incidence of abortions was found only in women who had delivered, on an average, three children before conization. That cervical incompetence due to excision of tissue did not account for early onset of labor is evident from the fact that only 18 of 130 deliveries were premature. Although the 13.8% incidence of prematurity is somewhat higher than the general incidence, it is noteworthy that the incidence of prematurity in these patients before conization was 18%.

The complication rate was not increased in term pregnancies, and in 90 of 101 cases delivery was spontaneous and uneventful. In only three cases (3%) was inadequate dilatation of the scarred cervix the indication for cesarean section. In the remaining eight cases, operative intervention was not related to prior conization.

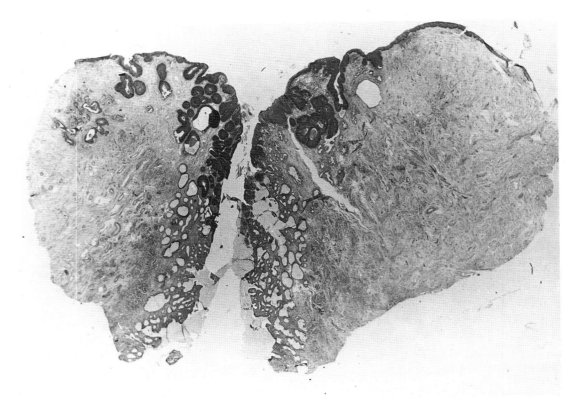

Fig. 20.4 15th week of gestation. Conization specimen with a carcinoma in situ (CIN III) on the ectocervix, in the lower and midcervical canal, and in a number of ectopic cervical glands, some of which are ectopic. On the left, a microcarcinoma 5 mm in diameter has originated in a gland, and reached 10 mm under the surface of the ectocervix. In the upper cervical canal, pregnancy-induced gland hyperplasia gives the thickened mucosa a honeycomb appearance

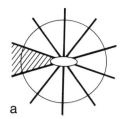

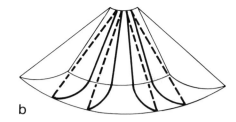

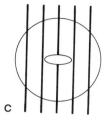

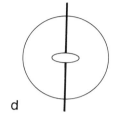

Histologic Processing of the Cone

The aim of histologic examination is twofold: (1) to assess the nature of the epithelial abnormalities, and (2) to determine if they have been completely removed. It is obvious that these goals are best achieved by detailed histologic assessment of the specimen, especially as far as completeness of excision is concerned. It is unwise for the pathologist to comment on the margins if only single sections are examined from blocks 2–3 mm thick. Reporting the margins as free under these circumstances may explain the relatively large number of "recurrences" following conization (2, 13).

The accuracy of histologic diagnosis depends on the handling of the specimen, the plane of sectioning, and the number of sections (5). Optimal fixation is essential. Dissection of the fixed specimen can take place in various ways. Some authors divide the specimen by radial incisions directed toward the external os or the canal in 8 to 12 sectors (Fig. 20.5 a). If the individual sector is processed in stepsections, as will be seen in the illustration, one obtains material oriented in unfavorable tissue planes. Although the number of sections may be quite large, this approach results in a very poor overview and has limited diagnostic value.

Opening the cone along the canal and dissecting the spread-out specimen into several blocks (Fig. 20.5 b) gives results similar to those of the radial method, but it may produce somewhat better overview sections. The best results by far are obtained by dissecting the fixed specimen using sagittal cuts. In this way, one can cut it into a variable number of blocks, as shown in Figure 20.5 c. At the clinic in Graz, the cone is bisected by a median sagittal cut (Fig. 20.5 d); which are embedded in their entirety (Fig. 20.6). The two blocks are then made into serial sections 200–300 μ apart, until the endocervical canal has disappeared. If lesions are still present, the two remaining blocks can be further processed. According to the size of the cone, 60–80 individual sections may be obtained (Fig. 20.5), thus providing a panoramic view of all existing lesions (Fig. 20.8).

Fig. 20.5 Dissection of the conization specimen. a Dissection using radial cuts. In one of the sectors, we show how the method by which it is processed must ultimately lead to unsuitable sections. **b** Dissection of the conization specimen that has been opened and rolled up. The result of this approach is similar to that in **a**. **c** Dissection of the conization specimen using a series of sagittal cuts. The resulting blocks can be cut from either side. **d** Dissection of the conization specimen using a median sagittal cut. Both blocks are evaluated from the cut surface laterally

20.6

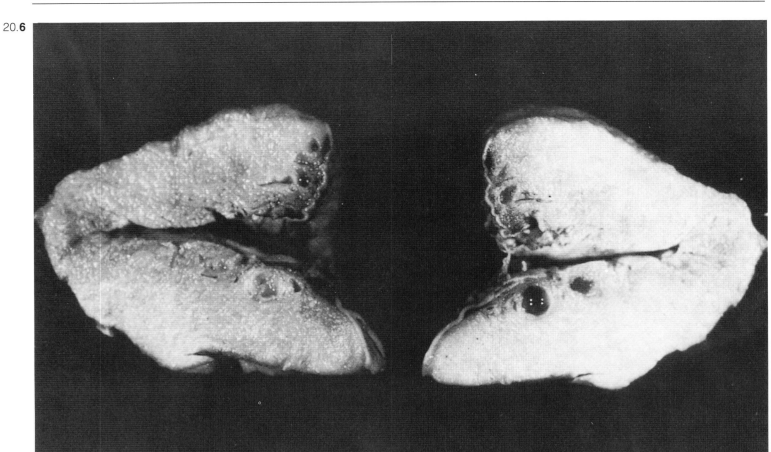

20.7

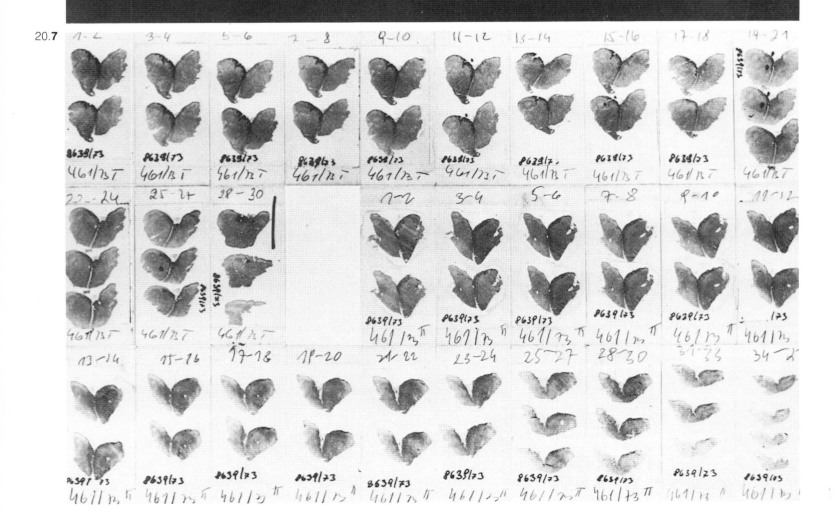

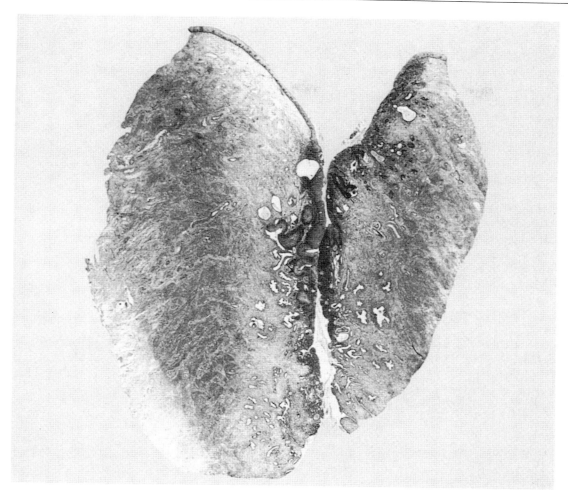

Fig. 20.**8   Single section from a conization specimen.** Note the carcinoma on the right, invading to a depth of 6 mm, exceeding the dimensions of a mircrocarcinoma. In addition, the glandular field of both lips is involved by carcinoma in situ (CIN 3) extending two-thirds up the canal. All margins of excision are free

◁ Fig. 20.**6   The fixed cone is divided into two.** Each half is embedded in toto and serially sectioned

◁ Fig. 20.**7   Serial sections from a conization specimen.** The empty space divides the two halves. There are altogether 57 individual sections in this case (from Obstet Gynecol 1977;49:641

References

1   Ahlgren M, Ingemarsson I, Lindberg LG, Nordquist SRB. Conization as treatment of carcinoma in situ of the uterine cervix. Obstet Gynecol 1975;46:135.

2   Bjerre H, Eliasson G, Linell F, Söderberg H, Sjöberg NO. Conization as the only treatment of carcinoma in situ of the uterine cervix. Am J Obstet Gynecol 1976;125:143.

3   Breinl H, Piroth H, Schuhmann R. Zur aktuellen Stellung der Konisation im Rahmen von Onkoprävention und Geschwulstdiagnostik an der Cervix uteri. Geburtshilfe Frauenheilkd 1976;36:507.

4   Burghardt E. Zur Operationstechnik der diagnostischen Konisation. Geburtshilfe Frauenheilkd 1963;23:548.

5   Burghardt E. Early histological diagnosis of cervical cancer. Philadelphia: Saunders, 1973.

6   Burghardt E. Albegger F. Zur Infiltrationstechnik der diagnostischen Konisation. Geburtshilfe Frauenheilkd 1969;29:1.

7   Ferguson JH, Brown GC. Cervical conization during pregnancy. Surgery 1960;111:603.

8   Holzer E. Fertilität, Schwangerschaft und Geburtsverlauf nach Konisation der Portio vaginalis uteri. Geburtshilfe Frauenheilkd 1972;32:950.

9   Holzer E. Die diagnostische Konisation der Portio vaginalis uteri während der Schwangerschaft. Geburtshilfe Frauenheilkd 1973;33:361.

10 Jones HW III, Buller RE. The treatment of cervical intraepithelial neoplasia by cone biopsy. Am J Obstet Gynecol 1980;137:882.

11 Kern G, Aslani A, Kern-–Bontke E, Gräfin zu Eulenburg H. Folgen der Zervixkonisation. Geburtshilfe Frauenheilkd 1967;27:879.

12 Kofler E, Philipp K. Schwangerschaft und Konisation wegen atypischer Epithelprozesse der Cervix uteri. Geburtshilfe Frauenheilkd 1977;37:942.

13 Larsson G. Conization for cervical dysplasia and carcinoma in situ: long-term follow-up of 1013 women. Ann Chir Gynaecol 1981;70:79.

14 Ober KG, Bötzelen HP. Technik, Vor- und Nachteile der Konisation der Cervix uteri. Geburtshilfe Frauenheilkd 1959;19:1051.

15 Rubio CA, Thomassen P, Kock Y. Influence of the size of cone specimens on postoperative hemorrhage. Am J Obstet Gynecol 1975;122:939.

16 Scott JW, Welch WB, Blake TF. Bloodless technique of cold knife conization (ring biopsy). Am J Obstet Gynecol 1960;79:62.

17 Sprang ML, Isaacs JH, Boraca CT. Management of carcinoma in situ of the cervix. Am J Obstet Gynecol 1977;129:47.

18 Van Nagell JR Jr, Parker JC, Hicks LP, Conrad R. England G. Diagnostic and therapeutic efficacy of cervical conization. Am J Obstet Gynecol 1976;124:134.

19 Wanless JF. Carcinoma of the cervix in pregnancy. Am J Obstet Gynecol 1971;110:173.

20 Wright CV, Davis E, Riopelle MA. Laser cylindrical excision to replace conization. Am J Obstet Gynecol 1984;150:704.

21
Subject Index